FITTING THE MIND TO THE WORLD

ADVANCES IN VISUAL COGNITION

Series Editors
Gillian Rhodes
Mary A. Peterson

Perceptions of Faces, Objects, and Scenes: Analytic and Holistic Processes
Edited by Mary A. Peterson and Gillian Rhodes

Fitting the Mind to the World: Adaptation and After-Effects in High-Level Vision
Edited by Colin Clifford and Gillian Rhodes

Fitting the Mind to the World

Adaptation and After-Effects in High-Level Vision

EDITED BY

Colin W.G. Clifford and Gillian Rhodes

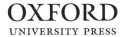

OXFORD

UNIVERSITY PRESS

Great Clarendon Street, Oxford OX2 6DP

Oxford University Press is a department of the University of Oxford.
It furthers the University's objective of excellence in research, scholarship,
and education by publishing worldwide in

Oxford New York
Auckland Cape Town Dar es Salaam Hong Kong Karachi
Kuala Lumpur Madrid Melbourne Mexico City Nairobi
New Delhi Shanghai Taipei Toronto

With offices in
Argentina Austria Brazil Chile Czech Republic France Greece
Guatemala Hungary Italy Japan South Korea Poland Portugal
Singapore Switzerland Thailand Turkey Ukraine Vietnam

Oxford is a registered trade mark of Oxford University Press
in the UK and in certain other countries

Published in the United States
by Oxford University Press Inc., New York

A catalogue record for this title is available from the British Library

Library of Congress Cataloging in Publication Data (attached)

Fitting the mind to the world: adaptation and after-effects in high-level vision/edited
by Colin W.G. Clifford and Gillian Rhodes. 1st ed. (Advances in visual cognition; 2).

Includes bibliographical references and index.
1. Visual pathways. 2. Visual cortex. 3. Visual perception.
4. Neuroplasticity. I. Clifford, Colin W.G. II. Rhodes, Gillian.
III. Advances in visual cognition (Oxford, England).
QP383.15.F565 2005   612.8'4–dc22   2005003249

Typeset by Cepha Imaging Pvt. Ltd., Bangalore, India
Printed in Great Britain
on acid-free paper by
Biddles Ltd., King's Lynn

ISBN 0-19-852969-4 (Hbk.:alk paper.)   978-0-19-852969-9 (Hbk.)

10 9 8 7 6 5 4 3 2 1

Preface

Adaptation phenomena provide striking examples of perceptual plasticity and offer valuable insight into the mechanisms of visual coding. Psychophysical aftereffects have aptly been termed the *psychologist's microelectrode* (Frisby 1980) because of their usefulness in investigating the coding of sensory information in the human brain. The broad relevance of adaptation is illustrated by its increasing use to study more cognitive aspects of vision such as the mechanisms of face perception and the neural substrates of visual awareness. This book brings together a collection of studies from international researchers demonstrating the brain's remarkable capacity to adapt its representation of the visual world in response to changes in its environment.

A major theme of the book is that adaptation at all stages of visual processing serves a functional role in the efficient representation of the prevailing visual environment. Information about the visual world is coded in the rate at which neurons fire. However, neurons can only respond over a certain range of firing rates. Adaptation of the way in which neurons code visual information tends to make optimal use of this limited response range. These principles are well-established at the level of light adaptation in the retina. However, it is only relatively recently that researchers have started to look for analogous behaviour at the higher levels of the visual system. This book is the first to bring together evidence that adaptation in high-level vision, as at the lower levels, serves to fit the mind to the world.

C.W.G.C.

and **G.R.**

Contents

Section III Attention and awareness

Contributors

David Alais, Department of Physiology, University of Sydney, NSW 2006, Australia. alaisd@physiol.usyd.edu.au

Derek H. Arnold, Department of Psychology & Institute of Cognitive Neuroscience, University College London, 26 Bedford Way, London WC1H 0AP, UK. derek.arnold@ucl.ac.uk

Randolph Blake, 512 Wilson Hall, 111 21st. Avenue South, Nashville, TN 37201, USA. randolph.blake@vanderbilt.edu

Igor Bondar, Institute of Higher Nervous Activity and Neurophysiology, Russian Academy of Sciences, Butlerova Street 5a, 117485 Moscow, Russia. igor.bondar@tuebingen.mpg.de

Colin W.G. Clifford, School of Psychology, Griffith Taylor Building (A19), The University of Sydney, NSW 2006, Australia. colinc@psych.usyd.edu.au

David J. Field, Department of Psychology, 246 Uris Hall, Cornell University, Ithaca, NY 14853-7601, USA. djf3@cornell.edu

Kalanit Grill-Spector, Department of Psychology, Jordan Hall, Building 420, Room 414, Stanford University, Stanford, CA 94305, USA. kalanit@psych. stanford.edu

Sheng He, Dept of Psychology, University of Minnesota, 75 E. River Rd., Minneapolis, MN 55455, USA. sheng@umn.edu

Michael R. Ibbotson, Centre for Visual Sciences, Research School of Biological Sciences, Australian National University, Canberra 2601, ACT, Australia. ibbotson@rsbs.anu.edu.au

Emma Jaquet, School of Psychology, University of Western Australia, Stirling Highway, Crawley, WA 6009, Australia. jaquee01@tartarus.uwa.edu.au

Linda Jeffery, School of Psychology, University of Western Australia, Stirling Highway, Crawley, WA 6009, AUSTRALIA. linda@psy.uwa.edu.au

Zoe Kourtzi, Max Planck Institute for Biological Cybernetics, Spemannstrasse 38, 72076 Tuebingen, Germany. zoe.kourtzi@tuebingen.mpg.de

David A. Leopold, National Institutes of Health, Unit on Cognitive Neurophysiology and Imaging, 49 Convent Drive, Bldg 49, Room B2J1, MSC 4415, Bethesda, Maryland 20892, USA. leopoldd@mail.nih.gov

Elinor McKone, School of Psychology, Australian National University, ACT 0200, Australia. Elinor.McKone@anu.edu.au

Gillian Rhodes, School of Psychology, University of Western Australia, Stirling Highway, Crawley, WA 6009, Australia. gill@psy.uwa.edu.au

Rachel Robbins, School of Psychology, Australian National University, ACT 0200, Australia. Rachel.Robbins@anu.edu.au

Satoru Suzuki, Department of Psychology, Northwestern University, 2029 Sheridan Rd., Evanston, IL 60208, USA. satoru@northwestern.edu

Frans A.J. Verstraten, Helmholtz Research Institute, Utrecht University, Psychonomics Division, Heidelberglaan 2, NL-3584 CS Utrecht, The Netherlands. F.A.J.Verstraten@fss.uu.nl

Nicholas J. Wade, Department of Psychology, University of Dundee, Dundee, DD1 4HN, Scotland. n.j.wade@dundee.ac.uk

Michael A. Webster, Department of Psychology/296, University of Nevada, Reno, Reno NV 89557, USA. mwebster@unr.nevada.edu

John S. Werner, Department of Ophthalmology, 4860 Y Street, Suite 2400, UC-Davis Medical Center, University of California, Davis, Sacramento, CA 95817. jswerner@ucdavis.edu

David Whitney, Group for Action and Perception, Department of Psychology, University of Western Ontario, London, Ontario N6A 5C2, Canada. dvw@uwo.ca

Qasim Zaidi, Professor of Vision Sciences, SUNY College of Optometry, 33 West 42nd St., New York, NY 10036, USA. qz@sunyopt.edu

Fitting the Mind to the World: Introduction

COLIN W.G. CLIFFORD AND GILLIAN RHODES

Adaptation is a characteristic of systems as diverse as economies, ant colonies and, of particular interest to us here, brains. It is a fundamental property of neurons in our brain, with moment to moment impact on our perception of the world. Perceptual adaptation occurs when a perceptual system alters its operating properties in response to changes in its inputs. This adjustment can occur over a wide range of time scales. Some forms of visual adaptation, such as accommodation of the lens to viewing distance (see Wade & Verstraten, this volume) are so rapid as to escape our notice. Other forms of adaptation occur over seconds or minutes, and can produce dramatic aftereffects, such as the waterfall illusion, tilt aftereffects (see Clifford, this volume), and distortions in the appearance of shapes (see Suzuki, this volume) and faces (see Leopold & Bondar; Rhodes *et al.*; Webster *et al.*, this volume). The perceptual learning of a fine discrimination, on the other hand, tends to occur over days, weeks, or even years. The development of an individual human visual system takes years. Finally, evolution has been refining vision for millions of years, through a process of adaptation by natural selection. Despite their very different time frames, these changes can all be thought of as forms of adaptation which share a common function: to fit the mind to the world. At a computational level, of course, the mechanisms that produce this fit may be quite different in each case. This volume focuses on adaptation which produces reversible changes over the relatively short time frames of seconds or minutes, partly because this is the time frame that has been most extensively studied by psychologists, and partly because it has such dramatic effects on our perceptual experience.

Of all the adaptive systems one could study, none is more personal to us than the seat of consciousness itself, the brain. If the eyes are the windows to the soul then, in modern neuroscience, the visual system has become very much the window to the brain, allowing us to probe its workings with carefully controlled stimulation. We now know intricate details of the chemical cascade through which our photoreceptors transduce photons of light into electrical signals. However, we still have a long way to go before we understand fully how our brain processes these signals at higher levels to recover information about the structure of our environment. If we understand how brains solve the problems of vision then we might be able to use this understanding to build intelligent robots capable of seeing in a similar way. Moreover, given that a large proportion of our cortex is dedicated to visual processing, there is always the hope that anything we can learn about the operation of the visual system might prove relevant to our understanding of cortical processing in general as well as bringing us one step closer to an explanation of how activity in our brains gives rise to the experience of conscious perception.

Central issues addressed in this volume are what functional significance, if any, adaptation and aftereffects have, what the underlying mechanisms are, and how adaptation affects our experience of the world. The book is divided into three sections. Section I deals with the phenomenology, function, and neural mechanisms of adaptation at the lower levels of the visual system, reviewing the foundations upon which our knowledge of adaptation at higher levels has been built and introducing functional ideas about adaptive coding in the context of motion processing, spatial vision, and colour perception. Section II highlights how our perception of complex visual patterns, including faces and their socially salient attributes of identity, emotion, and gender, are adaptively coded relative to dynamically established norms. Artificially biasing the diet of faces to which we are exposed rapidly resets those norms, demonstrating just how plastic our perception of these most human qualities really is. Section III illustrates the ingenious ways in which adaptation can be used as a technique to establish whether and at what levels of the visual system a stimulus has been processed. In some cases, it appears that processing can continue deep into the brain of the observer in the absence of any conscious awareness of the stimulus. In other situations, processing and perception correlate very closely in their time course as though what is perceived is an on-line monitor of the underlying neural processing. Adaptation can also tell us about the way in which voluntary attention to a stimulus affects processing of that stimulus.

In Chapter 1, Ibbotson reviews what is known about the biophysical and physiological basis of adaptation and the relationship between adaptation at the neural and perceptual levels. He focuses on adaptation to motion and to luminance contrast, the light intensity relative to the mean in surrounding areas. While contrast adaptation and motion adaptation have traditionally been considered as distinct phenomena, Ibbotson argues that the underlying mechanisms may in fact be closely related.

Although it is common to talk of the neural substrate of a particular perceptual phenomenon or illusion, Ibbotson stresses that adaptation to contrast and to motion may well occur at multiple sites along the visual processing hierarchy. The idea that a single perceptual aftereffect may be the result of adaptation at various stages of the visual system is also emphasized in Chapter 7 by Leopold and Bondar. This distributed locus for adaptation creates problems for single-cell investigations of adaptation, since it becomes hard to distinguish whether adaptation observed at a given site is occurring *de novo*, or whether it is simply inherited by virtue of adaptation at earlier processing stages. Similar issues also arise in the interpretation of brain imaging data employing the fMRI adaptation paradigm described in Chapter 6 by Kourtzi and Grill-Spector, since adaptation of the fMRI response in a given cortical region can reflect either adaptation at that site or adaptation amongst afferent neurons elsewhere in the brain.

In the motion domain, it seems that one way to tap into different levels of processing is through the use of different test stimuli. Psychophysical evidence indicates that, after prolonged exposure to a moving stimulus, the motion after-effects elicited by static versus flickering test stimuli appear to be mediated at different levels of the motion processing hierarchy (Nishida & Ashida 2000). Ibbotson points out that the use of stimuli designed to stimulate different processing stages may be a profitable strategy for studying adaptation in other visual domains.

While the motion aftereffect appears superficially maladaptive, an example of inappropriate perception of a stationary stimulus, it may in fact be the fingerprint of a generally beneficial process. Take as an example the process of light adaptation, which allows us to see over vast ranges of levels of illumination. One of the few situations in which we are aware of the process of light adaptation is when we move from bright sunlight to darkness or vice versa, in which case we may experience a few seconds of near blindness as our visual system adapts to the new light level. This example illustrates the idea that aftereffects may represent instances where our visual system is functioning in its normal way but the environment is in some sense extreme or abnormal. Similarly, our visual systems are presumably in a continual state of adaptation to the prevailing distribution of image motion signals, although we only become aware of this adaptation after prolonged inspection of a particular motion gives rise to a motion aftereffect.

Accounts of visual adaptation have typically taken one of two forms, those that view adaptation as a limitation of the system and those that view it as an active, functional process (see Clifford, this volume). On the one hand, the reduction in neuronal responsiveness resulting from prolonged stimulation has been described as neuronal fatigue, as if maintaining a high level of responding was somehow tiring out the neuron and reducing its effectiveness in representing information (e.g. Sutherland 1961). On the other hand, adaptation has been described as a form of gain control whereby the stimulus–response mapping of individual neurons or populations of neurons is dynamically adjusted to match the prevailing stimulus environment (e.g. Ullman & Schechtman 1982). Although this is an important conceptual distinction, it can be hard to distinguish passive fatigue from active gain control at the single neuron level as both typically entail a reduction in response to the adapting stimulus over time.

One way in which adaptive gain control can be experimentally identified using single-cell recording is by testing at a range of stimulus levels to establish unadapted and adapted response functions for the attribute in question.

For example, the contrast response function of neurons in primary visual cortex is typically found to shift laterally through adaptation rather than to exhibit reduced responsiveness across the entire contrast range (Ohzawa *et al.* 1982), consistent with a change in the dynamic range of the neuron to more closely match the stimulus contrasts sampled by the neuron in the recent past. This result clearly supports the view that adaptation is an active process serving a functional role in vision.

Possibly the clearest example of a functional benefit of adaptation in the visual cortex is found in motion perception. During prolonged exposure to a stimulus drifting at a constant velocity, the perceived speed of the stimulus tends to decrease. While underestimating the absolute speed of a stimulus would appear to be maladaptive, the ability to discriminate small changes in speed around the adapting level actually improves over the course of adaptation (Clifford & Langley 1996; Bex *et al.* 1999). Thus, the process of motion adaptation can be seen as sacrificing information about the absolute speed of a stimulus for enhanced differential sensitivity.

In Chapter 9, Webster, Werner, and Field emphasize that examples of such clear improvements in perceptual performance through adaptation are few and far between. However, the enhancement of differential speed sensitivity through motion adaptation has been observed in species as diverse as the fly and the humans. Given that the speed at which the visual image moves across our retinas is in a large part determined by our own locomotion through the environment, it would be redundant for our visual system to continually remind us how fast we are running (or, for an insect, how fast it is flying). Instead, it would be more efficient to use the available neural bandwidth to transmit information about *changes* in motion to enable us to control our movement by compensating for any deviations from the current velocity.

In Chapter 2, Clifford describes how some of the functional ideas about adaptation introduced at the single neuron level by Ibbotson in Chapter 1 can be extended to apply to the coding of stimulus attributes by a population of neurons. At the level of a single neuron, shifting the dynamic range to match the prevailing stimulus distribution can be thought of as a means of reducing the neuronal bandwidth devoted to signalling redundant information about unchanging components of the stimulus and thus increasing the effective bandwidth available to code changes in stimulation. While some degree of redundancy is desirable to overcome noise in the signal transmission process, the functional goal of adaptation has often been characterized as reducing redundancy in the neural representation towards this optimal level (e.g. Barlow & Foldiak 1989). For a stimulus attribute whose representation is distributed across a population of neurons, the redundancy of the representation can be reduced by adaptively decorrelating or orthogonalizing neuronal responses (e.g. Barlow & Foldiak 1989; Zaidi & Shapiro 1993).

Clifford shows that applying these functional ideas to the coding of visual attributes such as direction of image motion and spatial orientation can account for superficially maladaptive aftereffects in the spatial and motion domains.

He also argues that although the specialized processing of form and motion in the human visual system involves distinct cortical regions, parallels in the perceptual phenomenology between the two domains suggest that similar computational principles might apply to both.

Clifford shows how the analogy between adaptive coding in the form and motion domains correctly predicts an aftereffect in spatial vision whereby adaptation to oriented structure generates the illusion of the perpendicular orientation in a randomly structured test. He also argues that the same functional principles that appear to underlie adaptation to visual motion and to local image structure can help us understand the adaptive coding of attributes discussed in later chapters of this volume such as colour, shape, properties of faces, and aspects of auditory stimuli.

In Chapter 3, Wade and Verstraten take a historical and somewhat more philosophical approach to the phenomenon of adaptation. They point out that while one of the central themes of this book is the functional role of adaptation, this is not the route that has historically been followed by students of adaptation. Instead, probably because of their perceptually compelling nature, study has traditionally focused on superficially maladaptive aftereffects. However, in common with several other chapters in this volume, Wade and Verstraten themselves propose that aftereffects are in fact evidence of a continual process of visual recalibration.

Wade and Verstraten describe their chapter as a selective history of adaptation, and they have selected to trace the history of scientific interest in three forms of adaptation over quite different timescales. Accommodation, the change in curvature of the lens as a function of viewing distance, is a rapid process occurring over hundreds of milliseconds. Motion adaptation has a time course of seconds. Adaptation to optical distortions, for example through the wearing of prisms, is typically studied over minutes or even days!

Wade and Verstraten distinguish three ways in which the term *adaptation* is used in the study of vision. These they label procedure, process, and perception. Adaptation as procedure refers to the experimental methods used. Adaptation as process refers to activity at the neural level. Adaptation as perception refers to the phenomenological experience. Implicitly, many of the chapters in this volume are attempting to use the procedure of adaptation to better understand the processes of adaptation and relate these processes to the perceptual phenomena of adaptation. It is clearly important to make explicit the conceptual distinctions between these three definitions of *adaptation*.

In Chapter 4, Zaidi discusses the role of adaptation in colour constancy. Colour constancy enables us to recognize objects on the basis of their surface reflectance properties despite changes in the level and spectral composition of the illumination. Extracting invariant properties of objects for the purpose of object recognition is usually considered the domain of high-level vision. Thus it seems appropriate that a book on adaptation in high-level vision should contain a chapter on colour constancy alongside those on higher level aspects of spatial vision such as shape perception and the recognition of complex visual patterns.

Colour constancy is an inverse problem in which the surface reflectance of an object has to be inferred from the spectral composition of light reaching the eye. The spectral composition of this light is the result of a multiplicative interaction between the illuminant and the surface of the object. It is the surface reflectance profile of an object that we recognize as its colour. To solve the problem of colour constancy our visual system must essentially factor out the contribution of the illumination to the spectral composition of light reaching the retina. Solving the problem is of great survival value for species with trichromatic vision and understanding how the solution is obtained is of real practical interest in the field of machine vision, especially for machines such as mobile robots that are designed to operate in natural environments under a wide range of illumination conditions.

Colour constancy requires the visual system to take into account contextual information in recovering the colour of an object. It is not sufficient simply to know the spectral composition of light coming from a surface in order to recognize that surface by its colour since this fails to disambiguate information about the surface from characteristics of the illumination. In principle, the contextual information could be spatial, obtained by using the gamut of light coming from the whole visual scene to estimate and hence discount the illuminant, or temporal. Zaidi shows that it is primarily temporal, with colour constancy in human vision achieved in a large part by spatially local adaptation which effectively allows colour at any given location in the visual field to be coded relative to the recent history of stimulation in that region.

Next we move to Section II (Chapters 5–9), which deals explicitly with adaptation in high-level vision. In Chapter 5 Suzuki demonstrates how adaptation and aftereffects can be used to investigate the neural coding of high-level shape features, such as aspect ratio, curvature, taper, skew, and convexity. He has discovered that rapid sequences of briefly presented adapt and test stimuli generate aftereffects that are robust to changes in size and position. Such aftereffects cannot be due to adaptation of low-level shape coding mechanisms because these are retinotopically organized. His method therefore isolates the effects of adaptation in relatively high-level shape coding mechanisms.

Suzuki outlines a hierarchy of shape coding based on this work. At low levels of the visual system, he proposes that form is coded using *central-tendency coding*, with the form of a feature signalled by the central tendency of a population of cells, consisting of subgroups or channels that are systematically tuned to different values of that feature. For example, orientation would be coded by a population of cells, with subgroups tuned to different orientations which span the range of possible orientations. For a given stimulus, orientation is signalled by the central tendency of activation within this population. He suggests that this well-known coding system is also used for higher-level shape coding. His argument builds on the claim that 'the psychophysical signature of central-tendency coding' is repulsive aftereffects. For example, after viewing a line tilted slightly to the left, a vertical line appears tilted slightly to the right. He reviews a series of experiments from his own laboratory which show similar repulsive aftereffects for a variety of high-level shape features.

Suzuki suggests that the function of central-tendency coding may be to enable the coding of subtle discriminations between very similar stimuli. Such coding would be especially useful for stimuli with similar structure, such as faces, and he notes that repulsive aftereffects have indeed been found for a variety of face features (see also Chapters 6–9 in this volume). He also suggests that this form of coding may be acquired with expertise and perceptual learning, which leads to the interesting prediction that experts, but not novices, with homogeneous categories (e.g. birds, dogs) may show repulsive aftereffects for those categories. In the case of high-level shape features, he speculates that experience using features such as skew and taper as cues to 3-D shape might result in the development of central-tendency coding for such features. On this view, infants would not be expected to show repulsive aftereffects for these features. It would be interesting to see if that were the case.

Suzuki also suggests that high-level shape coding is characterized by a special form of central-tendency coding, namely *opponent coding*. In opponent coding, two distinct populations of cells code values above and below, respectively, some category boundary. He argues that the coding of all high-level shape features could be structured in this way, because all vary between two extreme ends, with a neutral point or category boundary in the middle. For example, skew, taper, and curvature all switch from one direction to its opposite about a point of symmetry, aspect ratio switches from elongation along one axis to elongation about an orthogonal axis, and convexity switches from convex to concave across a null point. He suggests that the null point or category boundary can be considered a '*norm*', because it represents the average of the two extreme ends of the continuum. The same idea is developed explicitly for face coding in Chapter 8 by Rhodes *et al*. More general arguments for the computational and metabolic efficiency of opponent coding can be found in Chapter 9 by Webster, Werner, and Field.

In Chapter 6, Kourtzi and Grill-Spector describe how adaptation over short time frames (seconds), can be combined with brain imaging to study visual representations in the primate brain. This fMRI-adaptation approach, developed by Grill-Spector and her colleagues, exploits the fact that the fMRI response is reduced by repeated presentation of the same stimulus, which they attribute to suppression of stimulus-specific neurons. Therefore, if a change in a stimulus dimension causes an increased response or 'rebound' from adaptation, then the population of neurons must be selective for, or code, that property. If adaptation remains constant across a change, then the population coding must be invariant to that property. This method is more sensitive than the conventional fMRI approach, which compares activation to different kinds of stimuli by averaging across voxels in relatively large regions, because it is potentially able to detect a rebound response in a subset of neurons within a voxel. Thus, while functional differences within such regions are unlikely to be seen using the conventional approach, they may be detected using the fMRI-adaptation paradigm.

Kourtzi and Grill-Spector demonstrate the power of this new method in a series of elegant studies reviewed in their chapter. Using it they have shown that neurons in both V1 (peripheral) and V2 (central) code global shape (defined by contour collinearity), and that the lateral occipital complex (LOC, a region in lateral occipital cortex extending anteriorly into the temporal lobe) codes object shape independent of the low-level image features (e.g. shading, contour) used to define the shape. They have also used fMRI-adaptation to address a long-standing question in visual cognition, namely how we can recognize objects despite the infinite set of viewpoints from which they can be seen. Traditionally, two competing solutions to this problem have been proposed. In one, the problem is solved by abstracting 3-D, object-centred (view-invariant) representations. In the other, the problem is solved by having a set of 2-D image-based (view-specific) representations. Kourtzi and Grill-Spector found that adaptation was not invariant to rotation around the vertical axis in either the fusiform (anterior LOC) or lateral occipital (LO) regions of the LOC, suggesting that view-specific representations of objects (including faces) are coded in these regions. Clearly this method has enormous potential for furthering our understanding of how visual information is coded at all levels of the visual system.

In Chapter 7, Leopold and Bondar begin with a critical analysis of what we can expect to learn from aftereffects – what can they tell us about the neural basis of perception? Despite the fact that aftereffects occur for many simple stimulus attributes, such as tilt or direction of motion, they argue that these aftereffects cannot be understood in terms of simple feature-based adaptation, such as adaptation of orientation-tuned neurons in V1 in the case of the tilt aftereffect. Instead, they propose that aftereffects reflect adaptation of the entire visual system and that their interpretation may not be straightforward.

That said, however, they go on to show that aftereffects in the perception of facial identity can tell us something very interesting indeed about how faces are visually coded. The basic finding is that perception of identity is facilitated by a brief adaptation to a face's opposite, known as its anti-face, which, in a multidimensional face space whose dimensions represent the information used to distinguish faces, lies diametrically opposite the target face on a vector passing through the norm or average face. This opponent aftereffect points strongly to norm-based coding of faces, whereby the attributes of a face are coded relative to an appropriate norm or average face. Norm-based coding emerges strongly as a theme in this collection both for faces and for high-level shape (see Chapters 5, 8, and 9).

Leopold and Bondar also report new data showing the same face identity aftereffect in a monkey. This result raises the possibility that norm-based coding is a fundamental feature of an evolutionarily old face processing module. Alternatively, the authors suggest that it could be a general mechanism for coding complex patterns, with norms functioning as implicit reference points for coding the structure of such patterns.

In Chapter 8, Rhodes and colleagues continue the discussion of face aftereffects and how they may shed light on the ways the visual system solves the difficult computational problem of distinguishing faces, which all share the same basic configuration. Like Leopold and Bondar (Chapter 7) they suggest that norm-based coding would provide an elegant solution to the problem. They begin with a brief review of face processing, its neural substrates, and the likely roles of innate mechanisms and experience in the development of our face perception skills. They then review a variety of aftereffects in face perception, for identity, face shape, gender, race, and expression, which highlight the plasticity of face perception and suggest the dynamic adjustment of face norms, in response to changes in the population of faces experienced. These norms may function as reference points against which the distinctive aspects of individual faces can be coded.

Rhodes *et al.* then consider a possible functional role for adaptation in face processing, namely enhanced discrimination of faces either around the adapting point, or the new norm. Although enhanced discrimination would appear to be a useful consequence of calibrating face coding mechanisms to the statistics of the environment, none was found. They go on to discuss some new work suggesting that face dimensions with greater real-world variation are easier to adapt than ones with lesser variation, which suggests that face aftereffects might prove useful in exploring the dimensions of face-space. Finally, they describe a neurally plausible model of prototype-referenced opponent coding of faces, analogous to that proposed by Suzuki (Chapter 5) for shape coding. In the model, distinct neural populations code above-average and below-average values on the various dimensions used to discriminate faces.

In Chapter 9, Webster, Werner, and Field consider how adaptation can help us understand the phenomenology of vision, the subjective experience of seeing. They argue that the visual environment, and our adaptation to it, largely determines our visual experience. Therefore, viewers who share the same visual environment will have similar visual experience, whereas those who inhabit different visual environments will have a different visual experience. The argument is that adaptation normalizes visual coding to the stimuli we see, which ensures efficient coding by calibrating neural responses to fit the range of stimuli experienced. This could be done by adapting to the average stimulus value and representing stimuli that deviate from the average, i.e. by norm-based coding (for similar views see Chapters 5, 7, and 8 in this volume). Such coding is metabolically and computationally efficient, because the system responds primarily to rare rather than common stimuli. It also makes salient those stimuli that deviate from the current norm or state of adaptation. Therefore, what is visually salient to a person, i.e. their phenomenal experience, depends on their state of adaptation, and ultimately on their visual environment. An important corollary of this argument is that to understand visual experience, we must understand the statistics of the environment.

The authors present examples from colour vision and the perception of blur to demonstrate how a shared environment may be more important in shaping visual experience than physiological differences between the visual systems of observers. The good news is that physiological changes associated with aging have surprisingly little impact on visual experience, although the bad news is that they certainly affect performance.

Webster and his colleagues also consider the functions of adaptation. At the most basic level, they argue that adaptation calibrates neural responses to the range of stimuli experienced and reduces redundancy in coding, thereby allowing flexible and efficient deployment of a limited neural response range to a changing visual environment. The authors consider a variety of specific mechanisms by which this calibration could be achieved. They also discuss the role of adaptation in generating perceptual constancies and the time frames over which adaptation operates, from the rapid calibration underlying many visual aftereffects to calibration over evolutionary time frames.

An obvious consequence of adaptation should be to enhance performance, so that discrimination is best for the most commonly encountered stimuli. Webster and his colleagues note that although such enhanced performance around the adaptation level has certainly been found in some domains (e.g. light adaptation), it has been surprisingly difficult to find in others. This observation leads them to consider the intriguing possibility that it is the phenomenal consequences of adaptation that may be particularly important. Certainly the most dramatic consequence of adaptation for an observer is the visual aftereffect it generates. It is the perception of a drifting riverbank, not the apparently decreasing speed of the river, that impresses us in the waterfall illusion. Webster and his colleagues propose that the increased visual salience of stimuli which deviate from the norm or adaptation level may play an important role in the deployment of attention. Unexpected stimuli often require evaluation and action, so that a mechanism which directs our attention to them would be very useful.

Finally, we move to Section III (Chapters 10–12), which deals with the use of adaptation to study attention and awareness. In Chapter 10, Blake and He critically review the use of adaptation as a tool to investigate the neural correlates of consciousness (NCC). Key to the use of adaptation in this way is the ability to dissociate phenomenal perception from physical stimulation by breaking down the one-to-one correspondence between the world and our perception of it that we all take for granted. One way to achieve this decoupling is to use adaptation to change the appearance of a subsequent stimulus. The same stimulus can be perceived quite differently after adaptation than before due purely to changes in the adapted state of the observer's visual system. Another way to decouple stimulation and perception is to investigate adaptation outside of awareness by using adapting stimuli that do not give rise to a conscious percept.

Unconscious adaptation is a means of probing what aspects of a visual stimulus can be processed, and what parts of the visual system stimulated, in the absence of awareness of that stimulus. This can be achieved by presenting the adapting stimulus at such a fine spatial scale that the spatial structure cannot be consciously resolved by the observer, by placing the stimulus in the observer's peripheral vision and surrounding or 'crowding' it with similar patterns, or by presenting the stimulus to one eye and a dissimilar pattern to the other eye such that 'binocular rivalry' is induced and perceptual awareness alternates every few seconds between the two patterns. In all cases there will be periods during which the stimulus is invisible to the observer but it still has access to at least some of the visual processing hierarchy and thus has the potential to generate adaptation at those processing levels.

Correlating the results of studies of unconscious adaptation with what is known about the physiological properties of neurons at various stages of the visual processing hierarchy has led to the conclusion that activity in primary visual cortex is not by itself sufficient for visual awareness (see Koch 2004). However, Blake and He urge caution in interpreting the results of such studies. First, they make the point that individual regions of the brain are not homogeneous but contain multiple layers and cell types. Thus, even if activity within some unspecified subset of the region's neurons is not sufficient for awareness then there is no guarantee that activity of other neurons in that region is not in fact sufficient for consciousness. Second, just as there may well be no one site of adaptation to a given visual attribute (see Chapters 1 and 7), Blake and He emphasize that there may be no one area that is by itself sufficient to support visual awareness. In that case, unconscious adaptation might still be observable in an area that formed part of a distributed NCC but could not serve as a NCC in isolation.

In Chapter 11, Alais continues with the theme of using adaptation as a tool within cognitive neuroscience, this time to investigate the mechanisms of visual attention. Focusing on the motion aftereffect, Alais reviews evidence from psychophysical and brain imaging studies showing that adaptation can be modulated by selective attention. The fact that aftereffects can be reduced in the absence of attention to the adapting stimulus shows that attention is not simply a high-level cognitive phenomenon but one that can influence low-level sensory processing. This would appear to argue strongly against models of late attentional selection, whereby visual processing runs almost to completion preattentively, instead favouring an early selection account.

However, Alais cautions against this interpretation as overly simplistic. Motion adaptation is not mediated at any single early stage of visual cortical processing. Instead, brain imaging studies suggest that the motion aftereffect involves adaptation in a network of distributed areas from V1 through to MT and beyond (e.g. Huk *et al.* 2001). Attentional modulation of motion processing appears to involve a similar distributed network, boosting neural responses to the attended motion and attenuating those to non-attended directions. While attentional modulation of motion processing has been observed at the earliest stage of cortical processing, V1 (e.g. Gandhi *et al.* 1999), this modulation may well be generated top-down through feedback from higher-level areas involved in decision making and planning.

Rather than viewing attention in terms of a dichotomy between early and late selection, Alais suggests that the existing data are better accounted for by the Attentional Load Theory (Lavie 1995) whereby the degree of processing of unattended stimuli depends upon the resources allocated to the attended task. When the attentional load is high, little processing power will remain for analysis of the unattended stimuli. When the attentional load is low, the unattended stimulus will be processed more deeply. In this way, Attentional Load Theory predicts that the results of attentional manipulations in adaptation experiments can resemble either early or late selection depending upon the demands of the task diverting attention from the adapting stimulus.

In Chapter 12, Arnold and Whitney describe how adaptation can be used to study the perceptual binding problem. The Binding Problem is the problem of how more or less independently processed perceptual attributes become associated or bound in the perception of unified objects. A binding problem exists not only between different sensory modalities, such as sight and sound, but also between attributes within a modality such as visually perceived colour, form, and motion. Indeed, Arnold and Whitney propose that similar processes may underlie binding between and within modalities.

An entertaining example of the power of binding between modalities to influence our perception is the ventriloquist effect, in which a person's voice is spatially mislocalized so as to be perceived as emanating from the mouth of a dummy. Adaptation to a consistent auditory–visual spatial offset has been shown to generate a 'ventriloquist aftereffect' (Recanzone 1998). The perceived position of a subsequent auditory stimulus is biased towards the location of the adapting visual stimulus, even when the auditory test stimulus is presented in isolation. Adaptation can also produce similar shifts in perceived position purely within the visual modality, supporting Arnold and Whitney's conjecture that binding within and between modalities involves similar processes. In functional terms, such processes are viewed as implementing a dynamic strategy of cue combination whereby information from multiple sources is adaptively weighted according to its reliability.

Twenty-five years after Frisby (1980) popularized aftereffects as the psychologists' microelectrode, they remain a powerful tool for understanding perception. This collection of chapters showcases what we have learned about the coding of visual information, from the study of visual aftereffects and the processes of adaptation that produce them. William James once commented that, 'Mind and world ... have been evolved together, and in consequence are something of a mutual fit' (James 1892/1984, p 11). The chapters in this volume show how the fit continues to be maintained within the timeframe of our daily lives.

References

Barlow, H.B., & Foldiak, P. (1989). Adaptation and decorrelation in the cortex. In R. Durbin, C. Miall & G. Mitchison (ed.), *The Computing Neuron* (pp. 54–72). Wokingham: Addison-Wesley.

Bex, P., Bedingham, S., & Hammett, S.T. (1999). Apparent speed and speed sensitivity during adaptation to motion. *Journal of the Optical Society of America A, 16*, 2817–24.

Clifford, C.W.G., & Langley, K. (1996). Psychophysics of motion adaptation parallels insect electrophysiology. *Current Biology, 6*, 1340–2.

Frisby, J.P. (1980). *Seeing: Illusion, Mind and Brain*. Oxford: OUP.

Gandhi S.P., Heeger D.J., & Boynton, G.M. (1999). Spatial attention affects brain activity in human primary visual cortex. *Proceedings of the Academy of Sciences USA, 96*, 3314–9.

Huk A.C., Ress, D., & Heeger, D.J. (2001). Neuronal basis of the motion aftereffect reconsidered. *Neuron, 32*, 161–72.

James, W. (1892/1984). *Psychology: Briefer Course.* Cambridge, MA: Harvard University Press.

Koch, C. (2004). *The Quest for Consciousness: a Neurobiological Approach.* Englewood, CO: Roberts & Co.

Lavie, N. (1995). Perceptual load as a necessary condition for selective attention. *Journal of Experimental Psychology: Human Perception and Performance, 21*, 451–68.

Ohzawa, I., Sclar, G., & Freeman, R.D. (1982). Contrast gain control in the cat visual cortex. *Nature, 298*, 266–8.

Nishida, S., & Ashida, H. (2000). A hierarchical structure of motion system revealed by interocular transfer of flicker motion aftereffects. *Vision Research, 40*, 265–78.

Recanzone, G.H. (1998). Rapidly induced auditory plasticity: The ventriloquism aftereffect. *Proceedings of the National Academy of Sciences, 95*, 869–75.

Sutherland, N.S. (1961). Figural after-effects and apparent size. *Quarterly Journal of Experimental Psychology, 13*, 222–8.

Ullman, S., & Schechtman, G. (1982). Adaptation and gain normalization. *Proceedings of the Royal Society of London, Series B, 216*, 299–313.

Zaidi, Q., & Shapiro, A.G. (1993). Adaptive orthogonalization of opponent-color signals. *Biological Cybernetics, 69*, 415–28.

Section I

Foundations

1

Physiological Mechanisms of Adaptation in the Visual System

MICHAEL R. IBBOTSON

1.1 Introduction

The most well-understood type of adaptation in the human visual system is light adaptation, which adjusts the sensitivity of the retina to different brightness levels. If one walks from bright sunlight into a dimly lit area or vice versa there is an initial period of near blindness while the visual system adapts to the new environment. At first glance light adaptation appears to reduce visibility; however, the adaptation process is in fact highly beneficial. Retinal ganglion cells, which are spiking neurons that form the output from the retina, are capable of coding about a 2-log unit change in brightness level in their firing rate. Despite this limitation, the eye actually operates over about 10 log units of light level. The light adaptation process continually resets the retina's sensitivity to match prevailing luminance levels and this largely occurs early in the retina, e.g. rods (Hood & Birch 1993) and cones (Malchow & Yazulla 1986). When in near darkness, it is best to spread the functional bandwidth, defined as the response region where a change in brightness will actually cause a change in firing rate, across a limited range of brightness levels. This provides high sensitivity at low brightness levels but leads to saturation for most high brightness values. Conversely, in bright sunlight, detecting small brightness changes at low intensities is of less importance, so the system readjusts itself to spread its functional bandwidth across a higher and broader range of light intensities. This process is a type of gain control, and is designed so that an enormous range of inputs can be mapped onto a restricted range of outputs (Rodieck 1998).

The present chapter will consider the physiological mechanisms that drive adaptation at higher processing levels in the nervous system. It will discuss the mechanisms that generate beneficial alterations in the way that contrast and motion are coded, both of which require several levels of processing beyond the photoreceptors. Adaptation to contrast and motion is normally observed as an alteration in the visual perception of those attributes following prolonged exposure to a given visual stimulus (Harris 1980; Graham 1989; Blakemore 1990; Mather *et al.* 1998). Perhaps the most striking example of higher-level adaptation in the visual system is the motion aftereffect (MAE). Following exposure to a stimulus moving in one direction, a stationary pattern appears to move in the opposite direction. This illusion can be readily observed in the natural world, which explains why Aristotle was able to describe the phenomenon as early as 330 BC. Robert Addams (1834) noted that after gazing at a waterfall, and then suddenly directing his eyes to the rocks immediately adjacent to the water, he saw the rocky face as if in motion upwards, and with an apparent speed equal to that of the descending water. This powerful illusion shows how adaptation can generate internal representations of the outside world which, at times, can produce inappropriate perception. However, as will be discussed in the following sections, while short-lived misrepresentations of the world can occur, under most circumstances the effects of adaptation are beneficial. This chapter will describe contrast and motion adaptation as separate phenomena. However, such divisions may be false, as the basic biophysical mechanisms are closely related.

1.2 Contrast Adaptation

Contrast is a measure of light intensity relative to the mean in surrounding areas and is usually expressed as the Michelson contrast, which is defined as the difference between the maximum and minimum luminance divided by their sum. Adaptation to a textured pattern increases the contrast needed to detect similar patterns, and decreases the apparent contrast of the pattern (e.g. Blakemore *et al.* 1973; Snowden & Hammett 1992; Ross & Speed 1996; Foley & Chen 1997). As with the reduced visibility that follows a sudden move between different brightness levels, the reduction in sensitivity to contrast appears at first to reduce the capacity to process visual scenes but, in the next section, it will be shown that this is only the case under restricted conditions.

1.2.1 Contrast Adaptation as Gain Control?

Just as with light adaptation, one proposed function of contrast adaptation is gain control (e.g. Movshon & Lennie 1979; Ohzawa *et al.* 1982, 1985). In this

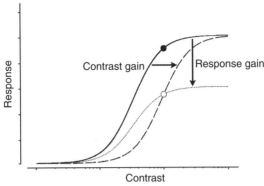

FIG. 1.1 The solid line shows a theoretical sigmoidal contrast response function
from a visual neuron in the non-adapted state. After a period of adaptation the theoretical
cell could either show a rightward shift in its response function along the contrast axis
(dashed line: contrast gain control) or a general compression in response to all contrasts (dotted line: attenuation in response gain). The black dot represents the response
to a given contrast in the unadapted state. The open circle shows the response to the
same contrast following changes to contrast gain or response gain, demonstrating the
importance of measuring full contrast response functions in the adapted state.

view, adaptation would adjust the sensitivity of cells to the range of contrasts
that they have experienced in the recent past. Accordingly, some psychophysical studies – but not all – have found an enhancement in performance associated with adaptation (Greenlee & Heitger 1988; Ross *et al.* 1993; Wilson &
Humanski 1993). In their classic papers on contrast gain control in the cat
visual system, Ohzawa *et al.* (1982, 1985) measured the contrast response functions of cells in the primary visual cortex (V1) of the cat while adapting them
to different contrast levels of stimulus gratings. In the unadapted state the cells
produced sigmoidal contrast response functions when spike rate was plotted as
a function of log-contrast (Fig. 1.1). During adaptation to a given mean contrast
the response functions shifted laterally along the log-contrast axis so that the
functional bandwidths of the cells were approximately centred on the mean
contrast level. These results demonstrate that a contrast-dependent change in
the gain of the contrast response function had occurred (Fig. 1.1). Similar findings of changes in contrast gain through adaptation have been reported in primate area V1 (Sclar *et al.* 1989). Importantly, few cells showed a large change
in response gain, which would lead to an overall reduction in response amplitude to all contrasts (Fig. 1.1).

1.2.2 The Site of Contrast Adaptation

For many years the type of contrast gain control described in psychophysical experiments (Blakemore *et al.* 1973; Snowden & Hammett 1992;
Ross & Speed 1996; Foley & Chen 1997) and in cortical neurons has been

thought to be an inherently cortical mechanism (Ohzawa *et al.* 1985; Sclar *et al.* 1989). This suggestion came originally from studies that reported little or no contrast gain control in the lateral geniculate nucleus (LGN), which is the main relay nucleus that provides input to the primary visual cortex in mammals (e.g. Ohzawa *et al.* 1985). The logical argument ran that if contrast gain control could not be observed in LGN but was present in V1 the effect must have cortical origins (Maffei *et al.* 1973; Movshon & Lennie 1979; Ohzawa *et al.* 1985; Sclar *et al.* 1985). Also, some of these studies reported partial interocular transfer of the contrast gain changes and, as information from the two eyes is first combined in cortex, this was used as evidence that contrast gain control was a cortical mechanism.

There is now evidence for contrast adaptation in the LGN (Sclar 1987; Shou *et al.* 1996; Sanchez-Vives *et al.* 2000*a,b*; Usrey & Reid 2000; Solomon *et al.* 2004). There is also evidence that contrast adaptation may occur, at least in part, as early as the retina because contrast adaptation strongly alters response sensitivity in monkey retinal ganglion cells (RGC) (Chander & Chichilnisky 2001). In salamander retina, substantial changes in stimulus contrast did not have detectable effects on the response properties of cones and horizontal cells, which eliminates the possibility that contrast adaptation relies on the mechanism of light adaptation in the cone transduction cascade (Baccus & Meister 2002). While photoreceptors and horizontal cells can be eliminated from the equation in salamander retina, Baccus and Meister (2002) did show that contrast-dependent changes occur in certain bipolar cells, some amacrine cells, and all RGCs studied in that retina. In summary, contrast-dependent changes in responsiveness occur in some retinal cells, certain cells in the LGN, and in the visual cortex. Some of the effects recorded in the cortex appear to be entirely cortical in origin while certain components of the adaptation appear to be inherited from earlier stages in the visual system (Sanchez-Vives *et al.* 2000*a*; Solomon *et al.* 2004). It appears that the large, general attenuation of neural responsiveness is generated intrinsically within cortical neurons but that certain stimulus-specific aspects of contrast adaptation may be derived from changes in the activities of pre-synaptic neurons (Sanchez-Vives *et al.* 2000*b*). More discussion relating to these latter mechanisms can be found in Section 1.4.

In conclusion, it appears that contrast adaptation occurs at multiple sites in the visual system and there appear to be species-specific differences in the location of adaptation (Solomon *et al.* 2004). For example, stimulation with high contrast gratings led to reductions in firing rate of 20 per cent in monkey retinal ganglion cells but 40–90 per cent in Salamander RGCs (Chander & Chichilnisky 2001), suggesting that adaptation is far stronger in salamander RGCs than in monkey cells.

1.2.3 Cellular Mechanisms

Carandini and Ferster (1997) found in neurons of the cat primary visual cortex (V1) that contrast adaptation is accompanied by a large (5–10 mV), long-lasting

(10–20 s) hyperpolarization. The resulting downward shift in the membrane potential versus contrast response functions leads in turn to a rightward shift in the contrast response functions obtained by measuring the mean firing rates of the cells (Fig. 1.2). Carandini and Ferster's data is the first to provide tangible evidence that intracellular changes in membrane potentials can lead to lateral shifts of the spiking output relative to stimulus contrast. Intracellular recordings from simple and complex cells in cat V1 demonstrate that repetitive stimulation with either a visual stimulus (sinusoidal grating) or intracellular injection of current generates a hyperpolarization that reduces the responsiveness of cells to subsequently presented visual stimulation or current injections (Mc Cormick *et al.* 1998; Sanchez-Vives *et al.* 2000*a,b*). The results suggest that the hyperpolarization observed in cat cortical neurons is generated by an intrinsic mechanism, which probably contributes to the general attenuation of responsiveness associated with contrast adaptation and also has a role in the lateral shifts in the contrast response functions obtained by measuring spiking output.

What are the biophysical mechanisms leading to the hyperpolarization observed in visual neurons? Intracellular *in vivo* and *in vitro* recordings in cat and ferret cortex suggest that the adaptation-induced hyperpolarization observed during contrast adaptation in V1 is associated with the activation of a Na^+-dependent K^+ current, with the possible contribution of an electrogenic Na^+/K^+ pump (Mc Cormick *et al.* 1998; Sanchez-Vives *et al.* 2000*a,b*). Retinal bipolar cells contain a strong Ca^{2+}-dependent K^+ conductance (Burrone & Lagnado 1997). This appears to have a role in driving contrast-dependent changes in neural activity in the retina because buffering Ca^{2+} in some bipolar cells disrupts contrast-driven effects (Rieke 2001). Adaptation in neurons of the fly optic lobe also appears to be driven by an activity-dependent K^+ conductance that hyperpolarizes the cells when an excitatory input raises intracellular levels of Ca^{2+} (Harris *et al.* 2000). Such observations have led Sanchez-Vives *et al.* (2000*b*) to propose a cellular model for contrast adaptation. High contrast stimuli generate action potentials and increased synaptic activity in visual neurons, which leads to an increase in intracellular Na^+/Ca^{2+}. In turn, this increased concentration activates sodium- and calcium-dependent outward K^+ currents. The outward movement of K^+ leads to a decrease in firing rate during stimulation and long-lasting after-hyperpolarization. This simple model can explain many of the observed effects relating to contrast adaptation. However, it is important to note that not all effects can be covered by such a basic model (see Section 1.4 for more discussion).

1.3 Motion Adaptation

Following exposure to a stimulus moving in one direction, a subsequently presented stationary pattern appears to move in the opposite direction. This illusion is referred to as the motion aftereffect (MAE) or, more poetically, as the waterfall illusion. The MAE *per se* probably has no functional value, but just as

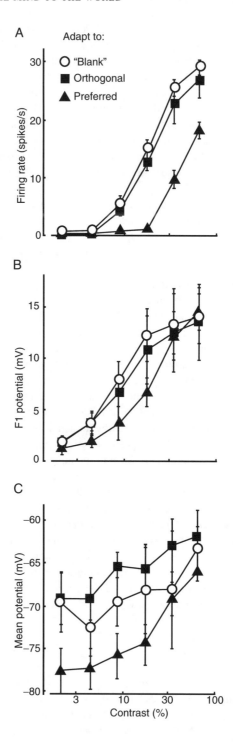

FIG. 1.2 (A) Contrast response curves derived from the mean firing rate of a neuron in cat V1 after adaptation to motion in the preferred (triangle), or orthogonal (square) directions and after exposure to a blank control stimulus (open circle). Following preferred direction adaptation the response function shifts rightwards along the contrast axis. (B) Contrast response functions under the same conditions derived from the amplitudes of the oscillatory responses of the membrane potential (intracellular recording) at the fundamental frequency to the movement of a grating stimulus. These changes in the membrane response show a slight change in the response function after preferred direction motion. (C) Response functions derived from the mean membrane potentials. These show that the responses after preferred direction motion are shifted downwards relative to controls, i.e. hyperpolarized. Error bars are twice the standard error of the mean over trials. Reprinted by permission from Neuropharmacology (37, 501–11) copyright (1998) Elsevier Publishers Ltd.

the period of blindness that follows a move from darkness into light reveals an underlying light adaptation mechanism, the MAE reveals an underlying motion adaptation mechanism.

1.3.1 Basics of the Motion Aftereffect

The most enduring theory to explain the MAE is the ratio model (Sutherland 1961), which is perhaps best described in its creator's words. 'The direction in which something is seen to move might depend upon the ratios of firing in cells sensitive to movement in different directions, and after prolonged movement in one direction, a stationary image would produce less firing in the cells which had just been stimulated than normally, hence apparent movement in the opposite direction would be seen to occur'. This descriptive model was later formalized by Moulden and Mather (1978). I will expand upon this basic notion in the sections that follow and look into the possible beneficial influences of motion adaptation. However, let us first establish the stimulus parameters that govern the MAE, as first rigorously examined by Wohlgemuth (1911). Once we know what stimuli give rise to the MAE, we can extrapolate that knowledge to identify the likely physiological mechanisms involved in motion adaptation.

When two moving patterns are presented either simultaneously (Verstraten et al. 1994) or alternately (Riggs & Day 1980) in different directions, say at 0° and 30° from the horizontal, only one coherent MAE is seen and it moves at 195°. That is, the illusory motion appears to travel in a direction opposite to the vector sum of the real motion directions. These findings could be the result of adaptation occurring at a level in the visual system where information about different directions has already been integrated. Such a concept led to the distribution-shift model for coding the direction of visual movement (Mather 1980). This model suggests that perceived direction might depend on the response distribution of all direction-selective neurons, which would then lead to an adaptation-induced shift in perceived direction if the distribution were altered by selective directional adaptation (Levinson & Sekuler 1976).

The strength of the MAE is strongly influenced by the temporal and spatial frequencies of moving patterns, i.e. the MAE is only observed if the spatial frequency and temporal frequency content of the pattern falls within certain defined limits. Pantle (1974) showed that the initial MAE speed and the MAE duration were maximal for grating patterns that were drifting at temporal frequencies of 2.5–5 Hz. These experiments were conducted with stimuli located in the centre of the visual field that subtended approximately 4.5° by 3.5°. Pantle used gratings with spatial frequencies of 3 and 6 cpd and both showed optimal initial MAE velocities and MAE durations at similar temporal frequencies, suggesting that the strength of the MAE was temporal frequency dependent and not speed dependent. Had the effect been speed dependent we would expect the optimum MAE strength to be correlated with a fixed speed, given by the ratio of the temporal and spatial frequency of the pattern.

Studies using translating gratings in isolated and centre-surround configurations have demonstrated that MAE strength scales with eccentricity (Murakami & Shimojo 1995). Wright and Johnston (1985) showed that the perceived MAE speed increases with eccentricity, in a manner approximating the change in cortical magnification with eccentricity (M-scaling: Rovamo & Virsu 1979). Eccentricity-dependent changes in MAE strength have been attributed to spatial inhomogeneities across the visual field, such as variations in receptive field size and spatial frequency tuning. Despite changes in spatial frequency tuning with eccentricity, Wright and Johnston (1985) found that the temporal tuning of the MAE was independent of spatial frequency and eccentricity. They found optimum MAE strength occurred at temporal frequencies of 5–10 Hz, which is close to that identified by Pantle (1974). Taken together, Pantle's and Wright and Johnston's results suggest that it is the number of contrast borders that pass over the receptive fields of the visual neurons per second that dictate the degree of adaptation, rather than the speed with which each contrast border moves. Maddess et al. (1988) showed that adaptation of neurons in cat cortex was also governed by the temporal frequency at which the contrast borders moved across the receptive fields of the cells. This physiological analysis supports the psychophysical observations. Taken together, the psychophysical and physiological data provide a clue that motion adaptation may be intricately linked to contrast adaptation and less so to speed-tuned motion processors.

Up to this point MAEs have only been discussed when the pattern following the period of motion is static. Relatively recently, an MAE with a range of different properties has been identified (von Grunau 1986; Mc Carthy 1993). The only difference in the way this MAE is generated is the type of test pattern used after the motion period. Rather than a static pattern, the use of a flickering pattern appears to reveal a different MAE, referred to as the flicker MAE, which might be generated by a different physiological mechanism (Nishida & Sato 1995). As outlined above, the MAE is temporal frequency tuned across a wide range of spatial frequencies. However, if flickering test stimuli are used instead of static patterns, the MAE is not dependent on temporal frequency. Rather, when MAE strength is plotted as a function of speed the peaks have approximately the same adapting speed of 5–8 degs/s for all spatial frequencies tested (Ashida & Osaka 1995). This result suggests that flicker MAEs are revealing a type of motion adaptation that is specific to the motion-processing pathway because only in that pathway is there a specific code measuring image speed (Perrone & Thiele 2001; Priebe *et al.* 2003). Recent investigations into the parameters governing the MAE in higher order motion processing suggest that human subjects can tap into one of two motion processing systems, one that is temporal frequency dependent and the other speed dependent (Price *et al.* 2004). These results reinforce the findings that adaptation can be speed dependent and that this must occur in a region of the brain specifically tuned to detect speed.

Other differences between the use of static and flickering stimuli relate to the types of motion that can produce an MAE. Everything outlined so far relates to MAEs produced by first-order motion, which is motion generated by the movement of spatial structures defined by luminance or colour. Motion can also be perceived with second- or higher-order structures, such as contrast modulation and texture borders (Cavanagh & Mather 1989). Second-order motion produces very weak MAEs when static test patterns are used. If flickering test patterns are used, the MAE generated by second-order motion can be quite strong. Nishida and Sato (1995) suggest that the flicker MAE is mediated at higher levels in the visual system. One strong argument for this theory is that flicker MAE shows complete interocular transfer independent of the type of motion used in the adaptation phase (Nishida *et al.* 1994). Static MAE also shows interocular transfer but usually only at around 60 per cent of its monocular strength (Barlow & Brindley 1963; Lehmkuhle & Fox 1976; Moulden 1980).

1.3.2 Physiological Explanations

Directional motion adaptation must arise in some way from the activity of direction-selective neurons in the visual system, which must play a role in generating the psychophysical phenomenon of the MAE. Direction-selective neurons are very common in the visual systems of all visual animals (for review, see Clifford & Ibbotson 2003). In many species direction-selectivity appears at levels very close to the photoreceptors. For example, directional bipolar cells and retinal ganglion cells are quite common in lower vertebrates (e.g. turtle: DeVoe *et al.* 1989). There is even evidence in the turtle retina that the distal end of some photoreceptors already show signs of directionality (Carras & DeVoe 1991; Criswell & Brandon 1992).

It is generally assumed that there are very few motion detectors in the human retina. This assumption is based on several findings. Non-human primate retina appears to have very few specifically motion sensitive neurons (DeMonasterio & Gouras 1975). Electroretinograms recorded from humans reveal that motion adaptation does not produce direction-specific effects (Bach & Hoffmann 2000). In contrast, visually evoked potentials recorded from the visual cortex show very strong direction-specific effects. This more direct evidence suggests that the great majority of motion-selective processing in primates occurs after the retinal ganglion cells. This being the case, one must assume that motion adaptation is also a post-retinal process in primates.

BARLOW AND HILL

While there is little evidence that primates have motion detectors in the retina, it was by recording the activity of retinal ganglion cells in the rabbit that the first clue to the physiological basis of the MAE was obtained. Barlow and Hill (1963) recorded the firing rates of direction-selective retinal ganglion cells during and following prolonged stimulation with a moving pattern. The initial responses when the image moved in the cell's preferred direction were strong but they declined gradually over the first 20 s to reach an approximately steady-state firing level (Fig. 1.3). When motion stopped, the firing rate fell below its baseline level and then recovered over the next 30 s. Motion in the opposite direction slightly reduced the cell's baseline firing rate but it returned to the baseline almost immediately after motion stopped (Fig. 1.3). Here was the first evidence that individual motion-sensitive cells altered their output in a way that fitted with Sutherland's (1961) ratio model. Remarkably, the time courses of recovery of the rabbit's retinal ganglion cells were similar to the perceptual experience of human MAEs. Clearly, it is a rather significant leap of faith to suggest that the activity of a rabbit retinal neuron could be directly related to human perception. Even so, at least neurons had been identified in a mammal that had the correct type of response to fit with existing theories relating to the MAE.

LINKING THE MAE WITH PHYSIOLOGICAL RECORDINGS

Prolonged motion stimulation causes a gradual reduction in firing output over a period of several seconds in most motion-sensitive cells (Barlow & Hill 1963; Ibbotson *et al.* 1998), including those in the visual cortex (e.g. Vautin & Berkley 1977). Motion adaptation also generates large, robust aftereffects with identified neural correlates in V1 (Hammond *et al.* 1988; Giaschi *et al.* 1993) and in higher areas of the monkey cortex (Petersen *et al.* 1985; van Wezel & Britten 2002). Hammond *et al.* (1988) assessed the time-course and recovery of responsiveness of cat V1 neurons following adaptation with moving bars, gratings, or textured fields. Results were compared with controls in which the adapting stimulus was replaced by a uniform field of identical mean luminance, and also assessed in relation to the strength and time course of adaptation. Firing rate declined to a steady-state during the first 30–60 s of adaptation and the induced aftereffects were direction-specific. The induced aftereffects appeared as attenuated responses to the direction of prior adaptation which lasted for 30–60 s after the motion adaptation stopped. Usually the aftereffects were restricted to driven activity with no consistent effects on the spontaneous discharge. The time courses and general properties of the cells support the conclusion that psychophysically measured MAEs and physiologically identified induced motion aftereffects are generated by cortical neurons.

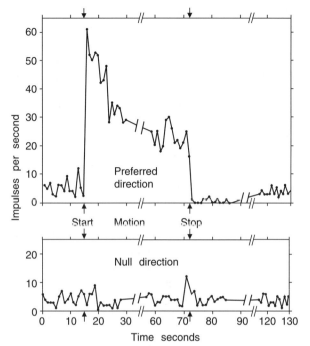

FIG. 1.3 Barlow and Hill (1963) experiment. Effects of stimulating a directionally selective unit in the rabbit retina for 1 minute by motion in the preferred and null directions. Impulses/second are plotted vertically, time horizontally. The maintained activity is suppressed following 1 minute of excitation by motion in the preferred direction. Motion in the null direction has no significant effect, the peak at 70 seconds being an artefact. Reprinted by permission from Nature (200, 1345–7) copyright (1963) Macmillan Publishers Ltd.

In non-human primates, direction-selective neurons in the primary visual cortex (V1) are tuned to specific spatial and temporal frequencies (Foster *et al.* 1985). In general, the range of spatiotemporal tuning observed in primate V1 neurons closely matches the tuning of the MAE, as described in Section 1.3.1. Foster *et al.* found that most neurons in V1 and some in V2 responded strongly at temporal frequencies up to 5.6–8.0 Hz, after which their responses dropped off. Having established that cells in the visual system have similar tuning properties to the MAE, it is now necessary to establish whether they adapt accordingly.

Area MT (middle temporal area) in the primate extra-striate cortex is the first brain area to specialize in motion processing and has a large proportion of direction-selective cells (Zeki 1974; Maunsell and van Essen 1983*a,b,c*). Most importantly, neural activity in MT is closely linked to the perception of motion (Newsome *et al.* 1989; Salzman *et al.* 1992; Thiele *et al.* 2000), as demonstrated by inactivating and by stimulating MT in animals trained to perform psychophysical tasks (Newsome & Pare 1988; Salzman & Newsome 1994). Inactivation impairs the ability to perform motion-related tasks (Newsome &

Pare 1988), while micro-stimulation of clusters of similarly direction-tuned MT cells allows the experimenter to bias an animal's perception of the direction of motion (Salzman & Newsome 1994). The human cortex contains an area that appears to be the homologue of MT in monkeys. The human homologue is referred to as area MT+ and lesions caused by strokes in this area of the brain lead to a greatly reduced perception of motion (Baker *et al.* 1991). Moreover, adaptation to moving patterns causes direction-specific reductions in the activity of MT+ (Huk *et al.* 2001; Tolias *et al.* 2001). Adaptation to moving patterns that produce strong perceptual MAEs has been shown to cause very substantial differential changes in activity in MT+ once attentional influences have been removed by using appropriate controls (Huk *et al.* 2001).

To date there are only a small number of studies that have attempted to correlate the activities of MT cells with the formation of MAEs. Petersen *et al.* (1985) recorded from cells in MT of the owl monkey and showed that motion in the preferred direction reduced the responses to subsequently presented stimuli. Conversely, motion in the anti-preferred direction enhanced the responses to subsequent test patterns moved in the preferred direction. This was for a long time the only experimental finding that had used long adaptation periods (20 s) that were similar in length to psychophysical MAE studies. Kohn and Movshon (2003) were the first to use prolonged stimulation of MT cells in such a way as to distinguish response adaptation from active gain control. They looked for active mechanisms by measuring the responses to a wide range of different test contrasts following the adapting motion period. They found that all MT neurons showed a significant shift in their contrast response functions following a period of motion adaptation in the preferred direction. The shift greatly reduced the responses of the neurons to subsequently presented low contrast stimulation but retained strong responses, with almost no loss in absolute firing rate, at high contrasts. As is the case for V1 neurons (Sclar *et al.* 1989), the adapted contrast response functions shifted laterally along the contrast axis such that the functional dynamic range of the cell was centred on the prevailing contrast. This result shows that 'motion adaptation' in MT is closely linked to contrast adaptation and is an active gain control process.

IS CONTRAST ADAPTATION IN MT LINKED TO MOTION PROCESSING?

As outlined earlier, models of the MAE suggest a stage of motion processing where the responses to stimuli moving in all directions are compared (Mather 1980). In terms of a back-and-forth motion along one axis, it is suggested that the responses to stimuli moving in one direction are subtracted from those moving in the opposite direction (Adelson & Bergen 1985; Simoncelli & Heeger 1998). This process might be implemented by MT cells because they are excited by motion in one direction and their spontaneous activity is inhibited by motion in the opposite, a process referred to as motion opponency (Snowden *et al.* 1991). To measure the effect of motion in the anti-preferred (AP) direction on MT cells, Kohn and Movshon (2003) recorded the responses of neurons to the simultaneous presentation of a combination of a low contrast (0.25) grating moving in the preferred direction and a grating moving in the anti-preferred direction, in which the contrast could be set between 0 and 0.75. The control experiment used the combined grating stimulus without any prior adaptation. At the highest combined contrast (preferred 0.25/AP 0.75) the inhibition generated by AP direction motion was stronger than the preferred direction excitation, so the overall response was 10 spikes/s below the cell's spontaneous firing rate (Fig. 1.4). When the AP and preferred direction gratings had equal contrasts (0.25), the cell's firing rate was equal to the spontaneous rate. Only when the contrast of the AP direction grating fell below 0.15 did the excitation generated by the preferred direction grating dominate the response. In fact, the response remained constant at around 40 spikes/s for all AP direction gratings that had contrasts < 0.15, suggesting that the inhibition generated at these low contrasts by the AP stimulus was not sufficient to have any impact on the response magnitude.

Kohn and Movshon plotted the responses as a function of the contrast of the AP direction grating and fitted the data with a curve (Fig. 1.4). One of the fitted parameters provided the contrast of the AP grating at which the response level was half-way between the maximum response and the spontaneous activity (C_{50}). In the control condition the C_{50} value occurred at contrasts close to 0.2. When the same experiment was repeated but this time with the combined gratings presented after prolonged AP direction motion, the response curve shifted

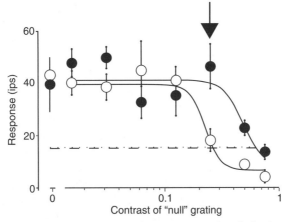

FIG. 1.4 Responses of an MT neuron to a low-contrast, preferred stimulus and a superimposed null grating of varying contrast before (open symbols, thin line) and after (closed symbols, thick line) null adaptation. Dashed and dotted line (overlying) indicate spontaneous activity before and after adaptation, respectively. Suppression observed at null contrasts of 0.25 and above was strongly reduced after adaptation. The evoked response to a 0.5 contrast counterphase grating (0.25 null grating and 0.25 preferred grating; vertical arrow) increased from 2 ips to 20 ips above the spontaneous rate. Also, at null grating contrasts above 0.25 the cell's response was no longer suppressed below the spontaneous rate. Reprinted by permission from Neuron (39, 681–91) copyright (2003) Elsevier Publishers Ltd.

to the right so that the C_{50} value was now at contrasts of 0.4–0.5 (Fig. 1.4). The response at the highest contrast combination (preferred 0.25/AP 0.75) was now equal to the spontaneous firing rate, showing that the AP direction inhibition was no longer sufficient to overpower the preferred direction excitation. The rightward shift in C_{50} indicates that the AP grating required more contrast to suppress the preferred direction excitation (Fig. 1.4). These results have been interpreted to mean that the gains of the neurons tuned to the AP direction are attenuated, thus reducing their ability to suppress the recorded cell's preferred direction response. It can be concluded that contrast gain control is built into the directional tuning mechanism of MT cells such that the contrast gain control revealed by physiological and psychophysical testing will appear as strongly direction-selective. The results point to a link between contrast and motion adaptation in that an additional direction-selective mechanism is imposed on the contrast adaptation that is presumably inherited from earlier non-directional processing stages (e.g. Solomon *et al.* 2004).

CORRELATES OF THE FLICKER MAE

Although MT neurons are direction-selective, most will generate a small response to static flickering stimuli such as a grating in which the dark and light bars periodically reverse their brightness polarity – a counterphasing grating. Following strong adaptation in the anti-preferred direction, MT neurons show an enhanced response to a counterphase grating (Kohn and Movshon 2003). Responses to counterphase gratings averaged 10 spikes/s without prior adaptation but increased to around 20 spikes/s after anti-preferred adaptation. Elevated firing rates in MT neurons signal motion in the preferred direction. Consequently an increase in the post-adaptation firing rate in the presence of static counterphasing gratings, following anti-preferred adaptation, will signal preferred direction motion, thus providing a direct correlate of the flicker MAE (e.g. Nishida & Sato 1995). When MT neurons are exposed to 40 s of anti-preferred motion and then briefly exposed to counterphase flicker every 2–3 s the response to the flickering patterns returns to preadaptation levels in around 18 s. The duration of the flicker MAE in humans is approximately 14 s (Ashida & Osaka 1994), showing a close similarity between the timing of physiological findings in the macaque monkey and psychophysical findings in humans.

1.3.3 Is There a Function for Motion Adaptation?

We have seen that light adaptation allows the visual system to efficiently code 10 log units of light level despite the output cells from the retina only having the capacity within a given adaptation state to transmit about 2 log units of brightness. Contrast appears to be coded in the visual system in a similar fashion. Is there a specific mechanism generating motion adaptation and what is its purpose?

EVIDENCE FROM MAMMALS

For humans, the perceived speed of an image moving at a constant speed declines as a function of stimulus duration in an exponential fashion (Goldstein 1957; Clifford & Langley 1996; Bex *et al.* 1999; Hammett *et al.* 2000). This decline in response mirrors the decline in response of some direction-selective neurons in the visual cortex of non-human primates, suggesting a link between physiologically measured adaptation and behavioural output. Such a decline in perceived speed appears to have little benefit as it throws away a quantitative measure of absolute image speed. However, psychophysical studies have shown that as the perceived speed of a constantly moving stimulus decreases, sensitivity to changes in speed are enhanced (Clifford & Langley 1996; Bex *et al.* 1999; Clifford & Wenderoth 1999). The speed increment thresholds remain proportional to perceived speed, so that as the perceived speed decreases, the ability to detect small changes about that speed increases. This finding provides evidence of a beneficial purpose for motion adaptation because it suggests that the representation of absolute speed may be sacrificed to improve differential sensitivity. Why is it important to enhance differential speed sensitivity? When travelling at a constant speed for prolonged periods (long-distance running or driving) it takes a lot of energy to code the absolute speed of travel, e.g. at optimal image speeds a neuron would have to fire at a high steady rate for the entire duration of the motion. It is more efficient to reduce the steady firing rate to a very low level, thus losing the absolute measure of speed, and use the full dynamic range of each cell to detect speed changes, which can signal a sudden decrease or increase in speed. By utilizing this information about change it is possible to use a simple negative feedback system to adjust for any alterations in image speed and return to the desired velocity (e.g. Ibbotson 1991). In information terms the absolute speed of travel becomes largely redundant because most of the information you need to sustain that speed through a negative feedback loop can be provided by selectively signalling change.

If cells adapt to motion in this way we would predict that following motion adaptation, the shape of a cell's speed-tuning function would depend on the motion (direction and speed) of the image in the recent past. Saul and Cynader (1989*a,b*) examined the influence of motion adaptation on responses of neurons in area 17 (V1) of the primary visual cortex of the cat. They recorded responses to motion before and after adaptation to moving gratings. They found that in the spatial domain, adapting at a given spatial frequency resulted in a broad reduction in responsiveness at spatial frequencies above and below the adapting frequency, often with a differential loss of sensitivity at low spatial frequencies (Saul & Cynader 1989*a*). In the temporal domain, adaptation generally shifted the preferred temporal frequencies of the cells. The most common result was that adaptation at a particular temporal frequency led to the maximal response attenuation at that same frequency, thus altering the shape of the overall tuning function (Saul & Cynader 1989*b*). Interestingly, the changes in temporal frequency tuning were direction-dependent. After preferred direction adaptation, response attenuation was greater at frequencies equal to or above the adapting frequency. After anti-preferred direction adaptation, attenuation was greatest at frequencies equal to or below the adapting level. While these results show that temporal and spatial frequency tuning changes in the visual cortex following adaptation, it is also noteworthy that this region is not a specialized motion processing area. It is possible that the adaptation effects observed in V1 are further refined in specialized motion processing areas further up-stream in the cat system, such as in the postero-medial suprasylvian area (PMLS), which is the approximate homologue of area MT in primate cortex (Dreher *et al.* 1996).

It might be expected in more specialized motion processing areas that when cells are exposed to high mean image speeds, responses to low velocities will be attenuated but that responses to high velocities will be released from saturation. One possible expectation is that the speed tuning functions will shift from the solid line (un-adapted) to the dashed line (post-adapted) in Fig. 1.5(A). This would lead to an effective rightward shift in the speed response functions relative to the speed axis rather than a simple change in response gain across all velocities (dotted line, Fig. 1.5(A)). Such a shift would allow an enhanced ability to distinguish between speeds in the middle range of the scale and potentially increase the overall range of speeds that can be coded.

Experiments have shown that speed gain control of this type does occur in some cells in the sub-cortical nucleus of the optic tract (NOT), which is an area of the mammalian brain that contains a very high proportion of motion-opponent, direction-selective neurons (Collewijn 1975a,b; Ibbotson *et al.* 1994). The NOT resides in the pretectum and its neurons are known to connect with the brain stem areas responsible for driving optokinetic responses (e.g. Collewijn 1975a,b). Recordings from the NOT of the marsupial wallaby have shown that many cells demonstrate a form of speed gain control (Ibbotson *et al.* 1998). Examples of the effect of preferred direction adaptation on the speed response functions of two NOT neurons are shown in Fig. 1.5(B,C). Before adaptation the spike rates of the cells increased steadily with image speed to the cell's maximum response, after which the spike rate fell again as speed increased. Following adaptation to gratings drifting in the preferred direction the responses of the neurons fell into two broad classes, those in which adaptation led to a change in response gain across all image velocities (Fig. 1.5(B)) and those in which the attenuation primarily occurred at low image velocities (Fig. 1.5(C)). In the first group, the optimum response (R_{max}) was reduced to values of 50–75 per cent of the preadapted level. In the second group, adaptation to drifting gratings dramatically attenuated the responses to low-speed motion while those close to the optimum speed generally showed only moderate reductions to 75–98 per cent of the unadapted R_{max} levels (Fig. 1.5(C)). The combination of attenuated low speed responses and small changes in R_{max} led to changes in the steepness of the speed response functions and rightward shifts in the inclining phases of the speed response functions. The NOT cells were also tested for changes in their contrast response functions following adaptation. It was found that cells that showed strong rightward shifts in their speed

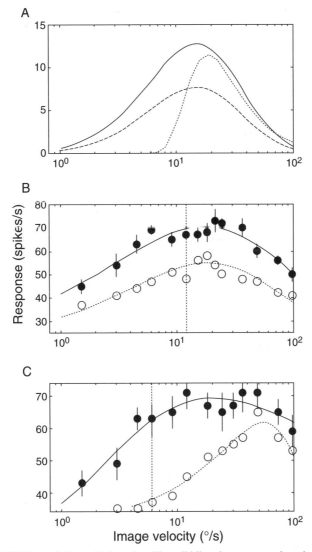

FIG. 1.5 (A) Theoretical speed adaptation. The solid line shows a non-adapted speed response function. The dotted line shows the possible result of speed gain control in which the rising phase of the function has shifted to the right along the speed axis. The dashed line shows what would occur if adaptation led to a reduction in response gain. (B, C) Each panel shows speed response functions for a single NOT neuron, measured before (filled symbols, solid line) and after (open symbols, dashed line) adaptation to motion in the preferred direction. The adapting speed is shown by the vertical dashed line in each panel. Error bars are standard deviations. (B) Response functions for a cell in which post-adaptation responses reveal a reduction in response gain. (C) Responses from a cell where the adapted response function shifts to the right along the speed axis (speed gain).

response functions also showed large shifts in their contrast response functions, suggesting a close link between motion and contrast adaptation. Investigations of this type are now underway in high-order motion-specialized regions of cat (PMLS) and primate (MT) cortex to see if and how the temporal frequency-specific effects observed in V1 (Saul & Cynader 1989*b*) are utilized to provide beneficial alterations in speed tuning in cortex.

EVIDENCE FROM INVERTEBRATES

The concept of active speed gain control appears to be widespread in the animal kingdom because evidence for it has also been identified in the motion-sensitive neurons in the optic lobe of the fly. The responses of a uniquely iden-tifiable, highly direction-selective neuron in the fly optic lobe have been shown to decline in spiking frequency during constant-speed stimulation. Maddess and Laughlin (1985) presented the fly cells with a moving pattern with a speed of 58°/s for 6.7 s. During this time the cell's spike rate fell from 320 spikes/s to 180 spikes/s in an exponential fashion. During the 6.7 s period, 16 equally spaced 39 ms speed changes of 23.5°/s were added to the speed of the image. The responses to changes in speed increased as the steady-state spike discharge decreased, suggesting that an increase in relative sensitivity accompanied the decrease in absolute sensitivity during adaptation. These results provide physi-ological evidence to support findings from human psychophysics, as outlined in the Section 'Evidence from mammals' (Clifford & Langley 1996). However, until such experiments are repeated in primate cortex we cannot draw precise comparisons between physiological and psychophysical results.

It is noteworthy that the same cell in the fly optic lobe was tested for poten-tial lateral shifts in its speed response function following adaptation to motion. It was found that the speed response function in the unadapted state increased almost linearly when response was plotted as a function of log-speed. The response range was from 100 to 300 spikes/s, covering a speed range of 3–80°/s. When the speed response function was measured after the cell had been adapted to constant motion at 58°/s the function shifted rightwards in such a way that a linear relationship was obtained on the semilogarithmic plot cov-ering a response range of 80–220 spikes/s, coding velocities ranging from approximately 20–100°/s. The results show that the cell shifts its speed sensi-tivity to match the prevailing adaptation speed in much the same way as some cells in wallaby NOT. Consequently, the cell is able to better signal changes in speed about the mean adapting speed.

1.3.4 Cellular Mechanisms

Returning to the primate cortex, evidence based on the non-transferability of adaptation from one region of an MT neuron's receptive field to another area suggests that MT inherits many of the adaptation effects we observe from earlier cortical sites, such as V1 (Kohn & Movshon 2003). In the section on contrast adaptation in V1 it was shown that contrast gain control could be partially explained by a post-synaptic hyperpolarization of the V1 cell's membrane potential (Carandini & Ferster 1997). This cannot be the case for the MT neurons because adaptation in one region of the receptive field would generate a hyperpolarization that should then influence the responses to all test stimuli in all parts of the cell's receptive field. It follows that contrast adaptation occurs via cellular changes in areas prior to MT and is then coded by the spiking output of those cells and sent to higher-order areas of the cortex. It is, however, possible that higher order properties of the stimulus such as the speed of movement, which is known to be coded in MT for the first time in the primate cortex (Perrone & Thiele 2001; Priebe *et al.* 2003), could drive a further level of adaptation. Until now, no cellular mechanism to identify such adaptation has been identified in MT neurons or in other motion specific areas of the mammalian brain.

1.4 Biophysical Mechanisms

1.4.1 Network Mechanisms

The results reviewed up to now show that contrast and motion adaptation adjusts the spiking capacity of cells, which can cause a shift in their contrast and speed response functions. These effects can be described as a form of gain control. Intracellular work relating to contrast adaptation suggests that (1) adaptation induces a hyperpolarization; (2) for cortical neurons at least, the hyperpolarization adjusts the spiking capacity of the cells; and (3) the associated shift in the response functions leads to the perceptual effects of adaptation. However, several studies indicate that the mechanisms underlying adaptation are more complex than this simple scheme. For example, it is possible to produce adaptation in a cell using a broader range of stimuli than those that drive a response (Maffei *et al.* 1973; Saul & Cynader 1989*a,b*; Bonds 1991). This result is difficult to explain based entirely on a general hyperpolarization within a given cell. In addition, some psychophysical experiments have shown that stimuli that do not excite psychophysically defined channels can adapt them (Blakemore *et al.* 1971; Dealy & Tolhurst 1974). As a result of these findings, a number of additional models have been proposed. To account for the psychophysical data, models were proposed that depend on narrowly tuned excitation and a more broadly tuned inhibition, the latter being modulated by the contrast in the recent past (Ross & Speed 1991; Wilson & Humanski 1993; Foley & Chen 1997). To account for the physiological data, Heeger (1992) proposed an extension of the normalization model of processing in primary visual cortex. In this model, cortical cells within a large local pool inhibit one another such that their outputs are scaled (normalized) by a neural representation of contrast (Heeger 1992; Carandini *et al.* 1997*a*, 1998*a*). If this inhibition had a long-term memory, the normalization model could be extended to account for the observed adaptation effects (Heeger 1992).

While the broad outlines of the psychophysical and physiological models are similar, they differ in the specifics of how adaptation would affect the broadly tuned inhibition. In some models, the strength of inhibition depends only on the recent contrast in the adapting stimulus (Ross & Speed 1991; Heeger 1992), while in others, it is primarily dependent on the contrast in the test stimulus, but is modulated by adaptation (Foley & Chen 1997). In Wilson and Humanski's (1993) model, the strength of inhibition results from intracortical feedback whose synaptic efficacy is influenced by adaptation.

How might it be possible to distinguish between these models? While adaptation to a given pattern reduces the responses of V1 neurons to all subsequently viewed test patterns, the reduction is quite specific, being strongest when the adapting and test patterns are identical. For example, adaptation to a stimulus tilted clockwise to a cell's preferred orientation depresses the response to that stimulus more than it depresses the response to orientations counter-clockwise to the preferred orientation (Marlin *et al.* 1988; Hammond *et al.* 1989; Saul & Cynader 1989*b*; Giaschi *et al.* 1993; Carandini *et al.* 1997*b*). Similar stimulus-specific adaptation affects have been observed in the spatial and temporal frequency domains (Movshon & Lennie 1979; Albrecht *et al.* 1984; Saul & Cynader 1989*b*). Specificity effects of this sort would be predicted by the psychophysical model of Wilson and Humanski, which assumes that adaptation increases the strength of synaptic inhibition coming from neurons that are strongly activated. By contrast, other models (Ross & Speed 1991; Foley & Chen 1997) would predict that adaptation increases the overall inhibition, and thus reduces the tuning curves in a non-specific fashion. Barlow and Földiák (1989) have proposed another model that would predict the specificity effects described above (also see: Barlow 1990). This model is based on an 'anti-Hebbian' mechanism, which increases the amount of mutual inhibition between cells that are simultaneously active, and ascribes a more fundamental cognitive role to adaptation than the control of gain. A test of these theories in monkey V1 gave results that favoured Barlow and Földiák's (1989) theory (Carandini *et al.* 1997*b*, 1998*a*). This study focused on the effects of adaptation to plaids composed of two moving gratings whose orientations were parallel to and orthogonal to the one preferred by a recorded cell. It was found that adaptation often increased the amount of cross-orientation suppression, in some cases even turning cross-orientation facilitation into suppression. This result suggests that adaptation can affect the interaction between the groups of neurons tuned to orthogonal orientations, either by increasing their mutual inhibition or by decreasing their mutual excitation.

1.4.2 Synaptic Mechanisms

An important limitation of the models considered up to now is their dependence on adaptation-induced inhibition. However, there is no direct evidence implicating synaptic inhibition in the phenomenon of adaptation. It has been noted that neuronal adaptation persists during the application of the $GABA_A$ antagonist bicuculline (DeBruyn & Bonds 1986; Vidyasagar 1990). This $GABA_A$ is known to have an important role in cortical inhibition (Sillito 1992). Although involvement of postsynaptic $GABA_B$ receptors has an impact on cortical processing (Allison et al. 1996), effects of blocking these receptors have in general been relatively small.

Instead of adaptation-induced inhibition, short-term depression in the strength of excitatory synaptic transmission has been proposed as a mechanism for adaptation (Varela et al. 1997; Chance et al. 1998; Chung et al. 2002). In the visual cortex, this type of depression has been shown to affect both intra-cortical and thalamocortical synapses (Stratford et al. 1996; Abbott et al. 1997; Gil et al. 1997; Varela et al. 1997). When modelling the components of short-term synaptic plasticity acting over a number of time scales, it was found that the time constant of one of the slower components, 10–20 seconds, is similar to those measured for contrast and motion adaptation in single-unit studies (Albrecht et al. 1984; Maddess et al. 1988; Giaschi et al. 1993).

Depression could occur either at geniculocortical synapses, or at intracortical excitatory synapses, or at both. It could account for several properties of adaptation (Chance et al. 1998), especially in the context of a recurrent network of excitation (Somers et al. 1996). Firstly, depression could explain the finding that antagonists to presynaptic glutamate autoreceptors, thought to mediate excitatory synaptic depression, reduce extracellularly measured adaptation effects (McLean & Palmer 1996). Secondly, synaptic depression is not dependent on firing of the adapted cell but on the activity in presynaptic neurons. As the tuning of the synaptic input to a cell is substantially broader than that of the spike responses (Jagadeesh et al. 1993; Nelson et al. 1994; Carandini & Ferster 1998), depression could explain why a broader range of stimuli than those that produce a spike response can evoke adaptation. Thirdly, some psychophysical (Lorenceau 1987) and physiological (Maddess et al. 1988; Saul & Cynader 1989a; Bonds 1991) experiments have revealed that the higher the temporal frequency of a visual stimulus the greater is the adaptation produced. Synaptic depression would predict this behaviour because at low temporal frequencies, the pause in firing that occurs during the 'off' phase of each stimulus cycle allows for some recovery from depression. However, in most cases psychophysics reveals a clear tuning for temporal frequency (see Section 1.3.1), with a particular frequency giving the largest effect. These results might be explained if the increase in adaptation with increases in temporal frequency is ultimately limited by the temporal filtering properties of the cells. That is, beyond a certain frequency the cell is not able to respond as strongly, so even though the stimulus is being presented ever more frequently the system can no longer adapt to the input.

There is a second possible synaptic mechanism, which is that adaptation induces a shunting inhibition in cortical neurons. Shunting inhibition would increase the membrane conductance of the cells. Carandini and Ferster (1997) found no significant change in membrane conductance associated with adaptation in cat cortical cells. However, it seems likely that these measurements may have been influenced by the resistance of the electrode (Borg-Graham *et al.* 1998; Carandini *et al.* 1998*b*). Electrode resistance and capacitance are both higher (and more difficult to measure) for *in vivo* patch recording than they are *in vitro*. This increases the electrode time constant to values near that of the cell itself, making it difficult to decompose the response to injected current pulses into the neuronal and electrode components.

1.5 Conclusions

In this chapter it has been shown that adaptation can have highly beneficial effects in terms of coding image contrast and speed. Experimental data have been presented based on extracellular recordings from a variety of species to support the notion that adaptation acts as a type of contrast gain control and in some cells also as a form of speed gain control. Interestingly, there appears to be a close association between strong contrast gain control and speed gain control. While no intracellular recordings have looked at the underlying mechanisms of speed gain control, a substantial body of work now exists to demonstrate some of the intracellular mechanisms that lead to contrast adaptation. Given that contrast and speed gain control appear to be linked, it is reasonable to conclude that the intracellular mechanisms may be similar. It is likely that the motion-related effects are superimposed on already existing contrast effects, which are inherited from earlier processing stages.

This chapter has provided an overview of recent concepts relating to the cellular, synaptic, and network mechanisms that are responsible for adaptation. Thirty years of research on adaptation has given us substantial information on the phenomenon. Based mostly on psychophysical data, researchers have proposed models that link perceptual effects to the function of single cells and synapses. The available models, however, make contradicting predictions, and the available data are not sufficient to constrain them. There are a number of links that need to be bridged before a complete theory can be formulated. For example, findings on synaptic function obtained *in vitro* need to be confirmed *in vivo*, and then linked clearly with their proposed influences on the adaptation of neuronal visual responses. The large body of literature on the physiology of adaptation in animals must in turn be linked definitively to perceptual adaptation phenomena in humans. We are only now beginning to understand the mechanisms of low-level adaptation, such as contrast gain control, and much research is required before physiological explanations can be found for higher-order adaptation phenomena such as those related to face perception (Webster & MacLin 1999).

Acknowledgements

The author would like to thank Dr Matteo Carandini for his assistance in preparing this chapter, particularly Section 1.4. He was offered co-authorship which was graciously declined. Thanks to Drs Crowder and Schröter for their assistance with the figures.

References

Abbott L.F., Varela, J.A., Sen, K., & Nelson, S.B. (1997). Synaptic depression and cortical gain control. *Science, 275,* 220–4.

Addams, R. (1834). An account of a peculiar optical phenomenon seen after having looked at a moving body. *London and Edinburgh Philosophical Magazine and Journal of Science, 5, 373–4.*

Adelson, E.H., & Bergen, J.R. (1985). Spatio-temporal energy models for the perception of motion. *Journal of the Optical Society of America A, 2,* 284–99.

Albrecht, D.G., Farrar, S.B., & Hamilton, D.B. (1984). Spatial contrast adaptation characteristics of neurones recorded in the cat's visual cortex. *Journal of Physiology (London), 347,* 713–39.

Allison, J.D., Kabara, J.F., Snider, R.K., Casagrande, V.A., & Bonds, A.B. (1996). GABAB-receptor-mediated inhibition reduces the orientation selectivity of the sustained response of striate cortical neurons in cats. *Visual Neuroscience, 13,* 559–66.

Ashida, H., & Osaka, N. (1994). Difference of spatial frequency selectivity between static and flicker motion aftereffects. *Perception, 23,* 1313–20.

Ashida, H., & Osaka, N. (1995). Motion aftereffect with flickering test stimuli depends on adapting speed. *Vision Research, 35,* 1825–33.

Baccus, S.A., & Meister, M. (2002). Fast and slow contrast adaptation in retinal circuitry. *Neuron, 36,* 909–19.

Bach, C., & Hoffmann, M.B. (2000). Visual motion detection in man is governed by non-retinal mechanisms. *Vision Research, 40,* 2379–85.

Baker, C.L., Hess, R.F., & Zihl, J. (1991). Residual motion perception in a "motion-blind" patient, assessed with limited-lifetime random dot stimuli. *Journal of Neuroscience, 11,* 454–61.

Barlow, H.B. (1990). A theory about the functional role and synaptic mechanism of after-effects. In C. Blakemore (ed.), *Vision: Coding and Efficiency* (pp. 363–75). Cambridge: Cambridge University Press.

Barlow, H.B., & Brindley, G.S. (1963). Inter-ocular transfer of movement after-effects during pressure blinding of the stimulated eye. *Nature, 28,* 1347.

Barlow, H.B., & Földiák, P. (1989). Adaptation and decorrelation in the cortex. In R. Durbin, C. Miall, & C. Mitchison (ed.), *The Computing Neuron* (pp. 54–72). Workingham: Addison-Wesley.

Barlow, H.B., & Hill, R.M. (1963). Evidence for a physiological explanation for the waterfall illusion and figural aftereffects. *Nature, 200,* 1345–47.

Bex, P., Bedingham, S., & Hammett, S.T. (1999). Apparent speed and speed sensitivity during adaptation to motion. *Journal of the Optical Society of America A, 16,* 2817–24.

Blakemore, C. (Ed.) (1990). *Vision: Coding and Efficiency.* Cambridge, UK: Cambridge University Press.

Blakemore, C., Carpenter, R.H.S., & Georgeson, M.A. (1971). Lateral thinking about lateral inhibition. *Nature, 234,* 418–19.

Blakemore, C., Muncey, J.P., & Ridley, R.M. (1973). Stimulus specificity in the human visual system. *Vision Research, 13,* 1915–31.

Bonds A.B. (1991). Temporal dynamics of contrast gain in single cells of the cat striate cortex. *Visual Neuroscience, 6*, 239–55.

Borg-Graham, L.J., Monier, C., & Frégnac, Y. (1998). Visual input evokes transient and strong shunting inhibition in visual cortical neurons. *Nature, 393*, 369–73.

Burrone, J., & Lagnado, L. (1997). Synaptic depression and the kinetics of exocytosis in retinal bipolar cells. *Journal of Neuroscience, 20*, 568–78.

Carandini, M., & Ferster, D. (1997). A tonic hyperpolarization underlying contrast adaptation in cat visual cortex. *Science, 276*, 949–52.

Carandini, M., & Ferster, D. (1998). The iceberg effect and orientation tuning in cat V1. *Investigative Ophthalmology and Vision Science, 39*, S239.

Carandini, M., Anderson, J., & Ferster, D. (1998b). Excitatory and inhibitory conductance changes in simple cells of cat visual cortex. *European Journal of Neuroscience, 10*, 331.

Carandini, M., Barlow, H.B., O'Keefe, L.P., Poirson, A.B., & Movshon, J.A. (1997b). Adaptation to contingencies in macaque primary visual cortex. *Philosophical Transactions of the Royal Society of London, Series B, 352*, 1149–54.

Carandini, M., Heeger, D.J., & Movshon, J.A. (1997a). Linearity and normalization in simple cells of the macaque primary visual cortex. *Journal of Neuroscience, 17*, 8621–44.

Carandini, M., Movshon, J.A., & Ferster, D. (1998a). Pattern adaptation and cross-orientation interactions in the primary visual cortex. *Neuropharmacology 37*, 501–11.

Carras, P.L., & DeVoe, R.D. (1991). Directionally asymmetric responses to motion in cones. *Investigative Ophthalmology and Vision Science, 32*, 906.

Cavanagh, P., & Mather, G. (1989). Motion: the long and short of it. *Spatial Vision, 4*, 103–29.

Chance, F.S., Nelson, S.B., & Abbott, L.F. (1998). Synaptic depression and the temporal response characteristics of V1 cells. *Journal of Neuroscience, 18*, 4785–99.

Chander, D., & Chichilnisky, E.J. (2001). Adaptation to temporal contrast in primate and salamander retina. *Journal of Neuroscience, 21*, 9904–16.

Chung, S., Li, X., & Nelson, S.B. (2002). Short-term depression at thalamocortical synapses contributes to rapid adaptation of cortical sensory responses in vivo. *Neuron, 34*, 437–46.

Clifford, C.W.G., & Ibbotson, M.R. (2003). Fundamental mechanisms of visual motion detection: models, cells and functions. *Progress in Neurobiology, 68*, 409–37.

Clifford, C.W.G., & Langley, K. (1996). Psychophysics of motion adaptation parallels insect electrophysiology. *Current Biology, 6*, 1340–42.

Clifford, C.W.G., & Wenderoth, P. (1999). Adaptation to temporal modulation can enhance differential speed sensitivity. *Vision Research, 40*, 4324–32.

Collewijn, H. (1975a). Direction-selective units in the rabbit's nucleus of the optic tract. *Brain Research, 100*, 489–508.

Collewijn, H. (1975b). Oculomotor areas in the rabbit's midbrain and pretectum. *Journal of Neurobiology, 6*, 3–22.

Criswell, M.H., & Brandon, C. (1992). Cholinergic and GABAergic neurons occur in both the distal and proximal turtle retina. *Brain Research, 577*, 101–11.

Dealy, R.S., & Tolhurst, D.J. (1974). Is spatial adaptation an after-effect of prolonged inhibition? *Journal of Physiology (London), 241*, 261–70.

DeBruyn, E.J., & Bonds, A.B. (1986). Contrast adaptation in the cat is not mediated by GABA. *Brain Research, 383*, 339–42.

DeMonasterio, F.M., & Gouras, P. (1975). Functional properties of ganglion cells of the rhesus monkey retina. *Journal of Physiology (London)*, *251*, 167–95.

DeVoe, R.D., Carras, P.L., Criswell, M.H., & Guy, R.G. (1989). Not by ganglion cells alone: directional selectivity is widespread in identified cells of the turtle retina. In R. Weiler, & N.N. Osborne (ed.), *Neurobiology of the Inner Retina* (pp. 235–46). Berlin: Springer-Verlag.

Dreher, B., Wang, C., Turlejski, K.J., Djavadian, R.L., & Burke, W. (1996). Area PMLS and 21a of cat visual cortex: two functionally distinct areas. *Cerebral Cortex*, *6*, 585–99.

Foley, J.M., & Chen, C.C. (1997). Analysis of the effect of pattern adaptation on pattern pedestal effects: a two-process model. *Vision Research*, *37*, 2779–88.

Foster, K.H., Gaska, J.P., Nagler, M., & Pollen, D.A. (1985). Spatial and temporal frequency selectivity of neurones in visual cortical areas V1 and V2 of the macaque monkey. *Journal of Physiology (London)*, *365*, 331–63.

Giaschi, D., Douglas, R., Marlin, S.G., & Cynader, M.S. (1993). The time course of direction-selective adaptation in simple and complex cells in cat striate cortex. *Journal of Neurophysiology*, *70*, 2024–34.

Gil, Z., Connors, B.W., & Amitai, Y. (1997). Differential regulation of neocortical synapses by neuromodulators and activity. *Neuron*, *19*, 679–86.

Goldstein, A.G. (1957). Judgements of visual speed as a function of length of observation time. *Journal of Experimental Psychology*, *54*, 457–61.

Graham, N.V.S. (1989). *Visual Pattern Analyzers*. New York: Oxford University Press.

Greenlee, M.W., & Heitger, F. (1988). The functional role of contrast adaptation. *Vision Research*, *28*, 791–7.

Hammett, S.T., Thompson, P.G., & Bedingham, S. (2000). The dynamics of speed adaptation in human vision. *Current Biology*, *10*, 1123–26.

Hammond, P., Mouat, G.S., & Smith, A.T. (1988). Neural correlates of motion after-effects in cat striate cortical neurones: monocular adaptation. *Experimental Brain Research*, *72*, 1–20

Hammond, P., Pomfrett, C.J.D., & Ahmed, B. (1989). Neural motion after-effects in the cat's striate cortex: orientation selectivity. *Vision Research*, *29*, 1671–83.

Harris, C.S. (1980). *Visual Coding and Adaptability*. New Jersey: Laurence Erlbaum Associates.

Harris, R.A., O'Carroll, D.C., & Laughlin, S.B. (2000). Contrast gain reduction in fly motion adaptation. *Neuron*, *28*, 595–606.

Heeger, D.J. (1992). Normalization of cell responses in cat striate cortex. *Visual Neuroscience*, *9*, 181–97.

Hood, D.C., & Birch, D.G. (1993). Light adaptation of human rod receptors: the leading edge of the human a-wave and models of rod receptor activity. *Vision Research*, *33*, 1605–18.

Huk, A.C., Ress, D., & Heeger, D.J. (2001). Neuronal basis of the motion aftereffect reconsidered. *Neuron*, *32*, 1161–72.

Ibbotson, M.R. (1991). Wide-field motion-sensitive neurons tuned to horizontal movement in the honeybee, *Apis mellifera*. *Journal of Comparative Physiology A*, *168*, 91–102.

Ibbotson, M.R., Mark, R.F., & Maddess, T. (1994). Spatiotemporal response properties of direction-selective neurons in the nucleus of the optic tract and dorsal terminal nucleus of the wallaby, *Macropus eugenii*. *Journal of Neurophysiology*, *72*, 2927–43.

Ibbotson, M.R., Clifford, C.W.G., & Mark, R.F. (1998). Adaptation to visual motion in directional neurons of the nucleus of the optic tract. *Journal of Neurophysiology*, *79*, 1481–93.

Jagadeesh, B., Wheat, H.S., & Ferster, D. (1993). Linearity of summation of synaptic potentials underlying direction selectivity in simple cells of the cat visual cortex. *Science, 262,* 1901–4.

Kohn, A., & Movshon, J.A. (2003). Neuronal adaptation to visual motion in area MT of the macaque. *Neuron, 39,* 681–91.

Lehmkuhle, S.W., & Fox, R. (1976). On measuring interocular transfer. *Vision Research, 16,* 428–30.

Levinson, E., & Sekuler, R. (1976). Adaptation alters perceived direction of motion. *Vision Research, 16,* 779–81.

Lorenceau (1987). Recovery from contrast adaptation: effects of spatial and temporal frequency. *Vision Research, 27,* 2185–91.

Maddess, T., & Laughlin, S.B. (1985). Adaptation of the motion-sensitive neuron H1 is generated locally and governed by contrast frequency. *Proceedings of the Royal Society of London: Series B, 225,* 251–75.

Maddess, T., McCourt, M.E., Blakeslee, B., & Cunningham, R.B. (1988). Factors governing the adaptation of cells in area 17 of the cat visual cortex. *Biological Cybernetics, 59,* 229–36.

Maffei, L., Fiorentini, A., & Bisti, S. (1973). Neural correlate of perceptual adaptation to gratings. *Science, 182,* 1036–38.

Malchow, R.P., & Yazulla, S. (1986). Separation and light adaptation of rod and cone signals in the retina of the goldfish. *Vision Research, 26,* 1655–66.

Marlin, S.G., Hasan, S.J., & Cynader, M.S. (1988). Direction-selective adaptation in simple and complex cells in cat striate cortex. *Journal of Neurophysiology, 59,* 1314–30.

Mather, G. (1980). The movement aftereffect and a distribution-shift model for coding the direction of visual movement. *Perception, 9,* 379–92.

Mather, G., Verstraten, F., & Anstis, S. (ed.) (1998). *The Motion Aftereffect: A Modern Perspective*. Cambridge, MA: MIT Press.

Maunsell, J.H., & van Essen, D.C. (1983a). The connections of the middle temporal visual area (MT) and their relationship to a cortical hierarchy in the macaque monkcy. *Journal of Neuroscience, 3,* 2563–86.

Maunsell, J.H., & van Essen, D.C. (1983b). Functional properties of neurons in middle temporal visual area of the macaque monkey. II. Binocular interactions and sensitivity to binocular disparity. *Journal of Neurophysiology, 49,* 1148–67.

Maunsell, JH., & van Essen, D.C. (1983c). Functional properties of neurons in middle temporal visual area of the macaque monkey. I. Selectivity for stimulus direction, speed, and orientation. *Journal of Neurophysiology, 49,* 1127–47.

McCarthy, J.E. (1993). Directional adaptation effects with contrast modulated stimuli. *Vision Research, 33,* 2653–62.

McCormick, D.A., Sanchez-Vives, M.V., & Nowak, L.G. (1998). Role of membrane properties in the generation of contrast adaptation in the visual cortex. *Investigative Ophthalmology and Vision Science, 39,* S238.

McLean, J., & Palmer, L.A. (1996). Contrast adaptation and excitatory amino acid receptors in cat striate cortex. *Visual Neuroscience, 13,* 1069–88.

Moulden, B. (1980). After-effects and the integration of patterns of neural activity within a channel. *Philosophical Transactions of the Royal Society of London Series B: Biological Sciences, 290,* 39–55.

Moulden, B., & Mather, G. (1978). In defence of a ratio model for movement detection at threshold. *Quarterly Journal of Experimental Psychology, 30,* 505–20.

Movshon, J.A., & Lennie, P. (1979). Pattern-selective adaptation in visual cortical neurones. *Nature*, *278*, 850–2.

Murakami, I., & Shimojo, S. (1995). Modulation of motion aftereffect by surround motion and its dependence on stimulus size and eccentricity. *Vision Research*, *35*, 1835–44.

Nelson, S., Toth, L., Sheth, B., & Sur, M. (1994). Orientation selectivity of cortical neurons during intracellular blockade of inhibition. *Science*, *265*, 774–7.

Newsome, W.T., & Pare, E.B. (1988). A selective impairment of motion perception following lesions of the middle temporal visual area (MT). *Journal of Neuroscience*, *8*, 2201–11.

Newsome, W.T., Britten, K.H., & Movshon, J.A. (1989). Neuronal correlates of a perceptual decision. *Nature*, *341*, 52–4.

Nishida, S., Ashida, H., & Sato, T. (1994). Complete interocular transfer of motion aftereffect with flickering test. *Vision Research*, *34*, 2707–16.

Nishida, S., & Sato, T. (1995). Motion aftereffect with flickering test patterns reveals higher stages of motion processing. *Vision Research*, *35*, 477–90.

Ohzawa, I., Sclar, G., & Freeman, R.D. (1982). Contrast gain control in the cat visual cortex. *Nature*, *298*, 266–8.

Ohzawa, I., Sclar, G., & Freeman, R.D. (1985). Contrast gain control in the cat visual system. *Journal of Neurophysiology*, *54*, 651–65.

Pantle, A. (1974). Motion aftereffect magnitude as a measure of the spatio-temporal response properties of direction-sensitive analysers. *Vision Research*, *14*, 1229–36.

Perrone, J.A. & Thiele, A. (2001). Speed skills: measuring the visual speed analyzing properties of primate MT neurons. *Nature Neuroscience*, *4*, 526–32.

Petersen, S.E., Baker, J.F., & Allman, J.M. (1985). Direction-specific adaptation in area MT of the owl monkey. *Brain Research*, *346*, 146–50.

Price, N.S.C., Greenwood, J., & Ibbotson, M.R. (2004). Tuning properties of radial phantom motion after-effects. *Vision Research*, *44*, 1971–9.

Priebe, N.J., Cassanello, C.R., & Lisberger, S.G. (2003). The neural representation of speed in macaque area MT/V5. *Journal of Neuroscience*, *23*, 5650–61.

Rieke, F. (2001). Temporal contrast adaptation in salamander bipolar cells. *Journal of Neuroscience*, *21*, 9445–54.

Riggs, L.A., & Day, R.H. (1980). Visual aftereffects derived from inspection of orthogonally moving patterns. *Science*, *208*, 416–8.

Rodieck, R.W. (1998). *The First Steps in Seeing*. Sunderland, Massachussets: Sinauer.

Ross, J., & Speed, H.D. (1991). Contrast adaptation and contrast masking in human vision. *Proceedings of the Royal Society of London: Series B*, *246*, 61–9.

Ross, J., & Speed, H.D. (1996). Perceived contrast following adaptation to gratings of different orientations. *Vision Research*, *36*, 1811–18.

Ross, J., Speed, H.D., & Morgan, M.J. (1993). The effects of adaptation and masking on incremental thresholds for contrast. *Vision Research*, *33*, 2051–6.

Rovamo, J., & Virsu, V. (1979). An estimation and application of the human cortical magnification factor. *Experimental Brain Research*, *37*, 495–510.

Salzman, C.D., & Newsome, W.T. (1994). Neural mechanisms for forming a perceptual decision. *Science*, *264*, 231–7.

Salzman, C.D., Murasugi, C.M., Britten, K.H., & Newsome, W.T. (1992). Microstimulation in visual area MT: effects on direction discrimination performance. *Journal of Neuroscience*, *12*, 2331–55.

Sanchez-Vives, M.V., Nowak, L.G., & McCormick, D.A. (2000a). Membrane mechanisms underlying contrast adaptation in cat area 17 in vivo. *Journal of Neuroscience*, *20*, 4267–85.

Sanchez-Vives, M.V., Nowak, L.G., & McCormick, D.A. (2000b). Cellular mechanisms of long-lasting adaptation in visual cortical neurons in vitro. *Journal of Neuroscience*, *20*, 4286–99.

Saul, A.B., & Cynader, M.S. (1989a). Adaptation in single units in visual cortex: 1. The tuning of aftereffects in the temporal domain. *Visual Neuroscience*, *2*, 609–20.

Saul, A.B., & Cynader, M.S. (1989b). Adaptation in single units in visual cortex: 2. The tuning of aftereffects in the spatial domain. *Visual Neuroscience*, *2*, 593–607.

Sclar, G., Ohzawa, I., & Freeman, R.D. (1985). Contrast gain control in the kitten's visual system. *Journal of Neurophysiology*, *54*, 668–75.

Sclar, G., Ohzawa, I., & Freeman, R.D. (1987). The effects of contrast on visual orientation and spatial frequency discrimination: a comparison of single cells and behavior. *Journal of Neurophysiology*, *57*, 773–86.

Sclar, G., Lennie, P., & DePriest, D.D. (1989). Contrast adaptation in striate cortex of macaque. *Vision Research* 29, 747–55.

Shou, T., Li, X., Zhou, Y., & Hu, B. (1996). Adaptation of visually evoked responses of relay cells in the dorsal lateral geniculate nucleus of the cat following prolonged exposure to drifting gratings. *Visual Neuroscience*, *13*, 605–13.

Sillito, A.M. (1992). GABA mediated inhibitory processes in the function of the geniculo-striate system. *Progress in Brain Research*, *90*, 349–84.

Simoncelli, E.P., & Heeger, D.J. (1998). A model of neuronal responses in visual area MT. *Vision Research*, *38*, 743–61.

Snowden, R., & Hammett, S. (1992). Subtractive and divisive adaptation in the human visual system. *Nature*, *355*, 248–50.

Snowden, R.J., Treue, S., Erickson, R.G., & Andersen, R.A. (1991). The response of area MT and V1 neurons to transparent motion. *Journal of Neuroscience*, *11*, 2768–85.

Solomon, S.G., Peirce, J.W., Dhruv, N.T., & Lennie, P. (2004). Profound contrast adaptation early in the visual pathway. *Neuron*, *42*, 155–62.

Somers, D.C., Todorov, E.V., Siapas, A.G., & Nelson, S.B. (1996). Contrast adaptation effects modeled as thalamocortical and intracortical synaptic transmission changes. *Society for Neuroscience Abstracts*, *22*, 643.

Stratford, K.J., Tarczy-Hornoch, K., Martin, K.A.C., Bannister, N.J., & Jack, J.J. (1996). Excitatory synaptic inputs to spiny stellate cells in cat visual cortex. *Nature*, *382*, 258–61.

Sutherland, N.S. (1961). Figural after-effects of apparent size. *Quarterly Journal of Experimental Psychology*, *13*, 222–8.

Thiele, A., Dobkins, K.R., & Albright, T.D. (2000). Neural correlates of contrast detection at threshold. *Neuron*, *26*, 715–24.

Tolias, A.S., Smirnakis, S.M., Augath, M.A., Trinath, T., & Logothetis, N.K. (2001). Motion processing in the macaque: revisited with functional magnetic resonance imaging. *Journal of Neuroscience*, *21*, 8594–601.

Usrey, W.M., & Reid, R.C. (2000). Visual physiology of the lateral geniculate nucleus in two species of new world monkey: Saimiri sciureus and Aotus trivirgatis. *Journal of Physiology*, *523*, 755–69.

van Wezel, R.J.A., & Britten, K.H. (2002). Motion adaptation in area MT. *Journal of Neurophysiology*, *88*, 3469–76.

Varela, J.A., Sen, K., Gibson, J., Fost, J., Abbott, L.F., & Nelson, S.B. (1997). A quantitative description of short-term plasticity at excitatory synapses in layer 2/3 of rat primary visual cortex. *Journal of Neuroscience, 17,* 7926–40.

Vautin, R.G., & Berkley, M.A. (1977). Responses of single cells in cat visual cortex to prolonged stimulus movement: Neural correlates of visual aftereffects. *Journal of Neurophysiology, 40,* 1051–65.

Verstraten, F.A., Fredericksen, R.E., Grusser, O.J., & van de Grind, W.A. (1994). Recovery from motion adaptation is delayed by successively presented orthogonal motion. *Vision Research, 34,* 1149–55.

Vidyasagar, T.R. (1990). Pattern adaptation in cat visual cortex is a cooperative phenomenon. *Neuroscience, 36,* 175–9.

von Grunau, M.W. (1986). A motion aftereffect for long-range stroboscopic apparent motion. *Perception and Psychophysics, 40,* 31–8.

Webster, M.A., & MacLin, O. (1999). Figural aftereffects in the perception of faces. *Psychonomic Bulletin and Review, 6,* 647–53.

Wilson, H.R., & Humanski, R. (1993). Spatial frequency adaptation and contrast gain control. *Vision Research, 33,* 1122–49.

Wohlgemuth, A. (1911). On the after-effect of seen movement. *British Journal of Psychology Monograph Supplement, 1,* 1–116.

Wright, M.J., & Johnston, A. (1985). Invariant tuning of motion aftereffect. *Vision Research, 25,* 1947–55.

Zeki, S.M. (1974). Functional organization of a visual area in the posterior bank of the superior temporal sulcus of the rhesus monkey. *Journal of Physiology (London), 236,* 546–73.

2

Functional Ideas about Adaptation Applied to Spatial and Motion Vision

Colin W.G. Clifford

2.1 Introduction

Functional ideas about adaptation have been motivated by two main considerations. First, the visual system must be self-calibrating in its mapping of environmental stimulation onto patterns of neural activity (Andrews 1964; Rushton 1965; Ullman & Schechtman 1982). Self-calibration is the property of a system to change itself in response to changes in the environment (recalibration) and to adjust to perturbations within the system in an unchanging environment (error-correction). Second, adaptation might tend to optimize the use of the limited dynamic range of the visual pathways for the coding of visual stimuli (Laughlin 1989, 1990). The dynamic range of the visual pathways is limited by the number of neurons and the variability of neuronal firing. Use of this limited range can be optimized by reducing the transmission of redundant information about unchanging aspects of the stimulus (Attneave 1954; Barlow 1961). Dynamic range optimization tends to reduce redundancy in the responses of individual sensory neurons, maximizing the effective bandwidth available for the transmission of novel information about the stimulus (Srinivasan *et al.* 1982; Clifford & Langley 1996*a*). The principle of redundancy reduction can be extended from single neurons to populations of neurons by a process alternatively described as adaptive decorrelation (Barlow & Foldiak 1989; Barlow 1990, 1997; Atick *et al.* 1993;

Muller *et al.* 1999) or response orthogonalization (Kohonen & Oja 1976; Zaidi & Shapiro 1993).

The functional considerations of self-calibration and redundancy reduction suggest that vision is a dynamic process, with adaptive mechanisms continually operating to match the coding employed to the statistical structure of the visual stimulation. The extent to which the mapping between stimulus and neural response is unchanging will reflect the degree of statistical stationarity within the environment (Andrews 1964). When the structure of the environment is changed, such as during a period of adaptation, the mapping adapts accordingly.

This chapter reviews psychophysical studies showing marked similarities between adaptation in the orientation and motion domains, and recent physiological studies revealing some important differences. From a computational perspective, the problem of extracting information from the image signal can be cast as the recovery of orientation information in various domains (Adelson & Bergen 1991), with motion considered as orientation in space-time (see Clifford & Ibbotson 2003), suggesting that common computational principles might underlie the processing of orientation and motion despite apparently distinct cortical substrates (Clifford 2002). If adaptive coding of different visual attributes (orientation and direction-of-motion) does indeed follow similar computational principles, then it is tempting to speculate that these principles might also be applicable to understanding adaptation in higher-level visual processing. Consequently, I hope that what is written here about adaptation in the processing and perception of orientation and direction-of-motion will be of relevance to subsequent chapters of this book dealing with adaptation to shape, faces, and other complex patterns.

2.2 Adaptation: Function or Fatigue?

An early account of the neural basis of perceptual aftereffects, which Barlow & Foldiak (1989) trace back to Exner (1894), was that adaptation satiates or fatigues cells sensitive to the adapting stimulus (Kohler & Wallach 1944; Sutherland 1961). When the period of adaptation ceases, the spontaneous discharge of the fatigued cells remains suppressed (Barlow & Hill 1963). This produces a bias away from the adapted stimulus in the response of the population of cells sensitive to the adapted stimulus dimension, giving rise to a perceptual aftereffect. So, after adaptation to leftwards tilt, a vertical grating will appear tilted rightwards (Blakemore 1973), and, after adaptation to a downwards-moving pattern, a static pattern will appear to drift upwards (Wohlgemuth 1911).

Before seeking a functional basis for perceptual aftereffects it is important to consider accounts based on neuronal fatigue, which do after all have the attraction of parsimony. We offer two principal lines of evidence against the fatigue hypothesis. Discussion of other factors arguing against neural fatigue as the mechanism of psychophysically observed adaptation, such as the storage of aftereffects (Wohlgemuth 1911; Spigel 1960; Wiesenfelder & Blake 1992), can be found in Mather and Harris (1998).

First, cortical adaptation has been found to show a degree of pattern specificity (Movshon & Lennie 1979), rather than simply depending on the adapting neuron's response rate as predicted by the fatigue hypothesis. Movshon and Lennie found that the loss of responsiveness of cells in cat primary visual cortex following grating adaptation can be specific to the spatial frequency of the adapting stimulus. Similar specificity has also been shown to stimulus orientation (Hammond *et al.* 1989) and temporal frequency (Saul & Cynader 1989). One possible explanation for Movshon and Lennie's results might be that complex cells, which formed the majority of their sample, are excited by simple cells with different spatial frequencies. In this case, the stimulus specificity of adaptation in the responses of a complex cell could simply reflect fatigue in a particular afferent simple cell. However, Movshon and Lennie discount this possibility for two reasons. First, the spatial frequency selectivity of simple cells is little different from that of complex cells (Movshon *et al.* 1978). Second, they observed spatial frequency specific adaptation in a simple cell. Movshon and Lennie thus concluded that pattern-specific adaptation reflects on the operation of a pattern-selective cortical mechanism.

The second argument against the fatigue hypothesis is that the effects of adaptation on perceived orientation are remarkably similar to the effects of a simultaneously presented inducing stimulus. Since the early work of Gibson (Gibson 1937*a*; Gibson & Radner 1937), a large body of literature has built up on the characteristics and determinants of the tilt aftereffect (TAE) and tilt illusion (TI). In the TAE, adaptation to an oriented stimulus biases the perceived orientation of a subsequently presented stimulus. In the TI, the presence of an oriented surround stimulus biases the perceived orientation of a simultaneously presented test. The two phenomena show a very similar dependence on the angle between the adapting (inducing) stimulus and the test (O'Toole & Wenderoth 1977). If we accept that the lateral interactions underlying the TI serve a functional role, then the similar phenomenology of the TI and TAE suggests that tilt adaptation also has a functional basis.

The phenomenology of the TAE can be summarized as follows (Fig. 2.1). Prolonged exposure to an oriented pattern affects the perceived orientation of a subsequently observed pattern (Gibson & Radner 1937). For adapting orientations between 0° and 50°, a vertical test appears to be repelled away from the adaptor in orientation, with the strongest effect occurring between 10° and 20°. For larger angles, there is a smaller attraction effect, such that a vertical test appears rotated towards the adaptor. The strongest attraction effect is observed between 75° and 80° (Wenderoth & Johnstone 1987), and occurs robustly when the display includes relatively large adapting gratings or long adapting and test lines (Gibson & Radner 1937; Kohler & Wallach 1944; Morant & Harris 1965). The existence of the attraction effect is a particular challenge to fatigue-based accounts (Coltheart 1971).

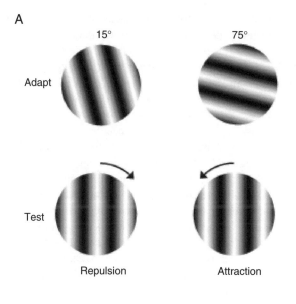

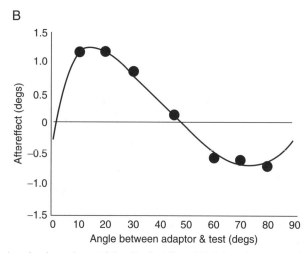

FIG. 2.1 Angular dependence of the tilt aftereffect. (A) Adaptation to a grating oriented at 15° to the vertical causes a subsequently viewed vertical test grating to appear tilted in the opposite direction – a repulsive aftereffect. If the adapting grating is oriented at 75° to the vertical then a smaller, attractive aftereffect is produced. (B) Magnitude of the tilt aftereffect as a function of the angle between adaptor and test. By convention, repulsive aftereffects are given positive sign. Data are redrawn from the first paper to describe the tilt aftereffect, Gibson and Radner (1937). The solid line shows a fit from the model described in Clifford *et al.* (2000).

The similarity between the TAE and TI suggests that similar mechanisms are involved (Wenderoth & Johnstone 1988). It is generally assumed that the TI is mediated by lateral interactions between orientation-tuned cortical neurons (Blakemore *et al.* 1970). Lateral inhibition and excitation have the capacity to regulate the gain of cortical circuits and sharpen tuning curves (Somers *et al.* 1995; Carandini & Ringach 1997; Adorjan *et al.* 1999). Adaptation-induced changes in response properties may play a similar functional role.

The search for a functional explanation of the TAE and other aftereffects dates back to the 'normalization' theory of Gibson (Gibson 1937*a,b*; Gibson & Radner 1937). According to the normalization theory, vertical and horizontal are norms of visual space. Prolonged inspection of a line tilted away from one of these norms (clockwise from vertical, say) will cause the nearest norm to shift in the direction of the adapting line (clockwise). After adaptation, a line at the orientation of the original norm (vertical) will appear rotated from the shifted norm in the opposite direction (anti-clockwise). However, the normalization theory is unable to account for the fact that the magnitude of attraction effects is smaller than that of repulsion effects (Gibson & Radner 1937; Morant & Mistovich 1960), or that adaptation to horizontal or vertical lines also generates a TAE for tilted test stimuli (Kohler & Wallach 1944). The latter observation, coupled with the fact that the angular dependence of the TAE is similar for vertical and oblique test stimuli (Mitchell & Muir 1976), suggests that consideration of relative rather than absolute orientation is the key to understanding the TAE.

I have recently proposed an explanation for the effects of adaptation on the perception of motion and orientation in terms of functional considerations underlying their cortical coding (Clifford *et al.* 2000). As described in detail here, psychophysical data on the effects of adaptation to orientation and motion are modelled through self-calibration and decorrelation (Barlow & Foldiak 1989) in their neural representations. I believe these principles will prove to be of general relevance in understanding the cortical coding of sensory information. The model is essentially an instantiation of the following axioms:

(1) our sensory systems map attributes of the environment onto patterns of neuronal responses;

(2) the range of responses is fixed, but the mapping is dynamic and adaptable;

(3) the mapping adapts to 'optimize' the use of the fixed response range;

(4) the extent to which the mapping is unchanging reflects statistical stationarity in the structure of the environment;

(5) when the structure of the environment is changed, e.g. during a period of adaptation, the mapping adapts accordingly.

These ideas are implicit in previous functional accounts of adaptation (e.g. Barlow & Foldiak 1989; Atick *et al.* 1993). What is novel here is that these functional principles are embodied in a model from which quantitative predictions can be derived.

2.3 Representation of Motion by a Neuronal Population

While Gibson (1937b) considered the distinction between 'unilateral' sensory dimensions such as length or duration and 'bilateral' dimensions such as convex-concave or leftwards-rightwards, his theory did not deal explicitly with circular dimensions such as direction of motion and orientation. Under normalization theory, adaptation was viewed as the shift of linked norms (subjective horizontal and vertical) between which a certain amount of 'play' was permitted (Gibson & Radner 1937). As Coltheart (1971) points out, this explanation is rather *ad hoc*. Mather (1980) proposed a more appropriate representation in the context of the motion aftereffect (MAE). He suggested that the MAE was not simply due to a shift in balance along a single dimension (e.g. leftwards-rightwards motion), but was better represented as a shift in the response distribution of a population of units each preferentially tuned to one of the whole range of directions of motion (see also Levinson & Sekuler 1976).

Implicit in Mather's notion of a distribution shift is the idea that the speed and direction of motion can be coded in the responses of a population of direction-selective units. The principal neural substrate of the MAE in human visual cortex is believed to be the human homologue of monkey area MT (Tootell *et al.* 1995; He *et al.* 1998; Culham *et al.* 1999; Huk *et al.* 2001). The vast majority of neurons in MT are strongly direction-selective (Albright *et al.* 1984). The response properties of these direction-selective cells can be characterized in the form of direction-tuning curves (Fig. 2.2). The peak of the direction-tuning curve defines the cell's preferred direction-of-motion, while the width of the curve defines the cell's direction bandwidth. Figure 2.2 shows the response of one MT neuron as a function of the direction of stimulus motion (redrawn from Snowden 1994).

Under a simple population coding scheme, the perceived direction of motion is given by the direction of the weighted vector average of the preferred directions of the units responding to the stimulus, where each unit's weighting is proportional to its response above the spontaneous level. While some subsequent theoretical studies have used methods related to maximum likelihood, rather than simple vector averaging, to arrive at the population response (see Pouget *et al.* 2000, for a review), the important notion here is that perceptual quantities can be represented in the responses of populations of neurons. According to Mather's distribution-shift theory, adaptation affects the way in which stimulus motion is mapped onto the responses of a population of motion-sensitive units. The resulting population response vector no longer corresponds to the motion of the stimulus, giving rise to illusions such as the MAE (Fig. 2.3).

2.4 Double-angle Representation of Orientation

It is perhaps less obvious that a vector representation is appropriate for orientation than for motion, which is itself a vector quantity (although see Gilbert & Wiesel 1990; Vogels 1990). However, the fact that orientation is a circular quantity means

A

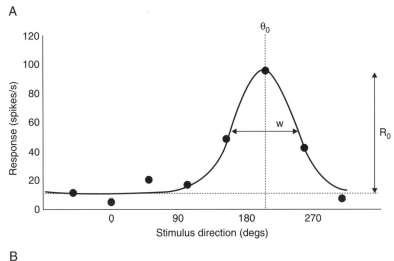

B

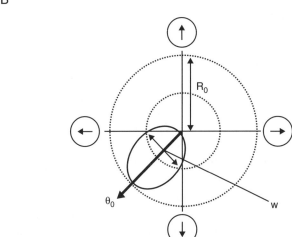

FIG. 2.2 Response of one MT neuron as a function of the direction of stimulus motion, redrawn from Snowden (1994). (A) The solid line shows the best-fit circular normal curve, a periodic function with a profile very similar to a Gaussian. The preferred direction of the neuron is defined as θ_0, while R_0 and w denote the peak response above baseline and the full-width at half-height (FWHH), respectively. For the cell shown here, $\theta_0 = 232°$, $R_0 = 86$ spikes/s, and $w = 78°$. (B) The same direction tuning curve represented on polar axes.

that there exist potential problems associated with a scalar representation. Orientation is a quantity that wraps around every 180°. Thus, if 0° corresponds to vertical then 180° is also vertical. This multivaluedness can be problematic. Let us assume that a vertically oriented stimulus excites two units, one whose preferred orientation is 1° right of vertical and one whose preferred orientation is 1° left (179°). If one unit signals 1° and another signals 179°, then what is the average

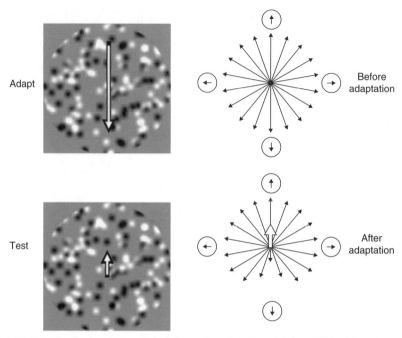

FIG. 2.3 Distribution shift model of the motion aftereffect (Mather, 1980). Adaptation to downwards motion causes a subsequently presented static stimulus to appear to drift upwards. Prior to adaptation, each of the population of direction-selective neurons is presumed to respond with a particular gain. Adaptation causes a reduction in the gain of the neurons responding most strongly to the adapting stimulus, such that the population response to a subsequent static test stimulus signals motion in the opposite direction, in this case upwards.

orientation being signalled? A scalar average of the two signals will give 90° (horizontal), not 0° or 180° (vertical). It is true that in this case the problem can be avoided by relabelling 179° as −1°, but this simply moves the discontinuity in scalar orientation values elsewhere and does not solve the problem.

Wrap-around issues can be avoided by representing the response of each orientation-tuned unit as a vector in a two-dimensional space, with the direction of the vector representing the unit's preferred orientation and the length of the vector representing the unit's response (Fig. 2.4). The responses of individual units can then be combined by a process such as vector averaging to give a population response vector. The direction of this vector represents perceived orientation.

Representing orientation in vector form brings out the potential similarity in coding of tilt and direction-of-motion (Fig. 2.5). Orientation wraps around every 180°, with horizontal and vertical as opposites, while direction-of-motion wraps around every 360°, with up and down as opposites. From this 'double-angle' representation for spatial orientation (Gilbert & Wiesel 1990), it follows that similar coding strategies underlying orientation and motion perception will

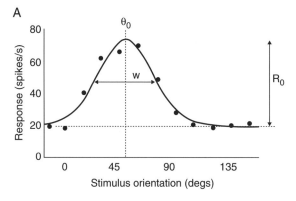

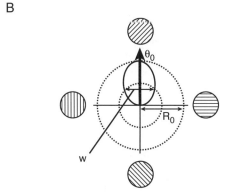

FIG. 2.4 Response of an orientation-selective neuron from area V4 in the ventral stream of primate visual cortex, redrawn from McAdams & Maunsell (1999). (A) The preferred orientation of the neuron is defined as θ_0, while R_0 and w denote the peak response above baseline and the full-width at half-height (FWHH), respectively. The best-fit circular normal function has parameters $\theta_0 = 49°$, $R_0 = 57$ spikes/s, and $w = 38°$. (B) The same orientation tuning curve represented on double-angle polar axes, such that a 360° rotation of the vector corresponds to a 180° rotation of the stimulus.

produce interactions in the motion domain at twice the angular difference to their orientation analogues, as observed psychophysically (Clifford 2002).

2.5 A Functional Model of Orientation and Motion Adaptation

The proposed model of adaptation (Clifford *et al.* 2000) rests upon several assumptions. Orientation is presumed to be encoded locally and retinotopically by patterns of neuronal responses. Exposure to an oriented adaptor can affect how the orientation of a subsequent test stimulus is mapped onto the responses of orientation-selective neurons. The model assumes that the mapping tends to optimize the use of a fixed neuronal response range for the encoding of orientation by adapting in two ways, which I term centring and scaling (Fig. 2.6).

A   B

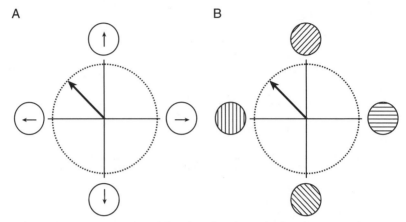

FIG. 2.5 Vector representation of direction of motion and orientation. (A) In the motion domain, the direction of the vector represents the direction of motion. (B) In the orientation domain, the direction of the vector codes for stimulus orientation. This is a 'double-angle' representation of orientation.

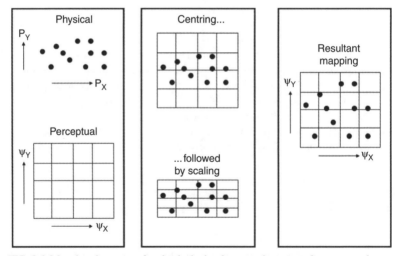

FIG. 2.6 Mapping the states of a physical stimulus onto the states of a perceptual system. The information about the stimulus that the perceptual system represents can be maximized if each state of the perceptual system occurs with equal frequency in response to the stimulus ensemble. Matching of the perceptual system to the stimulus requires that the response states of the perceptual system be centred on the prevailing stimulus distribution and scaled according to the variability along each stimulus dimension. The resultant mapping uses the full range of perceptual states to represent the prevailing stimulus distribution.

Centring and scaling are mechanisms by which the response of a population of neurons can be self-calibrating. Centring is adaptation to the mean of the prevailing stimulus distribution. It operates to set the zero-point of a population response, and is essentially equivalent to an error-correcting distribution shift (Andrews 1964; Mather 1980). Scaling is adaptation to variation within the prevailing stimulus distribution. It is one way in which adaptation might serve to decorrelate responses (Barlow & Foldiak 1989; Barlow 1990, 1997), and is equivalent to the transformation proposed by Atick *et al.* (1993) to underlie the effect of cortical adaptation on colour appearance. Both of these operations have a functional basis in maximizing the information content of the population response (Attneave 1954), and are analogous to the centring and scaling transformations applied to data prior to regression analysis (Draper & Smith 1998). In the language of control theory, centring is a form of additive (subtractive) gain control, while scaling is divisive (multiplicative) in nature.

In the orientation domain (Fig. 2.7(A)), centring serves to shift the population response away from the adapting orientation (the prevailing stimulus) and towards the opposite orientation (Fig. 2.7(B)) while scaling tends to equalize the response along different axes. If the adaptor is vertical, for example, then the adapting axis in the orientation domain is vertical-horizontal (Fig. 2.7(A)). Scaling then tends to equalize the amount of variation along the vertical-horizontal and left-right oblique axes (Fig. 2.7(C)). In combination (Fig. 2.7(D)), the effects of centring and scaling in the orientation domain can be used to model the effect of adaptation on subsequent orientation perception, as described in detail in Sections 2.9 and 2.10.

2.6 How Might Adaptation to the Mean and Adaptation to Variation be Realized in a Population of Neurons?

Clifford *et al.* (2000) proposed a simple neural model of how adaptation to the mean and adaptation to variation might be realized in a population of neurons. According to the model, adaptation to the mean is achieved by a reduction in the gain of the neurons responding most strongly to the adapting stimulus. This is essentially the 'distribution shift' model proposed by Mather (1980) (Fig. 2.3). At the level of single neurons, adaptation to the mean resembles neuronal fatigue in that the gain of neurons responding strongly during adaptation is suppressed. This is consistent with the known physiology of neurons from a range of cortical areas, and raises an interesting question. If the reduction in neuronal gain through adaptation looks like fatigue at the single neuron level but like adaptive gain control at the population level, which is the correct level of analysis for understanding the phenomenon? I have already made a case for considering adaptation as functional, rather than simply as a limitation of the system. However, it is also pertinent to note that the generation of neuronal action potentials ('spikes') is metabolically expensive (Laughlin *et al.* 1998). For a system with limited metabolic resources, a coding strategy in which neurons responded

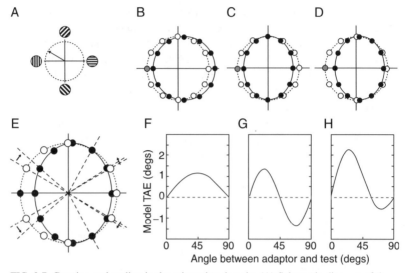

FIG. 2.7 Centring and scaling in the orientation domain. (A) Schematic diagram of the double-angle representation of spatial orientation. The population response is a vector in a two-dimensional space. The direction of this response vector represents perceived orientation. In this representation, horizontal and vertical are opposites. Thus, 180° in model space corresponds to 90° in perceived orientation. The effects of (B) centring, (C) scaling, and (D) centring and scaling in combination. White circles represent the response vector for a range of orientations in the unadapted state. Black circles show the response after prolonged exposure to the orientation denoted by the grey circle. Adaptation is modelled as a shift in the origin of the stimulus-response mapping and a rescaling of the adapting dimension. The geometry illustrated in (E) allows us to relate the perceived orientation of the test stimulus with and without adaptation. Predicted angular tuning functions of the tilt aftereffect due to the effects of (F) centring, (G) scaling, (H) a combination of centring and scaling. Redrawn from Clifford et al. (2000).

strongly to unchanging stimulation (as during periods of adaptation) would be wasteful of those resources. Thus, one could view adaptive gain suppression as a functional strategy to preserve or enhance information transmission in spite of biophysical limitations.

In the model proposed by Clifford et al. (2000), adaptation to variation is implemented as a tendency to increase the bandwidth of neurons tuned away from the adapting axis in the relevant domain. In the orientation domain, for example, if the adaptor is vertical then the adapting axis is vertical-horizontal (Fig. 2.7(A)). Adaptation to a vertical stimulus is then predicted to increase the orientation bandwidth of neurons tuned to oblique orientations. In this way, the population vector in response to stimuli similar to the adapting stimulus is pulled away from the population vector representing the adapting stimulus, tending to equalize the amount of response variation along the vertical-horizontal and left-right oblique axes in the orientation domain (Fig. 2.7(C)) despite the

A

B

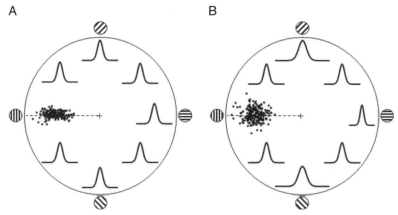

FIG. 2.8 Effects of systematic changes in neuronal bandwidth as a function of peak tuning relative to the adapting stimulus on the distribution of responses to the adaptor. (A) In the unadapted state, each model neuron in the population has equal orientation bandwidth. The distribution of population vectors (circles) relative to the origin of the orientation domain (cross) in response to a vertical stimulus in the presence of a small amount of neural noise is tightly clustered around the veridical orientation (dashed line). (B) Increasing the orientation bandwidth of model neurons tuned to oblique orientations and/or narrowing the bandwidth of neurons tuned around horizontal and vertical without changing the level of neural noise spreads out the distribution of population responses, increasing the range of perceived orientations elicited by vertical stimuli.

uneven stimulus distribution. In the presence of neuronal noise, these changes in bandwidth serve to increase the spread of population responses to the adapting stimulus. Clifford *et al.* (2000) also noted that reducing the breadth of filters tuned to the adapting orientation and its opposite might be an alternative or additional mechanism that would produce a similar result. Figure 2.8 illustrates the effects of systematic changes in neuronal bandwidth as a function of peak-tuning relative to the adapting stimulus on the distribution of responses to the adaptor.

2.7 Neurophysiological Evidence

At the time that Clifford *et al.* (2000) proposed their model there was no published evidence for a systematic effect of adaptation on neuronal bandwidth. Subsequent work has demonstrated such effects in orientation-selective cells of the primary visual cortex of cat (Dragoi *et al.* 2000) and monkey (Dragoi *et al.* 2002), and in direction-selective cells of monkey MT (Kohn & Movshon 2004). Interestingly, these bandwidth changes are not of exactly the form predicted by Clifford *et al.* (2000), nor do they show the same pattern across cortical areas.

Dragoi *et al.* (2000, 2002) measured the change in orientation selectivity of V1 neurons following adaptation as a function of the orientation difference between the adapting orientation and the neuron's preferred orientation in its unadapted state. They found that orientation selectivity increased monotonically with the absolute difference in orientation between preferred and adapting orientations (Fig. 2.9(A,B)). For neurons tuned close to the adapting orientation (0–40°), adaptation tended to decrease orientation selectivity, consistent with an increase in orientation bandwidth. For neurons tuned 70–90° from the adapting orientation, orientation selectivity tended to increase, consistent with a decrease in orientation bandwidth. In area MT, Kohn and Movshon (2004) found that adaptation actually decreased orientation bandwidth (increased selectivity) for neurons tuned close (0–60°) to the adapting direction, with no

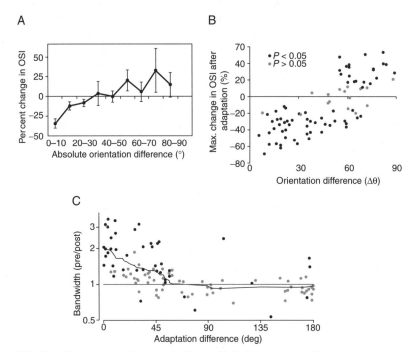

FIG. 2.9 Effect of adaptation on selectivity of individual neurons. Change in orientation selectivity (OSI) as a function of the angular difference between preferred orientation and the orientation of the adapting stimulus for neurons in primary visual cortex of (A) cat; (B) monkey. In both species, orientation selectivity decreases for neurons tuned close to the adapting orientation but increases for neurons tuned orthogonal to the adaptor. Reprinted with permission from Dragoi *et al.* (2000, 2002). (C) Change in direction selectivity of monkey MT neurons as a function of the adapting direction relative to the direction of the adapting stimulus (see Kohn and Movshon 2004). Direction selectivity increases for neurons preferring directions close (0–60°) to the adapting direction, with no clear effect on neurons tuned further away.

clear effect on neurons tuned further away (Fig. 2.9(C)). Thus, although the pattern of results in both V1 (Dragoi *et al.* 2000, 2002) and MT (Kohn & Movshon 2004) shows a systematic dependence of the breadth of tuning on difference in preferred tuning from the adaptor, there are marked differences between responses in the two regions.

In V1, orientation selectivity decreases for the strongly adapted neurons tuned close to the adapting orientation. In isolation, this effect would seem to tend to increase rather than decrease the correlation of population responses to the adapting stimulus. However, it is important to note that this effect typically does not occur in isolation but is accompanied by a reduction in gain (Dragoi *et al.* 2000) such that these neurons contribute only weakly to the overall population response. In MT, direction selectivity increases for neurons close to the adapting direction with little reduction in response gain (Kohn & Movshon 2004), tending to reduce the correlation of population responses to the adapting stimulus as predicted by Clifford *et al.* (2000), although the anticipated reduction in direction selectivity for neurons tuned further from the adapting direction of motion was not observed.

An additional effect of adaptation on the responses of both V1 and MT neurons is a shift in peak tuning (Muller *et al.* 1999; Dragoi *et al.* 2000, 2001, 2002; Kohn & Movshon 2004). Muller *et al.* (1999) found that the peak orientation tuning of complex cells, but not of simple cells, depended on the orientation of the adapting stimulus, although adaptation did affect the responsiveness of simple cells. They point out that their results are consistent with adaptation at the level of simple cells, which in turn drive complex cells. That account is entirely in accordance with the model proposed here, in which adaptation alters the responsiveness and orientation bandwidth of simple cells but not their peak tuning. However, Dragoi *et al.* (2000, 2001, 2002) found small but significant shifts in a large population of neurons in cat and monkey primary visual cortex, suggesting that shifts in peak tuning through adaptation are not restricted to complex cells. The reported shifts in peak tuning are unlikely to have major perceptual consequences if the largest shifts in peak response are accompanied by large reductions in gain.

An important difference between the effects of adaptation on neuronal responses in V1 and MT is the direction of the shifts in peak tuning. In V1, peak tuning is typically repelled away from the adapting stimulus (Muller *et al.* 1999; Dragoi *et al.* 2000, 2001, 2002). In MT, the shifts are predominantly towards the adapting direction of motion (Kohn & Movshon 2004). In MT the shifts in peak tuning are typically not accompanied by large reductions in peak responsiveness, suggesting that they may be of significance to perception.

While the effects of adaptation on the responses of MT neurons clearly differ from the specific predictions of Clifford *et al.* (2000), it is interesting to consider that they might still provide a means of implementing the functional principles of adaptation to the mean and adaptation to variation. MT neurons tuned around the adapting direction of motion show an average reduction in peak responsiveness of around 30 per cent (Kohn & Movshon 2004) consistent with adaptation to the mean at the population level. The effect of this reduction in gain is reinforced by the narrowing in direction bandwidth of neurons tuned around the adapting direction of motion (Kohn & Movshon 2004). Consequently, although reductions in peak responsiveness are modest, the area under the direction response function of neurons tuned around the adapting direction is markedly reduced. In combination, the reductions in responsiveness and direction bandwidth of neurons tuned around the adapting direction produce a shift in the distribution of responses consistent with adaptation to the mean at the population level.

The narrowing of direction bandwidth of MT neurons tuned around the adapting direction would also serve to repel the population response to stimuli close to the adapting direction away from the population vector representing the adaptor. This effect of bandwidth narrowing is reinforced by shifts in peak tuning towards the adapting direction. Together, the reduction in direction bandwidth of neurons tuned around the adapting direction and shifts in peak tuning towards the adaptor produce an effect on the population response consistent with adaptation to the variation. Thus, although the effects of motion adaptation on the responses of neurons in MT differ from the specific predictions of Clifford *et al.* (2000), they can still be interpreted within the functional principles of adaptation to the mean and adaptation to variation.

2.8 Implications for Coding

The plasticity in peak neuronal tuning evidenced by shifts in peak tuning does raise an interesting question about what exactly is being represented in the responses of V1 simple cells and MT neurons. In coding terms, simple cells are typically regarded as 'labelled lines'. That is to say, each neuron can be thought of as voting for its preferred orientation with a number of votes determined by the strength of its response. The votes from a population of neurons tuned to the full range of orientations are then combined as vectors to determine the stimulus orientation represented by that population. Under such a labelled line scheme, it is unclear how shifts in peak tuning would be interpreted. If the peak tuning of a neuron shifted while its label remained unchanged then, in its adapted state, the neuron would be voting for an orientation other than that to which it was currently most responsive. Alternatively, if the neuron's label changed along with its peak tuning (Sur *et al.* 2002) then the neuron would presumably have to inform efferent neurons of its new label.

The way out of this conundrum seems to be to accept that a labelled line scheme in which each neuron votes for its own preferred orientation is overly simplistic. While more sophisticated population coding schemes based on maximum likelihood have been proposed (Pouget *et al.* 2000), these lack the intuitive appeal of coding schemes in which the population response is determined from a linear combination of individual neuronal response vectors. However, the optimal linear estimation (OLE) scheme of Salinas and Abbott (1994) is a version of labelled line coding that relaxes the constraint that a neuronal label must match its peak tuning. Instead, the label (and weighting) attached to a neuron are determined not just by its own peak tuning but by the distribution of peak tunings of all the neurons in its population (Fig. 2.10). In the case where this distribution is uniform over the stimulus attribute being coded, OLE is equivalent to a traditional labelled line scheme (Salinas & Abbott 1994). However, in

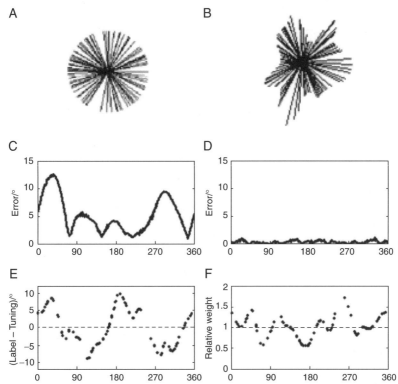

FIG. 2.10 Comparison of conventional labelled line coding and optimal linear estimation. (A) Preferred directions of 100 model neurons randomly sampled from a uniform distribution. All lines have equal length because, under a conventional labelled line scheme, the responses of all units are weighted equally. (B) Labels and weights assigned to the same 100 model neurons under optimal linear estimation. (C) Under the conventional labelled line scheme, any non-uniformity in the coverage of preferred directions produces systematic errors in the population's estimates of direction. (D) Corresponding errors under optimal linear encoding are an order of magnitude smaller. This advantage is produced by two factors. First, (E) the label assigned to each unit is no longer constrained to be the same as that unit's preferred orientation but also implicitly reflects the distribution of preferred orientations of other units in the population. In the example population shown here, differences of up to 10° are evident between the peak tuning of any individual unit and its label. Second, (F) the weight assigned to each unit's response is no longer constrained to be equal to the weights of all the other units.

cases where the distribution of peak tuning is not uniform, such as orientation coding in primary visual cortex where horizontally and vertically tuned cells predominate (Mansfield 1974), OLE produces accurate representations of stimulus orientation while a traditional labelled line scheme is subject to systematic biases (Salinas & Abbott 1994). Given that under OLE a neuronal label need not match its peak tuning, the observation that peak tuning can shift with adaptation is no longer a conundrum: the neuronal label can simply remain unchanged. While a thorough analysis of adaptive OLE has yet to be conducted, such an approach would seem valuable in that it retains much of the intuitive appeal and analytic tractability of traditional labelled line schemes while possessing the necessary flexibility to accommodate the existing physiological data on adaptation in the orientation domain.

2.9 Post-adaptation Perception: The TAE and DAE

The effects of adaptation to the mean and adaptation to variation, individually and in combination, are illustrated schematically in Fig. 2.7. Adaptation to the mean alone produces only repulsive interactions between stimuli of different orientations. Adaptation to variation can produce repulsion or attraction, depending on the angular difference between the oriented patterns in question. Together, the effects of adaptation to the mean and adaptation to variation generate an angular tuning function of the same form as that repeatedly observed psychophysically (Gibson & Radner 1937; Wenderoth & Johnstone 1987).

The direction aftereffect (DAE) (Fig. 2.11) is a motion analogue of the TAE whereby prolonged exposure to a moving pattern affects the perceived direction of subsequent motion (Levinson & Sekuler 1976; Patterson & Becker 1996; Schrater & Simoncelli 1998; Alais & Blake 1999; Rauber & Treue 1999). For angles up to around 100° between the directions of motion of the adapting and test patterns, the perceived direction of the test pattern tends to be repelled away from the adapting direction. The magnitude of this repulsion can be as much as 40° for adaptor-test angles of 30–40°. For angles larger than 100° between adapting and test directions, the perceived direction of the test tends to be attracted towards that of the adaptor (Schrater & Simoncelli 1998). The magnitude of this attraction effect is smaller than that of the repulsion, peaking at around 15° for angles of 150–160° between adapting and test directions.

The angular dependence of DAE reported is strikingly similar to that of the TAE. Notably, the 'critical' values for the DAE are consistently around twice those for tilt, with the peak repulsive and attractive effects occurring at adaptor-test angles of 30–40° and 150–160° for direction-of-motion (Schrater & Simoncelli 1998) as opposed to 10–20° and 75–80° for tilt (Gibson & Radner 1937). These data provide psychophysical support for the use of a double-angle representation for orientation (Gilbert & Wiesel 1990; Clifford *et al.* 2000) that allows direct comparison of angular tuning functions between the orientation and motion domains.

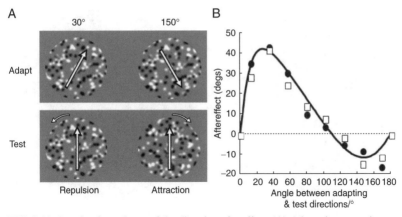

FIG. 2.11 Angular dependence of the direction aftereffect. (A) Adaptation to a stimulus moving at 30° to the vertical causes a subsequently viewed vertically moving stimulus to appear to move in an opposite oblique direction – a repulsive aftereffect. If the adapting stimulus is moving at 150° to the vertical then a smaller, attractive aftereffect is produced. (B) Magnitude of the direction aftereffect as a function of the angle between adaptor and test. By convention, repulsive aftereffects are given positive sign. Data for two observers are redrawn from Schrater and Simoncelli (1998). The solid line shows a fit from the model as described in Clifford *et al.* (2000).

2.10 Contextual Interactions in Time and Space

Wenderoth and Johnstone (1988) have previously shown that different factors affect the magnitude of the repulsive and attractive effects in orientation. For example, the presence of a surrounding frame during the test phase of the TAE abolishes the attractive effect while having little or no effect on the magnitude of the attractive effect (Kohler & Wallach 1944; Wenderoth & van der Zwan 1989). However, introducing a spatial separation between the location of an annular adapting stimulus and a concentric circular test stimulus has the opposite effect, reducing the magnitude of the repulsive but not the attractive TAE (van der Zwan & Wenderoth 1995). On the basis of this double dissociation, it has been suggested that the two effects might be mediated by different mechanisms. The functional decomposition of the tilt aftereffect into adaptation to the mean and adaptation to variation components is not equivalent to the phenomenological repulsive/attractive distinction. As can be seen from Fig. 2.7(F,G), the processes of adaptation to the mean and adaptation to variation both produce repulsion effects when the angle between adaptor and test is 15°, consistent with the observed TAE. However, with 75° between inducer and test, adaptation to variation produces attraction, consistent with the psychophysical effect, while adaptation to the mean produces repulsion.

A pair of processes with characteristics similar to adaptation to the mean and adaptation to variation has also been proposed to underlie the spatial analogue of the TAE, the tilt illusion (Fig. 2.12). The tilt illusion (TI) and TAE show a

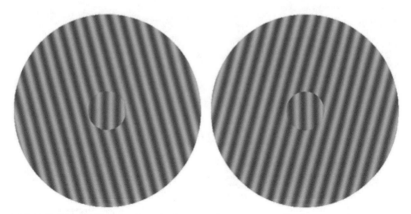

FIG. 2.12 The tilt illusion. A vertical test patch appears repelled in an orientation away from a surround oriented at 15°.

very similar dependence on the angle between the adapting (inducing) stimulus and the test (Gibson & Radner 1937; O'Toole & Wenderoth 1977). Wenderoth and Johnstone (1987, 1988) found that experimental manipulations designed to reduce low-level contributions to the TI (introducing a gap between test and inducer or using an inducer dissimilar in spatial frequency to the test) reduced the magnitude of the repulsion effect to the level of the attraction effect, as would be predicted if only a process of adaptation to variation were operating. Given that the TI and TAE are believed to engage similar mechanisms (Wenderoth & Johnstone 1988), this experimental observation supports the functional decomposition proposed here. The similar phenomenology of the TI and TAE suggests that the model proposed here may also be applicable to spatial inter-actions in the coding of orientation (Clifford *et al.* 2000; Smith *et al.* 2001), and more generally that contextual interactions in time and space may engage similar mechanisms and serve similar functions.

2.11 Post-adaptation Detection

I have demonstrated earlier (Clifford 2002) that the similarity of the effects of adaptation on the perception of orientation and motion described in Section 2.9 extends to the detection and discrimination of those attributes. Following adaptation to a grating, contrast detection thresholds are elevated in an orientation-specific manner, with the peak loss in sensitivity coinciding with the adapting orientation (Gilinsky 1968; Blakemore & Campbell 1969; Regan & Beverley 1985). Motion adaptation impairs the detection of subsequent test stimuli in an analogous way (Levinson & Sekuler 1980; Raymond 1993*a*; Hol & Treue 2001),

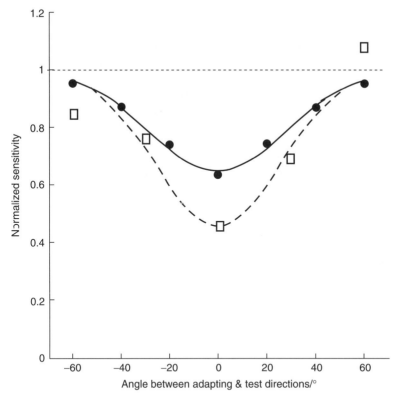

FIG. 2.13 Direction-specific adaptation of motion detection. Data are redrawn from
Raymond (1993*a*) (open squares) and Hol and Treue (2001) (filled circles). Sensitivity
to incoherent random dot motion is maximally reduced around the adapting direction
by 35–55%. The direction-specificity of the effect is well-fit by a Gaussian function
with a half-width at half-height of 30–34°.

with tolerance to noise in random dot motion maximally reduced around the
adapting direction by 35–55 per cent (Fig. 2.13).

This direction-specific loss in sensitivity shows complete inter-ocular transfer, demonstrating that it is of cortical origin (Raymond 1993*b*), and is well-fit
by a Gaussian function with a half width at half height (HWHH) of 30–34°.
It should be noted that the width of this function is not necessarily related to
the width of individual direction-tuning curves (Priebe & Lisberger 2002), but
presumably reflects lateral interactions in the population of direction-tuned
neurons. The assumption here is that motion detection is determined by the
responsiveness of the neuron most sensitive to the test direction. Thus, the
responsiveness of neurons tuned to the adapting direction will be reduced most,
with the reduction in responsiveness of any given neuron determined by the angle
between the adapting stimulus direction and that neuron's preferred direction.

2.12 Post-adaptation Discrimination

The effect of adaptation on orientation discrimination follows a characteristic angular tuning function such that discrimination performance around the adapting orientation improves (Regan & Beverley 1985; Clifford *et al.* 2001*a*) or remains unchanged (Barlow *et al.* 1976) but is markedly impaired for angles of 10–15° between adaptor and test. A similar pattern of results has been reported for the effect of motion adaptation on direction discrimination (Fig. 2.14), with direction discrimination around the adapting direction unimpaired (Hol & Treue 2001) or improved by 20–40% (Phinney *et al.* 1997; Clifford *et al.* 2001*b*) and discrimination thresholds for angles of 20–30° between adaptor and test raised by up to 60 per cent (Phinney *et al.* 1997; Hol & Treue 2001).

It has also been reported that adaptation to a grating orthogonal to the test orientation can improve orientation discrimination (Clifford *et al.* 2001*a*; Dragoi *et al.* 2002) and, analogously, that motion adaptation improves direction discrimination around the opposite direction of motion (Clifford *et al.* 2001*b*). As with orientation discrimination around the adapting orientation, not all studies

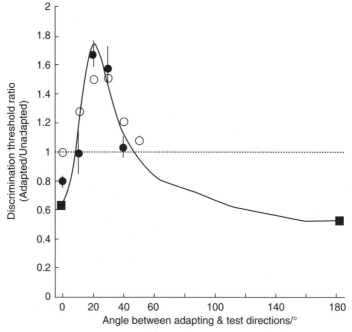

FIG. 2.14 The angular dependence of post-adaptation direction discrimination. Filled circles show data redrawn from Phinney *et al.* (1997); open circles from Hol and Treue (2001); filled squares from Clifford *et al.* (2001*b*). The solid line shows the fit from a model analogous to that proposed by Clifford *et al.* (2001*a*) for the effect of adaptation on orientation discrimination.

have found that orthogonal adaptation improves orientation discrimination (Westheimer & Gee 2002), possibly due to methodological differences (Clifford *et al.* 2003; Westheimer & Gee 2003). Electrophysiological data has shown that the response properties of neurons in primary visual cortex could support improvements in post-adaptation discrimination performance both parallel (Muller *et al.* 1999) and orthogonal (Dragoi *et al.* 2002) to the adapting orientation by decorrelating neuronal responses.

In the motion domain, the discrepancy between studies in the measured magnitude of the effect of adaptation on subsequent discrimination around the adapting direction remains mysterious. However, it is interesting to note from Fig. 2.13 that Hol and Treue (2001) also report smaller effects of adaptation on motion detection than did Raymond (1993*a*), suggesting that their adaptation paradigm might somehow be less powerful than those used in other studies.

While the angular tuning functions of the TAE and DAE can be modelled simply in terms of changes in the direction of the population response through adaptation, the magnitude of the population response must also be taken into account in order to model discrimination. The interaction of these two factors is illustrated in Fig. 2.15. Reducing the responsiveness of model neurons tuned close to the adapting direction has the effect of repelling the population

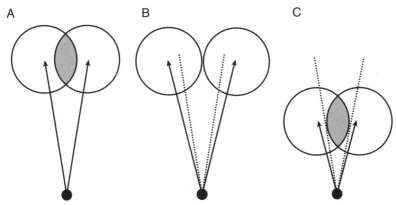

FIG. 2.15 Schematic illustrating the effects of adaptation on direction discrimination. (A) Discrimination between two directions of motion. The vectors represent the magnitude and direction of the unadapted population response to two stimuli. The circles represent the extent of variability in each population response, and the area of their overlap (grey region) is a metric of the difficulty of discriminating between the two directions. (B) Repulsion between the two population vectors reduces the area of overlap between the response distributions, such that the two directions of motion become easier to discriminate. (C) When the responsiveness of the individual neurons tuned around the adapting direction is reduced, response repulsion is accompanied by a reduction in the magnitude of the population response. This reduction in response magnitude increases the overlap of the two response distributions, thus tending to offset the effect of response repulsion.

response away from the adapting direction for subsequent nearby test directions (Fig. 2.15(B)), while leaving responses around the opposite direction unaffected. If discrimination required a certain mean difference in *perceived* direction, then this repulsion away from the adapting direction would suggest that a smaller *physical* difference in direction should be necessary to reach perceptual discrimination threshold around the adapting direction (compare Fig. 2.15(A,B)).

While such an account has been proposed for the effect of adaptation on orientation discrimination around the adapting orientation (Regan & Beverley 1985), it fails to explain improvements in discrimination remote from the adaptor (Clifford *et al.* 2001a,b; Dragoi *et al.* 2002). Moreover, reducing the response of individual neurons reduces the magnitude of the population response to directions around the adapting direction. This effective reduction in signal strength can be observed psychophysically in the form of elevated contrast detection thresholds around the adapting orientation (Gilinsky 1968; Blakemore & Campbell 1969; Regan & Beverley 1985) and elevated motion coherence thresholds around the adapting direction (Raymond 1993a; Hol & Treue 2001). When the reduced signal-to-noise ratio of the population response around the adapting direction is taken into account, we find that reduction in the responsiveness of model neurons tuned around the adapting direction can actually impair discrimination performance around the adapting direction (Fig. 2.15(C)).

The most marked impairments in discrimination performance, for orientations 10–15° from the adapting orientation and directions 20–30° from the adapting direction, are due to the reduced responsiveness of model neurons with preferred orientations or directions around that of the adapting stimulus. This is because these neurons have their highest differential sensitivity away from their preferred tuning. Differential sensitivity is highest where the slope of the neuronal response function is highest, not around its peak (Regan & Beverley 1985; Hol & Treue 2001).

2.13 Directional Tuning of the Effect of Adaptation on Perceived Speed

Adaptation can affect not only the direction of the population response vector but also its magnitude. In the motion domain, the direction of the population response vector represents the perceived direction of motion and its magnitude may be presumed to be monotonically related to perceived speed, although details of speed coding in the primate visual system are still a matter of intense debate (Perrone & Thiele 2002; Priebe *et al.* 2003). Psychophysically, as well as having marked effects on the perception of direction, motion adaptation has consistently been shown to effect perceived speed (Goldstein 1957; Carlson 1962; Rapoport 1964; Thompson 1981; Smith & Hammond 1985; Muller & Greenlee 1994; Clifford & Langley 1996a; Bex *et al.* 1999a; Clifford & Wenderoth 1999; Hammett *et al.* 2000). Smith and Hammond (1985) investigated the angular dependence of the effect of adaptation on perceived speed. They found that

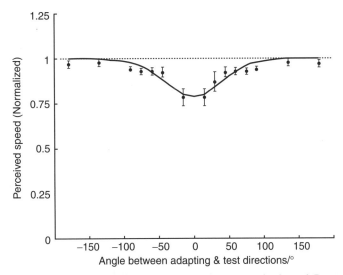

FIG. 2.16 Directional tuning of the effect of adaptation on perceived speed. Data are the mean from four subjects, redrawn from Smith and Hammond (1985), Fig. 4. The angular tuning function is well-fitted by a Gaussian function with a HWHH of 48°.

perceived speed was maximally reduced (by just over 20 per cent) when adaptor and test were parallel, while being almost unaffected for differences in adaptor and test directions of more than 90° when adaptor and test both moved at the same speed (2°/s). Data from their study are redrawn in Fig. 2.16.

The angular tuning function for the reduction of perceived speed through motion adaptation is well-fitted by a Gaussian function with a HWHH of 48°. This is comparable with the direction of tuning of threshold elevation (Fig. 2.13), which has a HWHH of 30–34° (Raymond 1993a; Hol & Treue 2001).

Motion adaptation has also been shown to affect subsequent speed discrimination performance (Clifford & Langley 1996a) such that speed discrimination thresholds remain proportional to perceived speed (Bex et al. 1999a; Clifford & Wenderoth 1999), at least for first-order motion if not for second-order (Kristjansson 2001). This is precisely the behaviour one would expect if speed discrimination depended not upon the adapted state of the population of neurons per se but simply upon the level of neuronal responses, and can thus be accounted for by the model without the need for any auxiliary assumptions.

In the orientation domain, the direction of the population response vector represents perceived orientation, and its magnitude may be presumed to code for perceived contrast. Thus, predictions can also be made about the effects of adaptation on the perception and discrimination of contrast, on which there is an extensive but not altogether coherent literature (Greenlee & Heitger 1988; Snowden & Hammett 1992; Ross & Speed 1996; Abbonizio et al. 2002; Barrett et al. 2002). Probably the most striking effect of adaptation on contrast perception is the decrease in perceived contrast over time of the adapting stimulus itself

(Hammett *et al.* 1994), analogous to the decrease in perceived speed observed in the motion domain as a function of adapting stimulus duration (Clifford & Langley 1996*b*; Bex *et al.* 1999*a*; Hammett *et al.* 2000). While the model of Clifford *et al.* (2000) does not contain explicit dynamics, it correctly predicts that the perceived contrast of a stimulus will be decreased after prolonged exposure (Fig. 2.7(E)).

2.14 Is there an Orientation Analogue of the MAE?

Prolonged exposure to a maintained motion stimulus has profound perceptual consequences. When fixation is transferred to a stationary pattern, illusory motion is seen in the direction opposite to the adapting motion but with little or no accompanying change in perceived position (Snowden 1998; Nishida & Johnston 1999). This 'motion aftereffect' (MAE) is distinct from the direction aftereffect (DAE) in that it is obtained with a static rather than a moving test stimulus. Given the other parallels in phenomenology between adaptation to orientation and motion described in this chapter, it seems reasonable to ask if the MAE has an analogue in the orientation domain (Clifford 2002).

First of all, let us establish what an orientation analogue of the MAE would be. The MAE is such that adaptation to any given direction of motion causes a subsequently presented static test stimulus to appear to move in the opposite direction. In the representation of Fig. 2.5(A), a static stimulus corresponds to the origin since, at this point, speed (the radial dimension) is zero and direction is undefined. The orientation analogue of the MAE is that a stimulus corresponding to the origin in the orientation domain (Fig. 2.5(B)) should be perceived to have an orientation opposite to that of the adapting stimulus. Opposite in the double-angle representation corresponds to a 90° difference in orientation, while the origin denotes a stimulus at which contrast (the radial dimension) is zero and orientation is undefined. Thus, an orientation analogue of the MAE would be that adaptation to a vertical pattern should give rise to an illusory percept of horizontal structure when a uniform (zero contrast) test field is presented.

While an aftereffect of perpendicular illusory structure was reported by McKay (1957) following adaptation to a high contrast grating, the illusory structure appeared not as static horizontal stripes but as particles streaming in horizontal motion. This fact, coupled with the observation that adaptation to rotary motion generates the percept of illusory lines at right angles to the motion, has been taken to suggest that the effect might be best understood as an interaction between orientation and motion processing rather than as a simple analogue of the MAE (Georgeson 1976).

If the effect of adaptation to a static oriented pattern is best explained as an interaction between the orientation and motion domains, why then is there no orientation analogue of the MAE when tested with a uniform field? While the double-angle representation of orientation suggests parallels between the coding of orientation and direction-of-motion, consideration of the speed-tuning properties of primate MT neurons suggests that the analogy between the two domains breaks down in the vicinity of their respective origins. The response of orientation-selective cortical neurons is typically a monotonically increasing, high-pass function of contrast (Sclar *et al.* 1990). At zero contrast, when no stimulus is present, the cell is by definition responding at its baseline rate. However, many direction-selective cells in primate MT show low-pass or broadband tuning for speed such that they respond to the slowest speeds tested in either the preferred or the anti-preferred direction (Lagae *et al.* 1993). These response properties are illustrated in Fig. 2.17.

Figure 2.17(A) illustrates that a static stimulus may elicit responses from directional cells tuned to opposite directions of motion. If the responsiveness of these cells is differentially affected by adaptation to motion in one of their preferred directions then the ratio of their responses to static stimuli will change such that there is a proportionally greater response from the neurons tuned to the direction opposite to the adapting motion. This is the code for slow motion in the direction opposite to that of the adapting stimulus and may constitute

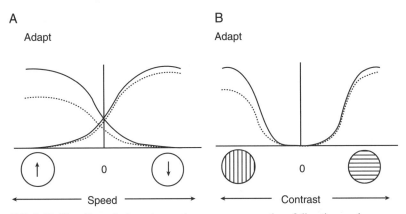

FIG. 2.17 The effect of adaptation on the response properties of direction- and orientation-selective neurons. (A) Illustration of the effects of adaptation on the response properties of direction-selective cells as a function of stimulus speed. In their unadapted state (solid lines), low-pass direction-selective neurons are responsive to static stimuli. Adaptation to upwards motion has a differential effect on the responsiveness of cells tuned to upwards and downwards motion (dotted lines). The greater reduction in responsiveness of the cell tuned to upwards motion biases the response to subsequent static stimuli, causing them to be perceived as drifting slowly downwards: a motion aftereffect. (B) Illustration of the effects of adaptation on the response properties of orientation-selective cells as a function of stimulus contrast. In both the unadapted state (solid lines) and after adaptation to a vertically oriented stimulus (dotted lines) the cells are unresponsive to zero contrast. This suggests that any aftereffects of adapting to a vertical stimulus on the perception of a subsequent zero contrast test field are due to interactions between orientation and motion processing rather than an orientation analogue of the motion aftereffect. Redrawn from Clifford (2002).

a neural correlate of the MAE. Figure 2.17(B) illustrates the effect of adaptation to an oriented stimulus on the contrast response functions of orientation-selective cells tuned to orientations parallel and perpendicular to the adapting orientation. Since these cells do not respond at zero contrast, the differential effect of adaptation on their response functions will not affect the coding of a zero contrast stimulus and no orientation analogue of the MAE will be produced.

2.15 A Negative Aftereffect of Spatial Pattern

While the classical MAE involves the illusory motion of a static test pattern, MAEs can also be observed by testing with dynamic patterns containing no net physical motion such as incoherent random dot kinematograms (Hiris & Blake 1992; Blake & Hiris 1993) and contrast-reversing patterns (Levinson & Sekuler 1975; von Grunau 1986). Incoherent random dot kinematograms (RDKs) contain no net motion as individual dots move in directions uniformly distributed over the whole 360° range. In the representation of Fig. 2.5(A), this corresponds to a circle centred on the origin, such that all directions are represented. The radius of the circle corresponds to the speed of motion of the individual dots. After adaptation to coherent motion, an incoherent RDK appears to drift in the opposite direction (Hiris & Blake 1992; Blake & Hiris 1993). To distinguish the effect from the MAE obtained with static test stimuli, I shall use the term 'dynamic MAE' to refer to the MAE observed with dynamic test stimuli such as incoherent RDKs.

To explain why no analogue of the classical MAE with a static stimulus is observed in the orientation domain, it was argued that the parallels between the two domains break down in the vicinity of their respective origins. Given that the test stimulus in the dynamic MAE is represented by a circle centred on the origin in the motion domain, rather than by the origin itself, we might predict that an analogue of the dynamic MAE would be observed in the orientation domain. What would an orientation analogue of the dynamic MAE be?

A circle centred on the origin in the orientation domain represents a stimulus containing equal amounts of all orientations. After adaptation to an oriented pattern, an analogue of the dynamic MAE according to the double-angle representation of orientation would be for a test stimulus containing equal amounts of all orientations to appear oriented perpendicular to the adaptor. To search for such an effect, Clifford & Weston (2005) used Glass patterns each consisting of a large number of dot pairs (Glass 1969; Glass & Perez 1973). To construct the adapting stimulus, one dot in each pair was positioned randomly within the stimulus and its partner was then positioned a fixed distance away in a direction defined by the particular pattern being generated. To construct the test stimulus, the direction of each partner dot was randomly determined such that the distribution of intra-pair orientations was statistically uniform.

Clifford & Weston (2005) found that, after adaptation to a concentric Glass pattern, the test stimulus appeared to contain predominantly radial

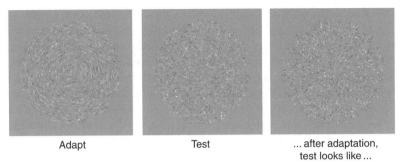

| Adapt | Test | ... after adaptation, test looks like ... |

FIG. 2.18 After adaptation to a 100 per cent coherent concentric Glass pattern, a test pattern of randomly oriented dot pairs (0 per cent coherence) appears to contain radial structure.

structure (Fig. 2.18). Similarly, after adaptation to a horizontal Glass pattern, the test appeared vertical. In both cases, the local orientation of the perceived structure in the test stimulus was perpendicular to the orientation of the corresponding region of the adaptor.

The aftereffect of adaptation to complex (radial or concentric) Glass patterns seems subjectively stronger than that to linear (horizontal or vertical patterns). Adaptation to complex patterns of motion has been shown to produce stronger aftereffects than adaptation to linear motion (Bex *et al.* 1999*b*), consistent with the involvement of high-level neurons selective for complex patterns of motion (Saito *et al.* 1986; Morrone *et al.* 1995). Thus, it could be that the aftereffect to Glass patterns is mediated at the level of complex form detection rather than at the level of local orientation coding. However, it has previously been shown that the percentage signal necessary for detection of complex Glass patterns is lower than that for linear patterns (Wilson & Wilkinson 1998). Thus, it could be that the subjectively weaker aftereffect for linear Glass patterns is due to lower sensitivity for linear than complex structure rather than to weaker adaptation. Indeed, when the magnitudes of the aftereffects to complex and linear Glass patterns were quantified in terms of subjective signal strength it was found that both were of the order of 30 per cent (Clifford & Weston 2005), similar in magnitude to the dynamic MAE (Hiris & Blake 1992; Blake & Hiris 1993).

These data suggest that the primary determinant of the aftereffect to Glass patterns is adaptation prior to the spatial pooling of local orientation signals. The prediction of this novel aftereffect is strong evidence that the human visual system employs similar strategies to code orientation and direction-of-motion.

2.16 Summary

Physiological evidence suggests that the processes underlying adaptation to motion and orientation involve different areas of the primate visual cortex and different patterns of change at the neuronal level. Activity in MT/MST has been shown to correlate with the psychophysical effects of motion adaptation (Tootell *et al.* 1995), while the processing of orientation appears to be distributed along the ventral pathway (Lennie 1998). Adaptation in V1 produces: (1) reductions in responsiveness around the adapting orientation; (2) decreases in selectivity around the adapting orientation but enhanced selectivity at remote orientations; and (3) shifts in peak tuning towards non-adapted orientations (Dragoi *et al.* 2000, 2002). In MT, adaptation to motion produces: (1) reductions in responsiveness around the adapting direction; (2) increases in selectivity around the adapting direction but little change at remote directions; and (3) shifts in peak tuning towards the adapted direction (Kohn & Movshon 2004). Despite these differences, evidence from studies employing psychophysical adaptation suggests that common computational principles underlie the coding of orientation and motion. Specifically, visual information appears to be adaptively coded in a manner that reduces redundancy and tends to make optimal use of the limited dynamic range of sensory neurons. While this chapter has focused on visual adaptation to orientation and motion, the principles of adaptive coding may prove general to other visual domains such as colour, shape, and face perception (see Chapters 4–9, this volume), and to other sensory modalities such as audition (Kashino & Nishida 1998).

Acknowledgements

This work was supported by a Queen Elizabeth II Fellowship to Colin Clifford from the Australian Research Council. I am grateful to Chris Benton, Szonya Durant, and Gill Rhodes for helpful comments on draft versions of this chapter and to Adam Kohn for sharing his data with me prior to publication, and for providing Fig. 2.9(C).

References

Abbonizio, G., Langley, K., & Clifford, C.W.G. (2002). Contrast adaptation may enhance contrast discrimination. *Spatial Vision, 16*, 45–58.

Adelson, E.H., & Bergen, J.R. (1991). The plenoptic function and the elements of early vision. In M.S. Landy & J.A. Movshon (ed.), *Computational Models of Visual Processing* (pp. 3–20). Cambridge, MA: MIT Press.

Adorjan, P., Levitt, J.B., Lund, J.S., & Obermayer, K. (1999). A model for the intracortical origin of orientation preference and tuning in macaque striate cortex. *Visual Neuroscience, 16*, 303–18.

Alais, D., & Blake, R. (1999). Neural strength of attention gauged by motion adaptation. *Nature Neuroscience, 2*, 1015–18.

Albright, T.D., Desimone, R., & Gross, C.G. (1984). Columnar organization of directionally selective cells in visual area MT of the macaque. *Journal of Neurophysiology, 51*, 16–31.

Andrews, D.P. (1964). Error-correcting perceptual mechanisms. *Quarterly Journal of Experimental Psychology, 16*, 104–15.

Atick, J.J., Li, Z.-P., & Redlich, A.N. (1993). What does post-adaptation appearance reveal about cortical color representation? *Vision Research, 33*, 123–9.

Attneave, F. (1954). Some informational aspects of visual perception. *Psychological Review*, *61*, 183–93.

Barlow, H.B. (1961). The coding of sensory messages. In W.H. Thorpe, & O.L. Zangwill (ed.), *Current Problems in Animal Behaviour* (pp. 331–60). Cambridge: Cambridge University Press.

Barlow, H.B. (1990). A theory about the functional role and synaptic mechanism of visual after-effects. In C.B. Blakemore (ed.), *Vision: Coding and Efficiency* (pp. 363–75). Cambridge: Cambridge University Press.

Barlow, H.B. (1997). The knowledge used in vision and where it comes from. *Philosophical Transactions of the Royal Society of London, Series B*, *352*, 1141–7.

Barlow, H.B., & Foldiak, P. (1989). Adaptation and decorrelation in the cortex. In R. Durbin, C. Miall, & G. Mitchison (ed.), *The Computing Neuron* (pp. 54–72). Wokingham: Addison-Wesley.

Barlow, H.B., & Hill, R.M. (1963). Evidence for a physiological explanation for the waterfall illusion and figural aftereffects. *Nature*, *200*, 1345–7.

Barlow, H.B., Macleod, D.I.A., & van Meeteren, A. (1976). Adaptation to gratings: no compensatory advantages found. *Vision Research*, *16*, 1043–5.

Barrett, B.T., McGraw, P.V., & Morrill, P. (2002). Perceived contrast following adaptation: the role of adapting stimulus visibility. *Spatial Vision*, *16*, 5–19.

Bex, P., Bedingham, S., & Hammett, S.T. (1999a). Apparent speed and speed sensitivity during adaptation to motion. *Journal of the Optical Society of America* A, *16*, 2817–24.

Bex, P.J., Metha, A.B., & Makous, W. (1999b). Enhanced motion aftereffect for complex motions. *Vision Research*, *39*, 2229–38.

Blake, R., & Hiris, E. (1993). Another means for measuring the motion aftereffect. *Vision Research*, *33*, 1589–92.

Blakemore, C. (1973). The baffled brain. In R.L. Gregory & E.H. Gombrich (ed.), *Illusion in Nature and Art* (pp. 8–47). London: Duckworth.

Blakemore, C., & Campbell, F. (1969). On the existence of neurones in the human visual system selectively sensitive to the orientation and size of retinal images. *Journal of Physiology*, *203*, 237–60.

Blakemore, C., Carpenter, R.H.S., & Georgeson, M.A. (1970). Lateral inhibition between orientation detectors in the human visual system. *Nature*, *228*, 37–9.

Blakemore, C., Muncey, J.P.J., & Ridley, R.M. (1973). Stimulus specificity in the human visual system. *Vision Research*, *13*, 1915–31.

Carandini, M., & Ringach, D.L. (1997). Predictions of a recurrent model of orientation selectivity. *Vision Research*, *37*, 3061–71.

Carlson, V.R. (1962). Adaptation in the perception of visual velocity. *Journal of Experimental Psychology*, *64*, 192–7.

Clifford, C.W.G. (2002). Perceptual adaptation: motion parallels orientation. *Trends in Cognitive Sciences*, *6*, 136–43.

Clifford, C.W.G., & Ibbotson, M.R. (2003). Fundamental mechanisms of visual motion detection: models, cells and functions. *Progress in Neurobiology*, *68*, 409–37.

Clifford, C.W.G., & Langley, K. (1996a). A model of temporal adaptation in fly motion vision. *Vision Research*, *36*, 2595–608.

Clifford, C.W.G., & Langley, K. (1996b). Psychophysics of motion adaptation parallels insect electrophysiology. *Current Biology*, *6*, 1340–2.

Clifford, C.W.G., & Wenderoth, P. (1999). Adaptation to temporal modulation can enhance differential speed sensitivity. *Vision Research*, *39*, 4324–32.

Clifford, C.W.G., Wenderoth, P., & Spehar, B. (2000). A functional angle on adaptation in cortical vision. *Proceedings of the Royal Society of London, Series B*, *267*, 1705–10.

Clifford, C.W.G., Ma Wyatt, A., Arnold, D.H., Smith, S.T., & Wenderoth, P. (2001a). Orthogonal adaptation improves orientation discrimination. *Vision Research, 41*, 151–9.

Clifford, C., Arnold, D.H., Ma Wyatt, A., & Wenderoth, P. (2001b). Opposite adaptation improves direction discrimination. *Investigative Ophthalmology and Visual Science, 42*, S532.

Clifford, C.W.G., Arnold, D.H., Smith, S.T., & Pianta, M.J. (2003). Opposing views on orthogonal adaptation: a reply to Westheimer & Gee (2002). *Vision Research, 43*, 717–19.

Clifford, C.W.G., & Weston, E. (2005). Aftereffect of adaptation to Glass patterns. *Vision Research, 45*, in press.

Coltheart, M. (1971). Visual feature-analyzers and after-effects of tilt and curvature. *Psychological Review, 78*, 114–21.

Culham, J.C., Dukelow, S.P., Vilis, T., Hassard, F.A., Gati, J.S., Menon, R.S., & Goodale, M.A. (1999). Recovery of fMRI activation in motion area MT following storage of the motion aftereffect. *Journal of Neurophysiology, 81*, 388–93.

Dragoi, V., Sharma, J., & Sur, M. (2000). Adaptation-induced plasticity of orientation tuning in adult visual cortex. *Neuron, 28*, 287–98.

Dragoi, V., Rivadulla, C., & Sur, M. (2001). Foci of orientation plasticity in visual cortex. *Nature, 411*, 80–6.

Dragoi, V., Sharma, J., Miller, E.K., & Sur, M. (2002). Dynamics of neuronal sensitivity in visual cortex and local feature discrimination. *Nature Neuroscience, 5*, 883–91.

Draper, N.R., & Smith, H. (1998). *Applied Regression Analysis*. New York: John Wiley & Sons.

Exner, S. (1894). *Entwurf zu einer physiologischen erklarung der psychischen erscheinungen*, Leipzig: Deuticke.

Georgeson, M.A. (1976). Antagonism between channels for pattern and movement in human vision. *Nature, 259*, 413–15

Gibson, J.J. (1937a). Adaptation, after-effect, and contrast in the perception of tilted lines. II. Simultaneous contrast and the areal restriction of the after-effect. *Journal of Experimental Psychology, 20*, 553–69.

Gibson, J.J. (1937b). Adaptation with negative after-effect. *Psychological Review 44*, 222–44.

Gibson, J.J., & Radner, M. (1937). Adaptation, after-effect, and contrast in the perception of tilted lines. I. Quantitative studies. *Journal of Experimental Psychology, 20*, 453–67.

Gilbert, C.D., & Wiesel, T.N. (1990). The influence of contextual stimuli on the orientation selectivity of cells in primary visual cortex of the cat. *Vision Research, 30*, 1689–1701.

Gilinsky, A. (1968). Orientation-specific effects of patterns of adapting light on visual acuity. *Journal of the Optical Society of America, 58*, 13–18.

Glass, L. (1969). Moiré effect from random dots. *Nature, 223*, 578–80.

Glass, L., & Perez, R. (1973). Perception of random dot interference patterns. *Nature, 246*, 360–2.

Goldstein, A.G. (1957). Judgements of visual velocity as a function of length of observation time. *Journal of Experimental Psychology, 54*, 457–61.

Greenlee, M.W., & Heitger, F. (1988). The functional role of contrast adaptation. *Vision Research, 28*, 791–7.

Hammett, S.T., Snowden, R.J., & Smith, A.T. (1994). Perceived contrast as a function of adaptation duration. *Vision Research, 34*, 31–40.

Hammett, S.T., Thompson, P.G., & Bedingham, S. (2000). The dynamics of velocity adaptation in human vision. *Current Biology, 10*, 1123–6.

Hammond, P., Pomfrett, C.J.D., & Ahmed, B. (1989). Neural motion after-effects in the cat's striate cortex: orientation selectivity. *Vision Research, 29*, 1671–83.

He, S., Cohen, E.R., & Hu, X. (1998). Close correlation between activity in brain area MT/V5 and the perception of visual motion aftereffect. *Current Biology, 8*, 753–9.

Hol, K., & Treue, S. (2001). Different populations of neurons contribute to the detection and discrimination of visual motion. *Vision Research, 41*, 685–9.

Hiris, E., & Blake, R. (1992). Another perspective on the visual motion aftereffect. *Proceedings of the National Academy of Sciences, USA, 89*, 9025–8.

Huk, A.C., Ress, D., & Heeger, D.J. (2001). Neuronal basis of the motion aftereffect reconsidered. *Neuron, 32*, 161–72.

Kashino, M., & Nishida, S. (1998). Adaptation in the processing of interaural time differences revealed by the auditory localization aftereffect. *Journal of the Acoustical Society of America, 103*, 3597–604.

Kohler, W., & Wallach, H. (1944). Figural aftereffects: an investigation of visual processes. *Proceedings of the American Philosophical Society, 88*, 269–357.

Kohn, A., & Movshon, J.A. (2004). Adaptation changes the direction tuning of macaque MT neurons. *Nature Neuroscience, 7*, 764–72.

Kohonen, T., & Oja, E. (1976). Fast adaptive formation of orthogonalizing filters and associative memory in recurrent networks of neuron-like elements. *Biological Cybernetics, 21*, 85–95.

Kristjansson, A. (2001). Increased sensitivity to speed changes during adaptation to first-order, but not to second-order motion. *Vision Research, 41*, 1825–32.

Lagae, L., Raiguel, S., & Orban, G.A. (1993). Speed and direction selectivity of macaque middle temporal neurons. *Journal of Neurophysiology, 69*, 19–39.

Laughlin, S.B. (1989). Coding efficiency and design in visual processing. In D.G. Stavenga, & R.C. Hardie (ed.), *Facets of Vision* (pp. 213–234). Berlin: Springer-Verlag.

Laughlin, S.B. (1990). Coding efficiency and visual processing. In C.B. Blakemore (ed.), *Vision: coding and efficiency* (pp. 25–31). Cambridge: Cambridge University Press.

Laughlin, S.B., de Ruyter van Steveninck, R.R., & Anderson, J.C. (1998). The metabolic cost of neural information. *Nature Neuroscience, 1*, 36–41.

Lennie, P. (1998). Single units and visual cortical organization. *Perception, 27*, 889–935.

Levinson, E., & Sekuler, R. (1975). The independence of channels in human vision selective for direction of movement. *Journal of Physiology (London), 250*, 347–66.

Levinson, E., & Sekuler, R. (1976). Adaptation alters perceived direction of motion. *Vision Research, 16*, 779–81.

Levinson, E., & Sekuler, R. (1980). A two-dimensional analysis of direction-specific adaptation. *Vision Research, 20*, 103–7.

Mansfield, R.J.W. (1974). Neural basis of orientation perception in primate vision. *Science, 186*, 1133–5.

Mather, G. (1980). The movement aftereffect and a distribution-shift model for coding the direction of visual movement. *Perception, 9*, 379–92.

Mather, G., & Harris, J. (1998). Theoretical models of the motion aftereffect. In G. Mather, F. Verstraten, & S. Anstis (ed.), *The Motion Aftereffect: A Modern Perspective* (pp. 157–185). Cambridge MA: MIT Press.

Mc Adams, C.J., & Maunsell, J.H.R. (1999). Effects of attention on orientation-tuning functions of single neurons in macaque cortical area V4. *Journal of Neuroscience, 19,* 431–41.

Mc Kay, D.M. (1957). Moving visual images produced by regular stationary patterns. *Nature, 180,* 849–51.

Mitchell, D.E., & Muir, D.W. (1976). Does the tilt aftereffect occur in the oblique meridian? *Vision Research, 16,* 609–13.

Morant, R.B., & Harris, J.R. (1965). Two different aftereffects of exposure to visual tilts. *American Journal of Psychology, 78,* 218–26.

Morant, R.B., & Mistovich, M. (1960). Tilt aftereffects between the vertical and horizontal axes. *Perceptual and Motor Skills, 10,* 75–81.

Morrone, M.C., Burr, D.C., & Vaina, L.M. (1995). Two stages of visual processing for radial and circular motion. *Nature, 376,* 507–9.

Movshon, J.A., & Lennie, P. (1979). Pattern selective adaptation in visual cortical neurones. *Nature, 278,* 850–52.

Movshon, J.A., Thompson, I.D., & Tolhurst, D.J. (1978). Spatial and temporal contrast sensitivity of neurones in areas 17 and 18 of the cat's visual cortex. *Journal of Physiology (London), 283,* 101–20.

Muller, R., & Greenlee, M.W. (1994). Effect of contrast and adaptation on the perception of the direction and speed of drifting gratings. *Vision Research, 34,* 2071–92.

Muller, R., & Greenlee, M.W. (1994). Effect of contrast and adaptation on the perception of the direction and speed of drifting gratings. *Vision Research, 34,* 2071–92.

Muller, J.R., Metha, A.B., Krauskopf, J., & Lennie, P. (1999). Rapid adaptation in visual cortex to the structure of images. *Science, 285,* 1405–8

Nishida, S., & Johnston, A. (1999). Influence of motion signals on the perceived position of spatial pattern. *Nature, 397,* 610–12

O'Toole, B., & Wenderoth, P. (1977). The tilt illusion: repulsion and attraction effects in the oblique meridian. *Vision Research, 17,* 367–74.

Patterson, R., & Becker, S. (1996). Direction-selective adaptation and simultaneous contrast induced by stereoscopic (Cyclopean) motion. *Vision Research, 36,* 1773–81.

Perrone, J.A., & Thiele, A. (2002). A model of speed tuning in MT neurons. *Vision Research, 42,* 1035–51.

Phinney, R.E., Bowd, C., & Patterson, R. (1997). Direction-selective coding of stereoscopic (Cyclopean) motion. *Vision Research, 37,* 865–9.

Pouget, A., Dayan, P., & Zemel, R. (2000). Information processing with population codes. *Nature Reviews Neuroscience, 1,* 125–32.

Priebe, N.J., & Lisberger, S.G. (2002). Constraints on the source of short-term motion adaptation in macaque area MT. II. Tuning of neural circuit mechanisms. *Journal of Neurophysiology, 88,* 370–82.

Priebe, N.J., Cassanello, C.R., & Lisberger, S.G. (2003). The neural representation of speed in macaque area MT/V5. *Journal of Neuroscience, 23,* 5650–61.

Rapoport, J. (1964). Adaptation in the perception of rotary motion. *Journal of Experimental Psychology, 67,* 263–7.

Rauber, H.-J., & Treue, S. (1999). Revisiting motion repulsion: evidence for a general phenomenon? *Vision Research, 39,* 3187–96.

Raymond, J.E. (1993a). Movement direction analysers: independence and bandwidth. *Vision Research, 33,* 767–75

Raymond, J.E. (1993b). Complete interocular transfer of motion adaptation effects on motion coherence thresholds. *Vision Research, 33,* 1865–70.

Regan, D., & Beverley, K.I. (1985). Postadaptation orientation discrimination. *Journal of the Acoustical Society of America A, 2,* 147–55.

Ross, J., & Speed, H.D. (1996). Perceived contrast following adaptation to gratings of different orientations. *Vision Research, 36,* 1811–18.

Rushton, W.A.H. (1965). Visual adaptation. *Proceedings of the Royal Society of London, Series B, 162,* 20–46.

Saito, H., Yukie, M., Tanaka, K., Hikosaka, K., Fukada, Y., & Iwai, E. (1986). Integration of direction signals of image motion in the superior temporal sulcus of the macaque monkey. *Journal of Neuroscience, 6,* 145–57.

Salinas, E., & Abbott, L.F. (1994). Vector reconstruction from firing rates. *Journal of Computational Neuroscience, 1,* 89–107.

Saul, A.B., & Cynader, M.S. (1989). Adaptation in single units in visual cortex: the tuning of aftereffects in the temporal domain. *Visual Neuroscience, 2,* 609–20.

Schrater, P.R., & Simoncelli, E.P. (1998). Local velocity representation: evidence from motion adaptation. *Vision Research, 38,* 3899–912.

Sclar, G., Maunsell, J.H., & Lennie, P. (1990). Coding of image contrast in central visual pathways of the macaque monkey. *Vision Research, 30,* 1–10.

Smith, A.T., & Hammond, P. (1985). The pattern specificity of velocity aftereffects. *Experimental Brain Research, 60,* 71–8.

Smith, S.T., Clifford, C.W.G., & Wenderoth, P. (2001). Interaction between first- and second-order orientation channels revealed by the tilt illusion: psychophysics and computational modelling. *Vision Research, 41,* 1057–71.

Snowden, R.J. (1994). Motion processing in the primate cerebral cortex. In A.T. Smith & R.J. Snowden (Eds.), *Visual Detection of Motion* (pp. 51–83). Academic Press.

Snowden, R.J. (1998). Shifts in perceived position following adaptation to visual motion. *Current Biology, 8,* 1343–5.

Snowden, R.J., & Hammett, S.T. (1992). Subtractive and divisive adaptation in the human visual system. *Nature, 355,* 248–50.

Somers, D.C., Nelson, S.B., & Sur, M. (1995). An emergent model of orientation selectivity in cat visual cortical simple cells. *Journal of Neuroscience, 15,* 5448–65.

Spigel, I.M. (1960). The effects of differential post-exposure illumination on the decay of the movement aftereffect. *Journal of Psychology, 50,* 209–10.

Srinivasan, M.V., Laughlin, S.B., & Dubs, A. (1982). Predictive coding: a fresh view of inhibition in the retina. *Proceedings of Royal Society of London, Series B, 216,* 427–59.

Sur, M., Schummers, J., & Dragoi, V. (2002). Cortical plasticity: time for a change. *Current Biology, 12,* R168–70.

Sutherland, N.S. (1961). Figural after-effects and apparent size. *Quarterly Journal of Experimental Psychology, 13,* 222–8.

Thompson, P. (1981). Velocity after-effects: the effects of adaptation to moving stimuli on the perception of subsequently seen moving stimuli. *Vision Research, 21,* 337–45.

Tootell, R.B.H., Reppas, J.B., Dale, A.M., Look, R.B., Serano, M.I., & Malach, R., *et al.* (1995). Visual motion after effect in human cortical area MT revealed by functional magnetic resonance imaging. *Nature, 375,* 139–41.

Ullman, S., & Schechtman, G. (1982). Adaptation and gain normalization. *Proceedings of the Royal Society of London, Series B, 216,* 299–313.

van der Zwan, R., & Wenderoth, P. (1995). Mechanisms of purely subjective contour tilt aftereffects. *Vision Research 35,* 2547–57.

Vogels, R. (1990). Population coding of stimulus orientation by striate cortical cells. *Biological Cybernetics, 64*, 25–31.

von Grunau, M.W. (1986). A motion-aftereffect for long-range stroboscopic apparent motion. *Perception and Psychophysics, 40*, 31–8.

Wenderoth, P., & Johnstone, S. (1987). Possible neural substrates for orientation analysis and perception. *Perception, 16*, 693–709.

Wenderoth, P., & Johnstone, S. (1988). The different mechanisms of the direct and indirect tilt illusions. *Vision Research, 28*, 301–12.

Wenderoth, P., & van der Zwan, R. (1989). The effects of exposure duration and surrounding frames on direct and indirect tilt aftereffects and illusions. *Perception and Psychophysics, 46*, 338–44.

Westheimer, G., & Gee, A. (2002). Orthogonal adaptation and orientation discrimination. *Vision Research, 42*, 2339–43.

Westheimer, G., & Gee, A. (2003). Opposing views on orthogonal adaptation: a response to Clifford, Arnold, Smith, and Pianta (2003). *Vision Research, 43*, 721–2.

Wiesenfelder, H., & Blake, R. (1992). Binocular rivalry suppression disrupts recovery from motion adaptation. *Visual Neuroscience, 9*, 143–8.

Wohlgemuth, A. (1911). On the after-effect of seen movement. *British Journal of Psychology Monograph Supplement, 1*, 1–116.

Wilson, H.R., & Wilkinson, F. (1998). Detection of global struture in Glass patterns: implications for form vision. *Vision Research, 38*, 2933–47.

Zaidi, Q., & Shapiro, A.G. (1993). Adaptive orthogonalization of opponent-color signals. *Biological Cybernetics, 69*, 415–28.

3

Accommodating the Past: A Selective History of Adaptation

Nicholas J. Wade and Frans A.J. Verstraten

3.1 Introduction

Adaptation occurs when there is adjustment to new conditions. In the context of perception, it refers either to changes with constant stimulation or to adjustments with varying stimulation. An example of the former is the change in the apparent intensity of a light source when observed for some time. A common instance of the latter is dark and light adaptation. If one goes to bed and turns off the lights, it is initially hard to see anything at all. However, after some time it seems that the eyes are adjusting to the new environment. This adjustment can be described in terms of a gain-control mechanism, comparable to an amplifier. If there are only a few portions of light – the so-called photons – their effects can be amplified such that the signal they produce leads to a percept. Also when turning on the lights after some time of sleep, the observer will not be able to see much – everything seems too bright. In that case the gain has to be turned down. Here, adaptation has a clear perceptual consequence. For both dark and light adaptation the gain control mechanism is a specific mechanism that enables an organism to operate under different circumstances, in this specific case different light conditions.

Adaptation to variation in light intensity has obvious functional advantages, and the same applies to other examples that have long been studied. One is adaptation of the dioptric state of the eye when changing focus to objects at different distances – now called accommodation. Unlike light and dark adaptation, accommodation involves motor as well as sensory components, and the process operates with great rapidity. The accommodative range changes throughout life, becoming very restricted after middle age. The adjustments required for such presbyopia take place over years, and so are not readily amenable to experimental enquiry. The strategy that has been adopted to examine similar long-term effects is to impose artificial modifications to the incoming patterns of light – by wearing prisms, mirrors, or lenses. Under these conditions the behavioural adaptations to rearranged sensory input can be investigated.

Between the levels of accommodation and prism adaptation are phenomena that have been intensively studied, but do not involve a motor component. They are visual aftereffects – changes in perceived properties of objects as a consequence of prolonged exposure to an unchanging stimulus. A visual aftereffect that has received considerable attention is in the motion domain. A static stimulus can appear to move following prolonged observation of constantly moving stimulus.

In this chapter we will examine three adaptation phenomena: accommodation, motion aftereffects, and adjustments to optical distortions. By examining these in a historical context, we hope to provide some useful pointers to studies of adaptation generally. Adaptation to objects at different distances from the eyes (accommodation) enables an animal to resolve its features adequately and to guide its actions appropriately. Adaptation to the constant characteristics of objects (like motion at a constant velocity) can increase sensitivity to objects moving at different velocities. Adaptation to optical distortions can reflect the longer-term adjustments in sensory–motor integration. Although this has been studied by imposing distortions (like optical inversion) on observers, it could be essentially the same process that accompanies growth in the size of the eyes or increases in their separation that occur during development. Before addressing these three phenomena, it is instructive to consider how the term 'adaptation' has been used and the ways in which it can be defined.

3.2 Defining Adaptation

A sensible strategy for psychologists to adopt is to investigate a phenomenon in terms of 'what is it good for and why has evolution incorporated such mechanisms in our brain?' In contrast to what one might think having read the examples above, the history of research on adaptation has not followed a functional path; it has not been driven by the question 'what is it good for?' One obvious reason for this is that studies of adaptation began long before ideas regarding evolution were established. That is, the phenomenal aspects of perceptual change were remarked upon initially, and their interpretations followed much later.

What could be a definition of adaptation that relates to the functions it serves? The following quotation, taken from a distinguished physiologist, seems to be a good starting point.

'Adaptation is "the continuous adjustment of internal relations to external relations".
A living organism may be regarded as a highly unstable system which tends to
undergo disintegrations as a result of any variation in its average environment [...]
Every activity in a living being must be not only a necessary sequence of some
antecedent change in its environment, but must be so adapted to this change as to
tend to its neutralization, and so to the survival of the organism.' (Evans 1945, p. 4)

At first sight, defining adaptation in terms of *a dynamic setting of the
operational range* is problematical when one considers another aspect that is
very often found in the adaptation literature, namely aftereffects. One famous
example of an aftereffect is the waterfall illusion, also known as the motion
aftereffect (MAE). It refers to the modification of motion perception following
prolonged observation of a regularly moving stimulus. When the movement is
stopped a static pattern will appear to move in the opposite direction (see Mather
et al. 1998 for a review). The term aftereffect implies an effect *after* something
has happened. Dynamic adjustments, however, are by definition an interaction
with the present environmental conditions, as in the case of light and dark
adaptation. Nonetheless, investigating the sequential aspects of adaptation
(aftereffects) has resulted in a more detailed understanding of adaptation
generally.

The term adaptation has been used widely but it has not been defined consistently. It has been applied to perception, to procedure, and to process. Applied
to perception, adaptation is the change experienced as a consequence of exposure to a stimulus. The exposure might be of short duration or it might take place
over a considerable period. In all cases, adaptation is said to take place when
there is some adjustment to the new pattern of stimulation. The characteristics
of perceptual change have not been consistently charted: they can be changes
in sensitivity (as with light and dark adaptation), biases in perception (as with
the MAE), or modifications in sensory–motor co-ordination (as in adjustment
to optical distortions). Moreover, the perceptual changes are sometimes recorded
simultaneously with or successively following stimulation. The latter has been
examined in greater detail than the former, largely because the procedures for
measuring successive effects are more securely based. Applied to procedure,
adaptation refers to the stimulus and timing characteristics that lead to changes
in perception and/or process. The standard procedure for establishing aftereffects is that of pre-test, adaptation, post-test: adaptation is inferred from the
differences between pre- and post-tests. Applied to process, adaptation occurs
when some measured or inferred physiological change takes place. Most
psychological studies are based on inferences about the process rather than
measurements themselves, although the inferences are linked to measures that
have previously been reported. These multiple features of adaptation are reflected
in the terms adopted. They include adaptation stimulus, recovery from adaptation, sensory adaptation, and top-up adaptation. If the term adaptation can be
applied to such varied phenomena and to the different ways in which they can
be examined, then questioning whether a single term should encompass them all
might be appropriate.

The process of adaptation is often inferred from psychological experiments rather than based on physiological measures. In this context, aftereffects have been likened to the neurophysiologist's microelectrode:

> 'Can sensory aftereffects help us to discover the sensory dimensions that are important to our own sense-organs and to our brain? Can they reveal, in other words, which attributes of a complex stimulus are singled out for neural analysis? If one suspects that a particular attribute of the stimulus is subject to specialised analysis, then the principle is to try to fatigue, or "adapt", selectively the neural mechanism tuned to detect that particular attribute. At its most naked, and within the privacy of the laboratory, the argument runs "If you can adapt it, it's there".' (Mollon 1974, p. 479)

This principle of fatigue or adaptation had been lurking within perception research for some time, and it has been eagerly adopted in the last three decades. For example, Frisby (1979) entitled a chapter of his book on vision: *Aftereffects: the psychologist's microelectrode*. He wrote that aftereffects 'give the psychologist a sensitive tool for probing the working of sensory mechanisms' (p. 89). Many psychologists have applied this tool to aftereffects but, like the physiologists' microelectrode, the sensory mechanisms it has probed appear increasingly complex.

3.3 Selection for a Selective History

This book is concerned with vision and in particular high-level vision. Hence, we will focus here on the history of visual phenomena with an eye for the high(er) level aspects. However, in order to understand the nature of adaptation, it is important to understand that there are different kinds of adaptation, as well as different ways of thinking about it. It would be possible to consider accommodation, light and dark adaptation, colour adaptation, movement adaptation, form adaptation, adaptation to prismatic displacements, and many other phenomena under this rubric. The three forms of adaptation we have selected – accommodation, adaptation to motion, and to optical distortions – reflect the wide range covered by this concept. The first and the last have a motor component whereas the MAE is generally considered to be a sensory phenomenon. The motor component in accommodation is reflexive whereas that in adaptation to optical distortions is under voluntary control. The physiological processes that are involved in the three phenomena are different although the differences have proved difficult to determine. Most is known about accommodation, much is inferred regarding MAEs, and investigations into the possible physiological changes that accompany adaptation to optical distortion are just commencing (see Linden *et al.* 1999). The psychological interest in the phenomena has also been grossly disparate. Accommodation has been examined principally as a possible source of distance information when viewing close objects. Studies of adaptation to optical distortions have been patchy since the time of Helmholtz (1867). They received a boost when Stratton (1896) described his experiences when viewing the world without inversion of the retinal image. In contrast the MAE has been studied intensively, particularly in the last four decades.

In addition to these many dimensions of difference, there is a wide temporal range over which the processes can operate. Accommodation is rapid: it requires only several hundred milliseconds for the lens to change its curvature in order to bring objects at different distances to focus on the retina. Adaptation to motion occurs over many seconds, but it is most readily expressed in the MAE following cessation of exposure to a moving stimulus. Adaptation to optical distortions takes place over minutes or days, depending on the nature of the distortion imposed. Shifts of visual direction, induced by prisms, can be recalibrated in minutes, whereas those involving inversion of the whole visual field require days.

3.4 Accommodation

Perceptual changes have been given a variety of names, of which adaptation was one, and they were rarely accorded precise definitions. For example, what we now call accommodation was long known as 'adaptation to distance'; Porterfield (1738) coined the term accommodation, although it was still referred to as adaptation to distance by some (e.g. Home 1794). Indeed, in many ways 'adaptation to distance' is a better, and more functional, description than 'accommodation'. It does reflect the manner in which it is possible to adapt the optical structures within the eye to focus on objects at different distances.

Accommodation or adaptation to distance is a process that reflects the functional definition given by Evans. In a historical sense, adaptation was the term applied to the adjustments of the eye required to focus on objects at different distances. The problem of accommodation became central to students of vision following Kepler's description of the dioptrics of the eye (see Smith 1998; Wade 1998). That is, Kepler showed that the retina was the receptive surface for vision and that light was refracted through the various transparent structures in the eye to focus on it; this raised the question of how the optical state could change. The equation of eye and camera further focused attention on the features of a camera that could afford focus over distances (see Wade & Finger 2001). It was known that cameras with pinhole lenses had a very long depth of field, whereas those with large apertures required a specific lens to focus on objects at a specific distance. Accordingly, the operation of a camera with a lens provided hypotheses about how accommodation might work in the eye: the eye could lengthen or the lens could move forward or backward in the eye. The possibility that the lens could change its curvature was entertained but rejected because no muscular fibres could be seen in an excised lens when observed under a microscope.

In 1793, the youthful Thomas Young, then a medical student, presented a paper concerned with some 'Observations on vision' to the Royal Society. In this Young argued, on logical rather than experimental grounds, that accommodation of the eye was achieved by changes in the curvature of the crystalline lens. He surveyed the many theories that had been proposed to account for the mechanism of accommodation, and dismissed most of them. He considered that variation in the curvature of the lens was the only interpretation consonant with the facts of accommodation, and he speculated as to the mechanism of this change by suggesting that the lens was muscular. His microscopic examination of a crystalline lens, taken from an ox, led him to the hypothesis that accommodation is mediated, 'by the ciliary processes to the muscles of the crystalline, which, by the contraction of its fibres, becomes more convex, and collects the diverging rays to a focus on the retina' (1793, p. 174). However, his conviction was based more on the logic of the argument than the anatomical evidence of muscle fibres. When he returned to the topic in 1801, he provided further evidence of the involvement of the lens in accommodation, and added more support to his hypothesis that the lens varied in curvature. However, he could not determine how this change took place.

The solution to the problem of accommodation was provided in the middle of the nineteenth century when Cramer (1853) and Helmholtz (1855) independently proposed that the lens was elastic and under tension. Helmholtz, in one of his *Popular Lectures*, reflected on the significance of accommodation in visual science when he noted: 'The mechanism by which this is accomplished... was one of the greatest riddles of the physiology of the eye since the time of Kepler ... No problem in optics has given rise to so many contradictory theories as this' (1873, p. 205). The conclusions reached by Helmholtz were the same as those of Cramer. Helmholtz summarized the mechanism by which accommodation is achieved succintly:

> 'On contraction, the ciliary muscle could pull the posterior end of the zonule forwards nearer the lens and reduce the tension of the zonule .... If the pull of the zonule is relaxed in accommodating for near vision, the equatorial diameter of the lens will diminish, and the lens will get thicker in the middle, both surfaces becoming more curved' (1924/2000, p. 151).

The variations in the power of accommodation with age were clarified by Donders (1864). Cramer, Helmholtz, and Donders all measured the curvature of the lens by means of an ophthalmometer: the sizes of Purkinje images were determined with accommodation on near and far targets (see Wade & Finger 2001). When the procedure for measuring this form of adaptation was established, the process by which the variations in lens curvature were achieved could be inferred.

Accommodation is a supremely functional process, but it is relatively rarely investigated by contemporary students of vision. The mechanism is reasonably well understood; it is confined mainly to the level of physiology, and does not reflect the higher level processes with which the book is concerned.

3.5 Adaptation to Motion

Adaptation to motion has a radically different history. There are in fact two aspects of motion adaptation that have been studied, although one has received much more experimental attention than the other, and they differ with respect to perception, procedure, and possibly process. Motion adaptation is perceived as a change in the apparent velocity of a constantly moving object. It is a simultaneous effect that has proved difficult to describe and even more difficult to measure. The procedures for recording the perceptual changes during adaptation are not well-established, although the process is commonly recorded physiologically. Changes in firing rates as a consequence of constant stimulation are grist to the physiologists' mill but changes in perception under similar circumstances have generally been eschewed by psychologists. The aftereffects of constant motion adaptation are more readily perceived and are more easily measured. The apparent motion of a stationary stimulus following exposure to a constantly moving one (called the motion aftereffect or MAE) is compelling and there are established procedures for measuring it. It is a successive effect which changes over time but this aspect is not so frequently measured. The procedure for determining the strength of the MAE is usually its duration, although other indices are used, too (see Pantle 1998). The MAE was described in antiquity. It was studied in detail from about the time that the process of accommodation was clarified (the mid-nineteenth century), and it remains at the heart of vision research. The process remains uncertain although close links have been made with the properties of single cells in the visual cortex called motion detectors (see Anstis *et al.* 1998). It has long been assumed that the processes involved in motion adaptation are the same as those for the MAE. There is evidence emerging to show that different processes are operating for adaptation and MAE, and the links to motion detectors are also being loosened.

Although we will focus on motion and its aftereffect, the issues considered are not restricted to motion. Similar phenomena of sensory adaptation occur in many modalities and dimensions within them, and cover a large number of phenomena – for instance, those concerning brightness, colour, and orientation. Coverage of these will be found in other chapters in this book.

Anstis (1986), among others, pointed out that there are several perceptual effects that result from looking at a moving pattern for some time. For example, while the pattern is still moving it may appear to slow down (e.g. Cords & von Brücke 1907; Thompson 1981). Wiesenfelder (1993) suggested that this has adaptive value, especially for animals capable of rapid movement. Adaptation could reduce the Weber fraction at high velocities, increasing the animal's ability to discriminate velocity. This principle has been demonstrated for motion sensitive neurons in insects (Maddess & Laughlin 1985) and for human motion perception (Clifford & Langley 1996). It is tempting to speculate that this mechanism is also involved in car driving, although the motion in this case is produced artificially. This 'adjustment to new motion conditions' seems to take time; it can be experienced rather easily, especially when slowing down. If, after some time of driving on a highway at say 120 kph, one returns to a 50-kph zone, the experienced velocity is much lower than that experienced at the same speed before such high velocities. One has to rely on the speedometer to maintain an acceptable car speed. Apparently the 'recalibration to a new environment' takes time. Other perceptual effects are evident once the adapting motion has stopped: velocity aftereffects (Thompson 1981), direction-specific adaptation (Sekuler & Ganz 1963), and the MAE, which is our focus here.

The MAE has a long history. Following its descriptions in antiquity by Aristotle and Lucretius (see Verstraten 1996) there do not seem to be any descriptions of the MAE until early in the nineteenth century when it was redis-covered frequently (see Wade & Verstraten 1998 for a detailed overview). The two most notable accounts were made by Purkinje (1820, 1825) and by Addams (1834). Purkinje first briefly described the MAE in an article concerned with visual vertigo. Addams observed what later became called the waterfall illusion (Thompson 1880) at the Falls of Foyers in northern Scotland (see Fig. 3.1).

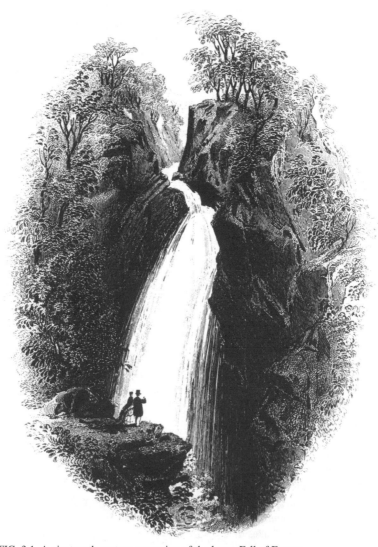

FIG. 3.1 A nineteenth century engraving of the lower Fall of Foyers.

Both Purkinje and Addams adopted an eye movement interpretation of the phenomenon.

Thompson (1877) extended the MAE to depth as well as direction, and MAEs in the third dimension were examined more systematically by Exner (1888) and von Szily (1905). Addams (1834) suggested that the motion of falling water could be simulated in the laboratory by moving stripes, but this was not put into practice until Oppel (1856) reached the same conclusion independently.

Nineteenth century studies of the MAE were reviewed by Wohlgemuth (1911). He confirmed many aspects of previous experiments showing that: motion over the retina is necessary to generate an MAE; the strength of the MAE is more marked with fixation; the MAE is restricted to the retinal area stimulated by prior motion; it immediately follows adapting motion and its visibility improves with practice; an MAE can be produced in each eye independently and what is seen with two eyes is a combination of the two monocular adaptations; adaptation of one eye transfers to the other; MAEs can be produced by a wide range of speeds, and by stroboscopic as well as real motion; following adaptation, motion can be seen with the eyes closed.

Wohlgemuth classified the previous interpretations into physical, psychical, and physiological. Eye movement explanations of MAEs were considered to be physical, but they could not accommodate the occurrence of oppositely directed MAEs visible simultaneously. Wohlgemuth devoted most attention to the physiological interpretations, particularly that advanced by Exner (1894). His own model was greatly influenced by Sherrington's (1906) theory of integration within the nervous system (see Wade & Verstaten 1998).

The models of Exner and Wohlgemuth were based on shrewd speculations regarding physiological processes. When the neurophysiology of vision became a little better understood, mainly as a consequence of electrophysiological recordings in the 1950s and 1960s, it greatly influenced models of motion detection and adaptation. These, in turn, fuelled the most intense phase of research on MAEs. This is discussed in detail in the chapter by Ibbotson in this volume (see also Niedeggen & Wist 1998) and here we will here only touch on this part of the recent history.

In 1963, Barlow and Hill explained the waterfall illusion in terms of visual processing by single cortical cells that were called motion detectors. They responded to stationary contours but most strongly to contours moving in a particular direction. Barlow and Hill provided support for earlier speculations by Sutherland (1961) towards the cause of MAEs. Consider what happens when an observer looks at the rocks by the side of a waterfall: the stationary rocks will have many contours, which will weakly stimulate motion detectors for all directions. For example, horizontal contours will excite different motion detectors for downward and upward movement, but the net effect of these would cancel. When the descending water is observed the downward motion detectors will be strongly stimulated, and if this stimulation is prolonged the motion detectors will adapt or fatigue – that is, their rate of firing will decrease. Subsequent observation of the stationary rocks will produce a different net effect: the adapted downward-motion detectors will exert less influence than the unadapted upward-motion detectors. Therefore, the signal from the rocks would be similar to one produced by contours moving slowly upwards, which corresponds to what is seen. Barlow and Hill (1963) suggested that MAEs, 'may result from the temporary imbalance of the maintained discharges of cells responsive to motion in opposite directions' (p. 1346). This so-called ratio model has been modified into a distribution-shift model by Mather (1980) in which neural activities for all directions are taken into account (see Clifford, this volume). A reason for this adjustment is that adaptation to motions in orthogonal directions results in MAEs that are in the opposite direction to the resultant (see also Riggs & Day 1980; Exner 1887, 1888; Borschke & Herscheles 1902; Verstraten *et al.* 1994).

Several studies, some of them very old, have provided evidence that makes an explanation based on motion detectors alone hard to defend. As early as 1878, Aitken reported that stimulation of the whole retina with linear motion during adaptation did not produce an MAE, a result which was confirmed by Wohlgemuth (1911): motion detectors are stimulated, yet no aftereffect is perceived. This only applies to linear motion since Reinhardt-Rutland (1987) did find MAEs following exposure to large spiral rotation. Day and Strelow (1971) directed attention to the importance of relative motion in the MAE by comparing equivalent adapting linear motions with and without a visible surround. Von Szily (1905) and Basler (1910) showed that an MAE can follow induced motion, and the interaction between induced motion and MAEs has been demonstrated by Anstis and Reinhardt-Rutland (1976), Reinhardt-Rutland (1981), and Swanston & Wade (1992). MAEs have been generated from the observation of stationary stimuli (Anstis 1990) and with 'phantom' gratings (Weisstein *et al.* 1977). The adequate stimulus for the MAE would appear to involve relative motion (Zöllner 1860), even if this is restricted to some arbitrary boundary within which the motion is displayed (see Wade *et al.* 1996).

3.6 Interpretations and Functional Significance

Motion adaptation has been interpreted mostly in terms of cortical motion detectors. It has basically been used as a tool to assist such inferences. A few attempts have been made to attribute functional significance to MAEs, mostly in the second half of the twentieth century. Earlier reports hardly refer, if at all, to a possible functional role for MAEs. One idea about the role of aftereffect is that it reflects the perceptual manifestation of a recalibration process (for other ideas, see Mather & Harris 1998; and Clifford, this volume).

An example of research that fits in the 'recalibration tradition' is an experiment by Harris *et al.* (1981). They proposed that the MAE arises as a result of a conflict between visual and vestibular information. Adaptation studies in laboratories typically involve a stationary observer looking at a moving pattern. According to Harris and his colleagues, this is not how the brain operates in more ecologically valid situations. A moving observer perceives motion for a prolonged time during which vestibular information is also available. They found that if the conflict is removed by adapting observers to motion that is related to their movements (e.g. by placing both the display and the observer on a moving trolley), the magnitude of the MAE was significantly reduced. That is, they examined MAEs in situations involving body movement thereby generating motion over the retina rather than presenting moving stimuli to static observers.

Consider the earlier mentioned aspects of car driving. Could the results of Harris *et al.* explain the fact that we hardly ever experience an MAE after driving a car? Since vestibular and visual information are not in conflict, there is hardly any aftereffect as a by-product. If recalibration is the important factor, it apparently happens rapidly and effortlessly. For car driving, especially when going from fast to slow speeds, one could argue that there is a kind of aftereffect, namely the underestimation of the car's speed. Maybe this is a perceptual manifestation of an ongoing (re)calibration process.

It would be interesting to relate motion adaptation to MAEs as phenomena based on the same principle, that of adjusting the operational range to the most sensitive setting – a (re)calibration process. However, motion adaptation is not related in a simple manner to MAEs: Wade *et al.* (1996) have demonstrated that motion adaptation can be closely related to localized motion detectors but the expression of the adaptation in the MAE depends upon the global structure of the test field. The same motion adaptation can yield different MAEs with differently structured test stimuli. MAEs can be compared to light and dark adaptation mechanisms which enable an organism to operate under a wide range of illuminations. The fact that we do not, or at least not very often, experience MAEs following driving can possibly be explained by perfect and fast calibration for ecologically valid conditions. Another explanation could be that the adapted neural substrates normally do not reach perceptual threshold. That is, it could be that the consequences of motion adaptation are present but they are not strong enough to be expressed perceptually.

Can we see an aftereffect as part of a constant process of recalibration or operational range optimization and avoid terms like *recovery from adaptation*? On this view, the visual system adapts to the prolonged stimulation and the adaptation is expressed via the test stimulus. For example, one challenge is to explain the many different kinds of aftereffects that have been reported, especially those that are phenomenologically different after exposure to the same adaptation conditions. That is, the expression of adaptation in the MAE is dependent upon the structure of the test pattern, so that different MAEs can result from the same adaptation (e.g. Nishida & Sato 1992; Wade *et al.* 1996; Wade & Salvano-Pardieu 1998; Verstraten *et al.* 1999; van der Smagt *et al.* 1999). The suggestion from such studies is that different processes might be sought for adaptation and aftereffect, and it is becoming increasingly unlikely that a single process will account for both components.

3.7 Adaptation to Optical Distortion

Adaptation to optical distortion is generally associated with radical rearrangements due to inverting the normally inverted retinal image. Adaptation to these changes typically requires days rather than minutes, and the spatial aftereffects last correspondingly longer than those described in the previous section. However, adaptation to less dramatic modifications of the visual input can be much faster and the aftereffects much shorter. Welch (1985) defined such an adaptation in the following way: '*a semipermanent change of perception or perceptual-motor coordination that serves to reduce or eliminate a registered discrepancy between or within sensory modalities or the errors in behavior induced by this discrepancy*' (Chapter 24, p. 3, original italics). Sensory adaptation and aftereffects like those of motion were explicitly excluded from this definition, which emphasizes the motor or functional aspects of adaptation. Experiments involving rearrangement have a moderately long history. For example, Helmholtz (1867), in his classic *Handbuch der physiologischen Optik*, applied distorting prisms to change the apparent direction of objects. The displacements were relatively small and the adjustment to them relatively rapid. He described it in the following way:

> 'Take two glass prisms with refracting angles of about 16° or 18°, and place them in a spectacle frame, with their edges both turned toward the left. As seen through these glasses, the objects in the field of view will all apparently be shifted to the left of their real positions. At first, without bringing the hand into the field, look closely at some definite object within reach; and then close the eyes, and try to touch the object with the forefinger. The usual result will be to miss it by thrusting the hand too far to the left. But after trying for some little while, or, more quickly still, by inserting the hand in the field and, under the guidance of the eye, touching the objects with it for an instant, then on trying the above experiment again, we shall discover that now we do not miss the objects, but feel for them correctly... Having learned how to do this, suppose we now take off the prisms and remove the hand from the field of view, and then, after gazing steadily at some object, close our eyes and try to take hold of it. We find then that the hand will miss the object by being thrust too far to the right; until after several failures, our judgement of the direction of the eyes is rectified again.' (Helmholtz 2000, p. 246)

Although Helmholtz did not conduct formal experiments on prism adaptation, he provided the essential conditions and results that have been obtained by subsequent researchers (see Welch 1978). Initially there is no compensation for the distortion, then the new spatial relations are learned, followed by an aftereffect when the distortion is removed. Adaptation to small changes is relatively rapid, and the aftereffects are short lived.

More dramatic distortions require longer periods for adaptation to occur. This was demonstrated by Stratton, who viewed the world with an upright retinal image (optically inverting the image before the inversion in the eye) and described his experiences over a period of days. Stratton's first study was published as a preliminary report in 1896, and theoretical aspects of it were discussed in a later note (1897*a*). He wore lenses in front of his right eye, with the left occluded, for a period of three days. At the time he was one of Wundt's students at Leipzig, and made the initial announcement of his experiment at the Third International Congress of Psychology, held at Munich in 1896. On his return to California he extended the experiment by wearing the lenses for eight days; the resulting experiences were described in two articles (1897*b,c*) published in *Psychological Review*.

The issue of concern was not with adaptation itself, but with the orientation of the retinal image. Nonetheless, the studies did lead to an examination of these longer term adjustments to radically different patterns of stimulation and sensory-motor coordination. Before Stratton, upright vision with an inverted retinal image was then typically accounted for by either projection or eye movement theories. Stratton posed the question: '*Is* the inverted image a necessary condition for our seeing things in an upright position? The method of approaching the problem was to substitute an upright retinal image for the normal inverted one and watch the result' (1896, p. 611). He was the watcher, that is, the only observer. At first, objects appeared inverted, perceptual–motor coordination was disrupted and there was a distinction between where objects were seen and where they were thought to be. 'By the third day things had thus been interconnected into a whole by piecing together the parts of the ever-changing visual fields' (p. 616). He did not report any aftereffects when the lenses were removed after three days, and he concluded that 'the difficulty of seeing things upright by means of upright retinal images seems to consist solely in the resistance offered by long-established previous experience' (p. 617).

The first experiment was conducted entirely indoors, but when he repeated it over eight days in California he ventured outdoors, too. The pattern of experiences was similar for the first three days, and the adaptation became more established thereafter. There were, however, aftereffects when the lenses were removed:

> 'On opening my eyes, the scene had a strange familiarity. The visual arrangement was immediately recognized as the old one of pre-experimental days; yet the reversal of everything from the order to which I had grown accustomed during the past week, gave the scene a surprising, bewildering air which lasted several hours. It was hardly the feeling, though, that things were upside down' (1897*c*, p. 470).

The theoretical lesson to be drawn from the longer study was essentially the same as that from the shorter one: 'harmony comes only after a tedious course of adjustment to the new conditions, and that the visual system has to build anew, growing from an isolated group of perceptions' (1897*c*, p. 471). Stratton (1899) disrupted the harmony between touch and sight in a further study that is cited less frequently. He wore a system of mirrors mounted on a harness that resulted in him seeing his body from above; this he experienced over a period of three days and found a similar course of adaptation. The conclusion was similar to that derived from the inversion experiments: 'The simplest explanation seems to me to be that a correspondence, point by point, between touch and sight, is built up associationally; and only by actual experience does a person learn what visual position corresponds to any given tactual position' (Stratton 1899, pp. 498–9). He then related this interpretation to cases in which sight had been restored in the blind, after the manner of Cheselden's patient (see Wade 1998).

The behavioural effects of adaptation to optical inversion have generally been confirmed in subsequent investigations, but whether the world subsequently looks upright has proved harder to resolve. Phenomenological reports have often proved confusing, as is evident from Kohler's (1964) work. He wore a variety of distorting optical devices for long periods and found that both perception and action adapted to the new spatial relations. In one study he wore a binocular mirror-device (which inverted the images on both eyes) continually for almost four months. Initially everything appeared inverted and all actions based on visual input were misguided. After a period of days and weeks his behaviour was no longer disrupted by the inverting mirrors: he was able to reach for objects appropriately and even carry out complex skills such as skiing. Throughout the weeks of adaptation he kept detailed protocols and records of his performance on perceptual–motor tasks. In some cases he described features (like smoke from a pipe) as being seen normally oriented whereas other objects remained apparently inverted. When the mirrors were removed long-lasting aftereffects were reported: the world was transformed once more, but recovery was quicker than adaptation had been.

'This experiment, the first of such long duration, was significant. In the first place, the aftereffects obtained were of optimal strength. In the second place, it gave rise to a number of peculiar aftereffects which I have already referred to as 'situational'. Not only curvatures, distortions, deviations, apparent movements, etc., were found to leave traces in the sensorium, but also the variations in intensity of these disturbances' (Kohler 1964, p. 39).

Kohler's experiments reawakened interest in visual adaptation to rearranged optical input and he added many new phenomena to its study, particularly gaze-contingent colour aftereffects. His observations led on to experiments on colour-contingent aftereffects by McCollough (1965). In a more recent study, Linden *et al.* (1999) examined four subjects wearing inverting optical devices for up to ten days. They presented psychophysical evidence to indicate that the perceptual world remained inverted throughout the period of adaptation, and brain-imaging (fMRI) indices displayed no changes in activity at early visual areas.

There is a general agreement about sensory–motor adaptation to optical distortions but less accord regarding any perceptual changes. A link might be made to contemporary distinctions between visual streams subserving action and perception (Goodale & Milner 2004). The motor component to sensory–motor adaptation can be recalibrated but it is not necessarily correlated with a perceptual change.

3.8 Concluding Remarks

The history of research on adaptation highlights problems of definition and interpretation. We have indicated how the term has been applied in several different ways–in terms of perception, procedure, and process. The same sequence can be said to apply to the investigation of adaptation. First the phenomena have to be experienced. That is, the initial stage is perception. Certain constant object properties, like colour, size, or motion, can be perceived to change under certain circumstances, like prolonged observation. These changes will be the source of interest, and the observational descriptions will lead to a more detailed experimental enquiry. It is likely that the more compelling phenomena will generate the greatest interest, which could be why aftereffects have received so much attention. Second, with the acceptance that a phenomenon can be considered as adaptation some method of adequately assessing it is required. This is the procedural phase. It is essential in terms of deriving reliable indices of the perceptual change. Again, aftereffects have provided a pre-test post-test paradigm that has proved reliable and has been widely adopted. Third, when the procedural issues are resolved, then an analysis of the process or mechanism can be undertaken. The majority of such studies have been based on inferences from behavioural measures regarding the underlying mechanisms rather than on direct recordings at the physiological level. Nonetheless, physiological indices are faced with the reverse problem of inference regarding the perception they are thought to mediate. Adaptation provides an arena in which these various levels of investigation and analysis can be gainfully explored (see Barlow 1990).

It is evident that adaptation to change can take many forms and it has been studied in many ways. We have selected three types of adaptation for discussion – accommodation, motion aftereffects, and adjustments to optical distortions. These reflect the range of phenomena to which the term has been applied, and they indicate the variety of interpretations that can be applied. The title of this book suggests that the brain's task is to fit the mind to the world. That is, the emphasis is on the functional aspects of behavioural benefits that accrue to adaptation. As a highly mobile organism and one that needs to operate under very different environmental conditions, this continuous adjustment seems to be essential for survival. These adaptations or sensitivity adjustments have many dimensions and we have chosen to make a distinction based on the time course over which adaptation occurs. The time course is less than a second for accommodation, seconds for aftereffects, and can require days for optical distortions. The question that arises then is whether a single term should be applied to these sorts of adaptation. The potential problem with using a single term is that it might suggest similar underlying processes involved in them. Such a conclusion cannot be drawn on our knowledge about the underlying mechanisms at this point. The process of perceptual adaptation is unevenly studied in these three phenomena. It is most clearly evident in the context of accommodation, where the optical stimulus for the muscular responses is known. The processes involved in adaptation and aftereffects can be related to known physiological processes, although there remain problems in linking adaptation to aftereffect. Relatively little is known about the processes underlying the long(er)-term adaptations to optical distortions. The thread connecting the last two is that the procedures applied to examining them both yield aftereffects.

One way to gain insight into how perceptual adaptation works, and how it affects our behaviour is to search for the neuronal substrates and the physiological processes involved. At a higher level of explanation, it is possible to consider that all kinds of adaptation are instances of adjusting some internal gain-control mechanism, irrespective of the exact underlying neural basis. With some exceptions, the history of studies of adaptation has not adopted the route of gain-control.

If a single process of continuous adjustment to new environmental conditions is discovered it would be most satisfying. However, it would have to cover a large number of adaptation effects. It is hoped that this book will stimulate renewed examination of these long known perceptual phenomena.

References

Addams, R. (1834). An account of a peculiar optical phænomenon seen after having looked at a moving body. *London and Edinburgh Philosophical Magazine and Journal of Science*, *5*, 373–4.

Aitken, J. (1878). On a new variety of ocular spectrum. *Proceedings of the Royal Society of Edinburgh*, *10*, 40–4.

Anstis, S. (1986). Motion perception in the frontal plane. In K.R. Boff, L. Kaufman, & J.P. Thomas (ed.), *Handbook of Perception and Human Performance: Sensory Processes and Perception* (Vol. 1, pp. 16-1–16-27). New York: Wiley.

Anstis, S. (1990). Motion aftereffects from a motionless stimulus. *Perception*, *19*, 301–6.

Anstis, S.M., & Reinhardt-Rutland, A.H. (1976). Interactions between motion aftereffects and induced movement. *Vision Research*, *16*, 1391–4.

Anstis, S., Verstraten, F.A.J., & Mather, G. (1998). The motion aftereffect. *Trends in Cognitive Science*, *2*, 111–17.

Barlow, H.B. (1990). A theory about the functional role and synaptic mechanism of visual aftereffects. In C. Blakemore (ed.), *Vision: Coding and Efficency* (pp. 363–75) Cambridge: Cambridge University Press.

Barlow, H.B., & Hill, R.M. (1963). Evidence for a physiological explanation of the waterfall illusion and figural aftereffects. *Nature*, *200*, 1345–7.

Basler, A. (1910). Über das Sehen von Bewegungen. V. Mitteilung. Untersuchungen über die simultane Scheinbewegung. *Archiv für die gesammte Physiologie des Menschen und der Thiere*, *132*, 131–42.

Borschke, A., & Hescheles, L. (1902). Über Bewegungsnachbilder. *Zeitschrift für Psychologie und Physiologie der Sinnesorgane*, *27*, 387–98.

Clifford, C.W.G., & Langley, K. (1996). Psychophysics of motion adaptation parallels insect electrophysiology. *Current Biolology*, *6*, 1340–2.

Cords, R., & von Brücke, E. (1907). Über die Geschwindigkeit des Bewegunsnachbildes. *Archiv für die gesammte Physiologie des Menschen und der Thiere*, *119*, 54–76.

Cramer, A. (1853). *Het Accommodatie vermogen der Oogen Physiologisch Toegelicht.* Haarlem: Loosjes.

Day, R.H., & Strelow, E.R. (1971). Reduction or disappearance of visual after effect of movement in the absence of patterned surround. *Nature, 230*, 55–6.

Donders, F.C. (1864). *On the Anomalies of Accommodation and Refraction of the Eye*. Trans. W.D. Moore. Boston: Milford House.

Evans, C. (1945). *Principles of Human Physiology*. London: J. & A. Churchill Ltd.

Exner, S. (1887). Einige Beobachtungen über Bewegungsnachbilde. *Centralblatt für Physiologie, 1*, 135–40.

Exner, S. (1888). Über optische Bewegungsempfindungen. *Biologisches Centralblatt, 8*, 437–48.

Exner, S. (1894). *Entwurf zu einer physiologischen Erklärung der psychischen Erscheinungen*. Vienna: Deuticke.

Frisby, J.P. (1979). *Seeing: Illusion, Brain and Mind*. Oxford: Oxford University Press.

Goodale, M.A., & Milner, D. (2004). *Sight Unseen: An Exploration of Conscious and Unconscious Vision*. Oxford: Oxford University Press.

Harris L.R., Morgan, M.J., & Still, A.W. (1981). Moving and the motion after-effect. *Nature, 293*, 139–41.

Helmholtz, H. (1855). Ueber die Accommodation des Auges. *Archiv für Ophthalmologie, 1*, 1–74.

Helmholtz, H. (1867). Handbuch der physiologischen Optik. In G. Karsten (Ed.) *Allgemeine Encyklopädie der Physik* (Vol. 9). Leipzig: Voss.

Helmholtz, H. (1873). *Popular Lectures on Scientific Subjects*. Trans. E. Atkinson. London: Longmans, Green.

Helmholtz, H. (1924). *Helmholtz's Treatise on Physiological Optics*. Vol. 1. Trans. J. P. C. Southall. New York: Optical Society of America.

Helmholtz, H. (2000). *Helmholtz's Treatise on Physiological Optics* (3 volumes). Trans. J.P.C Southall. Bristol: Thoemmes.

Home, E. (1794). Some facts relative to the late Mr. John Hunter's preparation for the *Croonian* lecture. *Philosophical Transactions of the Royal Society, 84*, 21–7.

Kohler, I. (1964). *The Formation and Transformation of the Perceptual World*. Trans. H. Fiss. New York: International Universities Press.

Linden, D.E.J., Kallenbach, U., Heinecke, A., Singer W., & Goebel, R. (1999). The myth of upright vision. A psychophysical and functional imaging study of adaptation to inverting spectacles. *Perception, 28*, 469–81.

Maddess, T., & Laughlin, S.B. (1985). Adaptation of the motion sensitive neuron H1 is generated locally and governed by contrast frequency. *Proceedings of the Royal Society of London B, 225*, 251–75.

Mather, G. (1980). The movement after-effect and a distribution-shift model for coding direction of visual movement. *Perception, 9*, 379–92.

Mather, G., & Harris, J. (1998). Theoretical models of the motion aftereffect. In G. Mather, F. Verstraten, & S. Anstis (ed.). *The Motion Aftereffect: A Modern Perspective* (pp. 157–185). Cambridge, MA: MIT Press.

Mather, G., Verstraten, F., & Anstis, S. (ed.) (1998). *The Motion Aftereffect: A Modern Perspective*. Cambridge, MA: MIT Press.

McCollough, C. (1965). Color adaptation of edge-detectors in the human visual system. *Science, 149*, 1115–16.

Mollon, J. (1974). Aftereffects and the brain. *New Scientist, February 21*, 479–82.

Niedeggen, M., & Wist, E. (1998). The physiologic substrate of motion aftereffects. In G. Mather, F. Verstraten, & S. Anstis (ed.). *The Motion Aftereffect: A Modern Perspective* (pp. 125–55). Cambridge, MA: MIT Press.

Nishida, S., & Sato, T. (1992). Positive motion aftereffect induced by bandpass-filtered random-dot kinematograms. *Vision Research, 32,* 1635–46.

Oppel, J.J. (1856). Neue Beobachtungen und Versuche über eine eigentümliche, noch wenig bekannte Reaktionsthätigkeit des menschlichen Auges. *Annalen der Physik und Chemie, 99,* 540–61.

Pantle, A. (1998). How do measures of the motion aftereffect measure up? In G. Mather, F. Verstraten, & S. Anstis (ed.), *The Motion Aftereffect: A Modern Perspective* (pp. 25–39). Cambridge, MA: MIT Press.

Porterfield, W. (1738). An essay concerning the motions of our eyes. Part II. of their internal motions. *Edinburgh Medical Essays and Observations, 4,* 124–294.

Purkinje, J. (1820). Beyträge zur näheren Kenntniss des Schwindels aus heautognostischen Daten. *Medicinische Jahrbücher des kaiserlich-königlichen öesterreichischen Staates, 6,* 79–125.

Purkinje, J. (1825). *Beobachtungen und Versuche zur Physiologie der Sinne. Neue Beiträge zur Kenntniss des Sehens in subjektiver Hinsicht.* Berlin: Reimer.

Reinhardt-Rutland, A.H. (1981). Peripheral movement, induced movement, and after-effects of induced movement. *Perception, 10,* 173–82.

Reinhardt-Rutland, A.H. (1987). Motion aftereffect can be elicited from large spiral. *Perceptual and Motor Skills, 64,* 994.

Riggs, L.A., & Day, R.H. (1980). Visual aftereffects derived from inspection of orthogonally moving patterns. *Science, 208,* 416–18.

Sekuler, R.W., & Ganz, L. (1963). Aftereffect of seen motion with a stabilized retinal image. *Science, 139,* 419–20.

Sherrington, C.S. (1906). *The integrative action of the nervous system.* Cambridge: Cambridge University Press.

Smith, A.M. (1998). Ptolemy, Alhazen, and Kepler and the problem of optical images. *Arabic Sciences and Philosophy, 8,* 9–44.

Stratton, G.M. (1896). Some preliminary experiments on vision without inversion of the retinal image. *Psychological Review, 3,* 611–17.

Stratton, G.M. (1897a). Upright vision and the retinal image. *Psychological Review, 4,* 182–7.

Stratton, G.M. (1897b). Vision without inversion of the retinal image. *Psychological Review, 4,* 341–60.

Stratton, G.M. (1897c). Vision without inversion of the retinal image. *Psychological Review, 4,* 463–81.

Stratton, G.M. (1899). The spatial harmony of touch and sight. *Mind, 8,* 492–505.

Sutherland, N.S. (1961). Figural after-effects and apparent size. *Quarterly Journal of Experimental Psychology, 13,* 222–8.

Swanston, M.T., & Wade, N.J. (1992). Motion over the retina and the motion aftereffect. *Perception, 21,* 569–82.

Szily, A. von. (1905). Bewegungsnachbild und Bewegungskontrast. *Zeitschrift für Psychologie und Physiologie der Sinnesorgane, 38,* 81–154.

Thompson, P. (1981). Velocity after-effects: the effects of adaptation to moving stimuli on the perception of subsequently seen moving stimuli. *Vision Research, 21,* 337–45.

Thompson, S.P. (1877). Some new optical illusions. *Report of the British Association for the Advancement of Science. Transactions of the Sections.* p. 32.

Thompson, S.P. (1880). Optical illusions of motion. *Brain, 3,* 289–98.

van der Smagt, M.J., Verstraten, F.A.J., & van de Grind, W.A. (1999). A new transparent motion after-effect [letter]. *Nature Neuroscience, 2,* 595–6.

Verstraten, F.A.J. (1996). On the *ancient* history of the direction of the motion aftereffect. *Perception, 25,* 1177–88.

Verstraten, F.A.J., Fredericksen, R.E., & van de Grind, W.A. (1994). Movement aftereffect of bi-vectorial transparent motion. *Vision Research, 34,* 349–58.

Verstraten, F.A.J., van der Smagt, M.J., Fredericksen, R.E., & van de Grind, W.A. (1999). Integration after adaptation to transparent motion: static and dynamic test patterns result in different aftereffect directions. *Vision Research, 39,* 803–10.

Wade, N.J. (1998). *A Natural History of Vision.* Cambridge, MA: MIT Press.

Wade, N.J., & Finger, S. (2001). The eye as an optical instrument. From *camera obscura* to Helmholtz's perspective. *Perception, 30,* 1157–77.

Wade, N.J., & Salvano-Pardieu, V. (1998). Visual motion after-effects: Differential adaptation and test stimulation. *Vision Research, 38,* 573–8.

Wade, N.J., Spillmann, L., & Swanston, M.T. (1996). Visual motion after-effects: Critical adaptation and test conditions. *Vision Research, 36,* 2167–75.

Wade, N.J., & Verstraten, F.A.J. (1998). Introduction and historical overview. In G. Mather, F. Verstraten, & S. Anstis (ed.), *The Motion Aftereffect: A Modern Perspective* (pp. 1–23). Cambridge, MA: MIT Press.

Weisstein, N., Maguire, W., & Berbaum, K. (1977). A phantom-motion after-effect. *Science, 198,* 955–8.

Welch, R.B. (1978). *Perceptual Modification. Adapting to Altered Sensory Environments.* New York: Academic Press.

Welch, R.B. (1985). Adaptation of space perception. In K.R. Boff, L. Kaufman, & J.P. Thomas (ed.), *Handbook of Perception and Human Performance: Sensory Processes and Perception* (Vol. 1., pp. 24-1–24-45. New York: Wiley.

Wiesenfelder, H. (1993). Visual motion after-effects: A comprehensive review and analyses (unpublished thesis; Vanderbilt University).

Wohlgemuth, A. (1911). On the after-effect of seen movement. *British Journal of Psychology, Monograph Supplement, 1,* 1–117.

Young, T. (1793). Observations on vision. *Philosophical Transactions of the Royal Society, 83,* 169–81

Young, T. (1801). On the mechanism of the eye. *Philosophical Transactions of the Royal Society, 91,* 23–88.

Zöllner, F. (1860). Über eine neue Art von Pseudoskopie und ihre Beziehungen zu den von Plateau und Oppel beschreibenen Bewegungsphänomenen. *Annalen der Physik und Chemie, 110,* 500–23.

4

The Role of Adaptation
in Color Constancy

QASIM ZAIDI

To function effectively in the world, people need to reliably identify objects and materials across illumination conditions. The subject areas known as lightness and color constancy deal with the identification of the mean and spectral reflectance of materials, respectively. Although, over time, the spectral and mean reflectance of a material can change, in many cases these physical properties are sufficiently stable to aid in identification. Physical properties of stimuli, however, are not available directly to observation, and need to be inferred from light inputs and neural transformations on these inputs. Even in those cases where reflectance is constant, physical inputs to the eye are altered by illumination conditions that include the mean and spectral radiance of the illuminant, and the source-object-sensor geometry. What are the neural transformations of the physical input that enable identification of like reflectances across different illumination conditions? Is adaptation a crucial neural transformation in this process? Is adaptation based on spatially extended scene statistics or on local information collated over time? These are the kinds of questions addressed in this chapter.

4.1 Adaptation and Lightness Identification for Real 3-D Objects under Natural Viewing Conditions

When viewing achromatic surfaces it is possible, in some instances, to separate the *lightness* of a surface from its *brightness*. Lightness is the mean reflectance,

103

where reflectance is the fraction of incident light reflected back by the surface, and is solely a property of the surface (Evans 1974). Brightness refers to apparent luminance, where luminance is the light reflected from the surface, and is thus a function of both the incident illumination and the surface reflectance. Perceived brightness differs from the physical quality of luminance because brightness is affected by adaptation (Craik 1938; Helson 1964) and by lateral interactions (Chevreul 1839; Zaidi 1999). Reflectance is also a physical quality, and the lightness of a surface is inferred either visually or cognitively by separating the information on the scene into environmental and material changes (Helmholtz 1962; Hering 1964).

Consider the demonstration in Fig. 4.1. Look at the four crumpled objects in the two compartments. Three of the objects are made of identical gray paper while one is made of a different shade of gray paper. The compartment on the right is receiving half the illumination of the compartment on the left. Which is the odd object? In order to correctly perform this task, you can first use brightness discrimination to select the compartment that contains the pair of objects with reflectances different from each other. However, once this compartment has been chosen, you have to identify the lightness within that compartment that is different from the two objects in the other compartment.

In Fig. 4.2, the two objects from the right compartment in Fig. 4.1 have been kept in the same place, while the two objects from the left compartment have been placed behind them to facilitate comparison under a single illuminant. It is clear from Fig. 4.2 that object 3 was the odd object, lighter than the other three. If you did not identify the object correctly, your response shows a failure of lightness constancy.

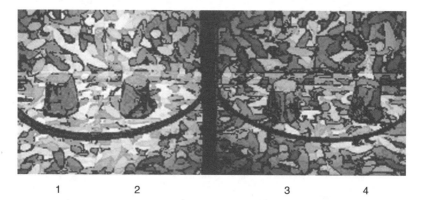

1   2   3   4

FIG. 4.1 Three of the crumbled objects are made of identical grey paper
and make up a *standard* set, while one *test* object is made of a different grey paper.
Backgrounds in the two compartments have the same reflectance distribution.
The compartment on the right is receiving half the illumination of the compartment
on the left. Which is the test object?

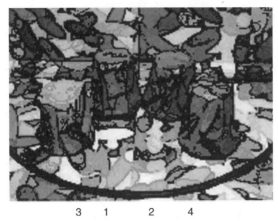

3   1   2   4

FIG. 4.2 For demonstration purposes, objects 1 and 2 from the left compartment
of Fig. 4.1 have been placed behind objects 3 and 4 in the right compartment.
When all four objects are under the same illumination, it becomes obvious that object 3
is the test object with a higher reflectance than the three identical standard objects.

Robilotto & Zaidi (2004) performed the experiment shown in Fig. 4.1 by
using real objects and lights, viewed binocularly with no constraints on eye-
movements. We used a method of constant stimuli and varied the lightness of
the test for each standard lightness. When the proportions of correct responses
are plotted against the reflectance difference between Standard and Test, the
proportions of correct "side" responses gives brightness discrimination psychometric functions, while the proportions of correct "object" responses give lightness identification psychometric functions. In order for the two functions to be
scaled on the same ordinate, detection and identification rates can be normalized
for guessing. Normalized response data for two hypothetical observers are shown
in Figs. 4.3(A) and (B). Dashed curves represent the proportions of side-correct
responses, and solid curves represent proportions of object-correct responses.
The top plot represents conditions where the Test object is under the brighter
illuminant, and the bottom represents conditions where the Test object is under
the darker illuminant.

What information is available in the display, and what is the best identification
performance that any visual system could achieve? Backgrounds in the two boxes
were made from the same materials, so they have similar statistics. The hypothetical observer represented by the curves in Fig. 4.3(A) calculates the mean
luminance of both backgrounds and the mean luminance of each of the four
cups, calculates the ratio of the luminances of the backgrounds, uses this as an
estimate of the ratio of the radiances of the illuminants, and applies the ratio to
the luminances of the objects to equate the reflectances of the three Standard
objects, and thus identifies the odd object. Because there is sufficient information
in the scene for this strategy of lightness identification, this observer's lightness
identification performance is limited only by the ability to discriminate within

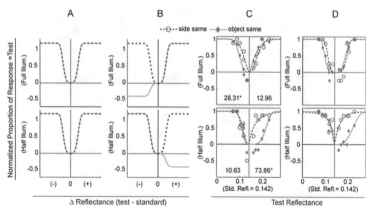

FIG. 4.3 Hypothetical observers and real data. Proportions of correct responses (corrected for guessing) are plotted versus the reflectance of the test. Dashed lines and open circles represent proportion of correct side responses (Brightness discrimination), while solid lines and filled diamonds represent proportion of correct object responses (Lightness identification). The top row represents conditions in which the test object is in the compartment under full illumination, while the bottom row represents conditions in which the test object is in the compartment under half illumination. The vertical line in each plot indicates the reflectance level of the standard set. (A) Responses of a hypothetical observer with perfect lightness identification limited only by discrimination. (B) Responses of a hypothetical observer based on picking the object most dissimilar in luminance. (C) Typical Lightness identification results. Psychometric curves were fit to both sets of data using maximum likelihood ratios. Under the hypothesis that identification responses across illuminants are limited only by the ability to discriminate among objects within the same illuminant, the incorrect object identification responses should be randomly distributed among the three Standard objects. The chi-squared values in each panel test this hypothesis with an asterisk denoting rejection of the hypothesis. (D) Typical normalized proportions of responses where the object chosen as most different in brightness was the object of odd reflectance.

illuminants, and the response functions for brightness discrimination and lightness identification are superimposed. If, however, an observer acted like a photometer, measured just the mean luminances of the four objects, and simply chose the object most different in luminance as the odd object, results would look like in Fig. 4.3(B). When a Test is under full illumination (top plot) and has a lower reflectance than the Standard, its luminance will be lower than the Standard in its compartment and closer to the luminance of the two Standards in the other compartment. When a Test is under half illumination (bottom plot) and has a higher reflectance than the Standard, its luminance will be higher than the Standard in its compartment and closer to the luminance of the two Standards in the other compartment. Under these types of conditions, for some values of Test reflectance at which brightness discrimination reliably identifies the correct side, the Standard on that side will be chosen as the odd object consistently and incorrectly. In Fig. 4.3(B), this is indicated by the curves below chance level, i.e. below zero normalized proportion correct.

Fig. 4.3(C) presents typical data from an observer. There seems to be an asymmetry in the data, as lightness identification seems to be systematically worse than brightness discrimination for lower reflectance Tests under full illumination and higher reflectance Tests under half illumination. Using a chi-squared test, the hypothesis that identification responses across illuminants are limited only by the ability to discriminate among objects within the same illuminant was rejected 10 out of 12 times for conditions where either Tests under full illumination were of lower reflectance than the Standards or where Tests under half illumination were of higher reflectance than the Standards, but only 1 out of 12 times for the other two conditions. The question thus arises whether a single perceptual strategy can account for failures and successes in lightness identification.

In the second experiment, we investigated whether observers were using a lightness-based strategy, or a brightness-based strategy. All stimuli and conditions remained the same, but instead of instructing the observers to choose the object with a different material, observers were asked to choose the object with a different brightness. Figure 4.3(D) shows the proportion of trials on which the Test object was chosen as most dissimilar in brightness. These curves are similar to the lightness identification curves, particularly in their asymmetry. Figure 4.4 plots the odd-brightness thresholds against the odd-lightness thresholds, and shows that reflectance values were similar for both observers. It is likely, therefore, that observers were using brightness dissimilarity to do the lightness identification task.

The lightness identification curves of the photometer-like observer discussed earlier do not resemble the measured curves except for similar directions of asymmetries. It is well-known that light adaptation affects brightness discrimination and appearance (Craik 1938; Helson 1964). Therefore, we tested

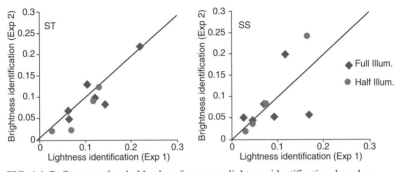

FIG. 4.4 Reflectance threshold values for correct lightness identification, based on lightness versus brightness dissimilarity.

whether a photometer-like observer could give results similar to our observers if we incorporated a mechanism of adaptation which computes the brightness of a stimulus as the product of its mean luminance and a scalar gain, where the gain is a monotonically decreasing function of mean luminance within a compartment (Hayhoe *et al.* 1987). The gain, G, for illumination, I, is governed by the free-parameter, κ, i.e. $G = \kappa/(\kappa + I)$.

Figure 4.5 illustrates hypothetical brightness dissimilarity responses based on this model for three different values of κ. If there were no adaptation ($\kappa = \infty$), judgments would be based solely on luminance values of the objects. As κ decreases, adaptation increases and less reflectance difference is needed for the object most different in reflectance to become the object most different in brightness. The model's brightness dissimilarity responses now start to approximate the reflectance identification responses of the observers, in particular the asymmetry in the curves with respect to the brightness discrimination curves, and the dip of a few points below chance.

Under everyday conditions, observers consistently judge surfaces as having a certain lightness or grayness. This subjective impression points out the tendency to use the physical property of reflectance in mental representations of surfaces. This phenomenological experience however is not sufficient evidence that the visual system has access to the reflectance or lightness of materials. For our 3-D objects, there are some conditions where lightness identification is limited solely by the limen of brightness discrimination, but in other conditions

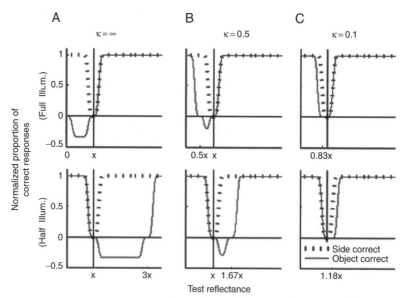

FIG. 4.5 Normalized proportion of correct responses, based on a model of brightness dissimilarity incorporating multiplicative adaptation. (*Left*), (*center*), and (*right*) represent models based on three levels of gain with decreasing *k* values. Standard reflectances are denoted by *x*.

lightness identification is considerably worse. We have shown that the same relative brightness based strategy reproduces both sets of results. This conclusion is based on the fact that the psychometric curves for lightness identification and brightness dissimilarity are systematically asymmetric relative to brightness discrimination curves measured simultaneously for the same objects, and this asymmetry can be predicted quantitatively from observers' choices of most dissimilar brightnesses, and qualitatively from the choices of a photometer-like model observer incorporating brightness adaptation. Note that reflectance dissimilarities are not asymmetric around the standard reflectance, so lightness percepts could not be the basis of the asymmetric brightness dissimilarity judgments in Fig. 4.3(D). The visual system may have evolved to identify object properties, but this identification can only be based on sensory information and transformations, and adaptation is a critical aid in correct identification.

4.2 Differences between Brightness and Color Information for Material Identification

In the generic case, illuminants differ not only in radiance, but also in spectral composition. When the spectrum of the illuminant changes, so do the spectra of lights reflected from surfaces. Just as the brightness of a surface is a function of the luminance of the light reflected from the surface, adaptation and surround effects; the perceived color of a surface is a function of the spectrum of the light reflected from the surface, adaptation and surround effects. The term color constancy describes the extent to which object colors appear unchanging despite changes in the spectral composition of the illumination (Helson *et al.* 1952; Land & McCann 1971; Land 1983; Kraft & Brainard 1999; Foster 2003). There exist good reasons to expect color to be better than brightness as a cue for material identification across illuminants. Zaidi (1998) showed an example where in a grey-level picture, bright leaves appear like they are under a brighter patch of light, whereas, in the color image, the leaves are revealed to have a light-yellow reflectance that is under the same illuminant as the surrounding area. The use of color information can thus supplement other strategies (Sinha & Adelson 1993) for separating reflectance changes from illuminant changes. More formally, Kingdom (2003) has shown that chromatic variations are used by the visual system to differentiate luminance variations that are due to shadows and shading from those that are due to surface reflectance. In addition, Sachtler and Zaidi (1992) showed that memory for chromatic qualities is superior to memory for gray levels: for short time intervals, memory thresholds for hue and saturation are almost as fine as discrimination thresholds, whereas memory for gray levels is considerably worse than discrimination. This raises the possibility that in the functionally important task of identifying similar objects dispersed across space and/or time, the color attributed to the objects may be vital. The appearance of a material can also be altered by color induction from the surround. In the case of brightness, the total induced effect is the weighted sum of surrounding effects, with areas closer to the material having greater weight. On the other hand, the total induced effect on the perceived color of a material is not the weighted sum of surrounding effects, and in fact is reduced drastically if there are high spatial-frequency chromatic variations in the surround (Zaidi *et al.* 1992).

4.3 Material Color Conversions due to Changes in Illuminant Spectra

In a situation where a spatially uniform light falls on flat surfaces of Lambertian reflectance (i.e. reflect light equally in all directions), the spectrum of the light incident on an observer's eye is the wavelength-by-wavelength multiplication of the illuminant spectrum and the surface reflectance spectrum at each point in the scene. In the human retina, the incident spectrum is absorbed by three types of cone photoreceptors, called L, M, and S for cones that are most sensitive to the Long, Middle, and Short wavelengths of the visible spectrum (Baylor *et al.* 1987). The outputs of the cones are combined by post-receptoral neurons into two classes of color signals (L versus M, and S versus $L+M$) and a luminance signal ($L+M$) (Derrington *et al.* 1984). These signals are transmitted to the cortex, where they are combined in a myriad of ways to subserve the many functions of the visual system.

Since the spectrum reflected from each surface is a multiplication of the illuminant and reflectance spectra, the effect of a change in illumination spectrum is different for each surface reflectance. The situation turns out to be simpler if, instead of changes in the spectra of light, one considers changes in the cone-coordinates. For sets of everyday objects, and natural and man-made illuminants, when the L- (or M-, or S-) cone-coordinate (Smith and Pokorny 1975) for each object under one illuminant is plotted against the L- (or M-, or S-) cone coordinate for that object under a different light, the points all fall close to a straight line through the origin (Dannemiller 1993; Foster & Nascimento 1994; Zaidi *et al.* 1997). The top row of Fig. 4.6 shows the L, M, & S cone absorptions calculated from the reflectance spectra of a sample of 280 natural and man-made materials (Chittka *et al.* 1994; Vrhel *et al.* 1994; Hiltunen 1996; Marshall 2000) under Zenith Skylight plotted against the values under Direct Sunlight (Taylor & Kerr 1941). Within each cone class, a change in the spectrum of the illuminant leaves signals from different objects unchanged in their relative positions with just local exceptions, i.e. the effect is to multiply all object cone-coordinates by the same constant. This systematic shift is most likely due to integration within fairly broad cone absorption spectra, because it exists even for spiky illuminant spectra, like fluorescent lights (Zaidi 2001). Nascimento *et al.* (2002) showed that these multiplicative shifts also hold for illuminant changes on natural scenes. The Macleod–Boynton (1979) chromaticity axes ($L/(L+M)$, $S/(L+M)$) provide a good representation of the post-receptoral color signals (L versus M, and S versus $L+M$). Zaidi *et al.* (1997) showed that when the effects of changes in illuminant spectrum are transformed to Macleod–Boynton coordinates, the $L/(L+M)$ chromaticities are shifted by an additive constant, whereas the

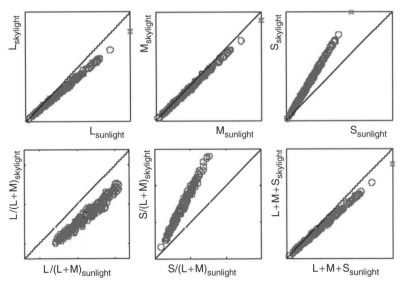

FIG. 4.6 Top row plots show excitations of L-, M-, and S-cones from each of 280 reflectance spectra rendered under two illuminants: zenith skylight on the ordinate and direct sunlight on the abscissa. Bottom row plots show excitations of post-receptoral chromatic and luminance mechanisms ($L/(L+M)$, $S/(L+M)$, and $L+M+S$) from the same stimuli. In each plot, the X represents the illuminant.

$S/(L+M)$ chromaticities are shifted by a multiplicative constant (bottom row of Fig. 4.6). The additive shift in $L/L+M$ is due to the extremely high correlation between L and M cone-coordinates for sets of surfaces under each illuminant (Zaidi 2001).

The situation above assumes that the color of each object is well-represented by a single triple of cone-coordinates. This assumption is valid for flat Lambertian surfaces of unvarying spectral reflectance lit by a uniform illuminant. However, most materials in the world have some surface texture and are not Lambertian, and most objects are not flat. Though good physics-based models for reflections from textured surfaces are extremely complex (Koenderink & van Doorn 1996), a decent approximation can be made by the assumption that for each facet, the total reflection is a weighted sum of the body reflection and the interface reflection (Oren & Nayar 1995), i.e. a weighted sum of the surface and illuminant cone-coordinates. Under this assumption, the affine transforms caused by illuminant changes for Lambertian surfaces also hold for rough surfaces if the source-object-sensor geometry is constant, e.g. if there is a change in the spectrum of the illuminant falling on a stationary scene, and the observer's viewpoint is unchanged (Zaidi 2001).

We will use the term "color conversion" (Helson 1938) to refer to changes in the spectra of the lights reflected from surfaces as the spectrum of the illuminant changes, and to subsequent changes at level of cone-absorptions. The term "neural transformation" refers to the receptoral and post-receptoral neural processes that serve to transform the perceived colors of objects under a test illuminant towards the colors of objects under a reference illuminant. The highly systematic nature of the color conversions described in Fig. 4.6, indicates that simple neural transformations could support color constancy, and the types of neural mechanisms that could, in principle, perform such transformations, range from automatic to volitional, and from peripheral to central.

In 1878, von Kries suggested that the invariance of color metamers to mean light level might be due to multiplicative gain control at the photoreceptor level, when these gains are set independently within each class of photoreceptor in inverse proportion to the local stimulation (von Kries 1878, 1905), i.e. a mechanism incorporating adaptation that computes the output of a cone as the product of its instantaneous input and a scalar gain, where the gain is a monotonically decreasing function of the mean input over time. Ives (1912) may have been the first to suggest an explicit mechanism for constancy under an illuminant change. He showed that the multiplicative factors that transform the *illuminant's* cone-coordinates to those of an equal energy illuminant also transform the cone-coordinates of *surfaces* to approximately their cone-coordinates under the equal-energy illuminant. Figure 4.6 helps to illustrate why this simple transform will work. The illuminants are plotted at the extreme end of the line of reflectances as crosses. Multiplying each cone-coordinate by the ratio of the illuminant cone coordinates will transform most surface cone-coordinates to the unit diagonal, thus equating neural signals under the two illuminants. Mathematically, the Ives transform consists of multiplying all cone-coordinates by the same diagonal matrix and has been widely analyzed in the computer vision literature where it is misnamed the von Kries transform. von Kries' original transform multiplies each local cone-coordinate by a scalar depending only on its *local* magnitude, and thus shifts all colors towards a neutral color (Vimal *et al.* 1987; Webster 1996) rather than achieving the required transformation to an equal energy illuminant.

4.3 Estimation of Illuminant Color

The Ives transformation relies on the visual system's ability to estimate the cone-coordinates of the illuminant. Since the illuminant itself is often not in the field of view, its cone-coordinates have to be estimated from scene statistics. Khang and Zaidi (2004) examined how observers extract the color of spectrally filtered spotlights that are cast on different variegated sets of materials. In an asymmetric spotlight matching technique, observers were asked to adjust the color of a Match spotlight moving over materials with uniform reflectance spectra, to match the color of a Standard spotlight moving on spectrally selective materials (Fig. 4.7, top left). Because the illuminated materials are different under the two spotlights, this match cannot be accomplished by point-by-point color matching, but instead requires matching the extracted colors of the illuminants. The only objects visible were those that fell under the spotlights. The spectra of the seven spotlights were obtained by double-passing equal energy light through

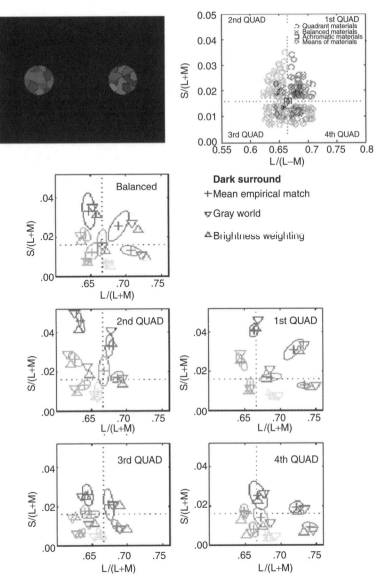

FIG. 4.7 (Top left) Red spotlight cast on green-yellow materials on the left and the same red spotlight on gray materials on the right. Observers were asked to estimate the color of the spotlight moving on chromatic materials and to match it by adjusting the color of the spotlight moving on gray materials. (Top right) MacLeod–Boynton chromaticities (under equal energy light) of the 240 materials used, which consisted of 6 sets of 40 materials, 4 sets of chromatic materials from each quadrant, one set of balanced chromatic materials, one set of achromatic materials. Colored diamonds indicate mean of each quadrant's materials, while the square and the gray diamond at the intersection of the horizontal and vertical dotted lines represent both the achromatic materials and the mean of the balanced chromatic materials. (Bottom) Mean chromaticities of the match spotlights (+), and predictions from a gray-world model (△) and a model that gives greater weight to the brighter materials (▽). The results are color-coded to correspond roughly to the appearance of the spotlight on the achromatic materials. (See also Plate 1 at the centre of this book.)

one of six Kodak CC30 color filters (Red, Green, Blue, Yellow, Magenta, and Cyan) (Kodak CC30, 1962) or through a Neutral Density filter with 70 per cent transmittance. The Standard spotlight moved over one of four sets of 40 materials from single quadrants of MacLeod–Boynton color space, or a fifth set equally balanced across quadrants (Fig. 4.7, top right), chosen from 4824 reflectance functions of flowers, leaves, fruits (Chittka *et al.* 1994), natural and man made objects (Vrhel *et al.* 1994), Munsell color chips (Hiltunen 1996), and animal skins (Marshall 2000). Match spotlights moved over 40 achromatic materials with reflectances equated to the balanced chromatic set. The simulation gave a vivid impression of spotlights moving over matte flat colored and achromatic surfaces in a dark scene. This experiment can reveal estimation strategies for illuminant color when only one illuminant is in the field of view, and there are no clues provided by highlights, shading and shadows. Since the patterns of results were similar for all three observers, we combined the results and calculated means and ±1 SD ellipses over all observers, and these are shown separately for each chromatic set in MacLeod–Boynton diagrams in Fig. 4.7 (bottom). For the chromatically balanced background, the ±1 SD ellipses included the veridical match. For the biased backgrounds, very few of the ellipses for the empirical matches contained the corresponding veridical matches. The mean empirical matches deviated from the veridical systematically in the direction suggesting a biasing effect of background chromaticities on illuminant estimation.

The simplest model for illuminant color estimation is the gray-world model, where estimates of the illuminant cone-coordinates are obtained by taking the means of all the cone-coordinates under the illuminant (Buchsbaum 1980). The veridicality of this estimate relies on the assumption that the mean surface reflectance is likely to be uniform. In Fig. 4.7, the predicted points from the gray-world hypothesis are close to the data points, and this model provides a reasonable, but not perfect, explanation for illuminant color estimation. The gray-world assumption is unlikely to be true for most natural scenes (Brown 1994; Webster & Mollon 1997; Webster 2002), so Golz & MacLeod (2002) have suggested that luminance-chromaticity correlations, e.g. luminance versus redness, may provide estimates that are less influenced by the set of reflectances available. Models for illuminant estimation, however, should incorporate the fact that high-intensity regions of scenes potentially contain more illuminant color information than do low-intensity regions. Tominaga *et al.* (2001) present the following thought experiment: The image of a black surface will have close to zero sensor responses under any illuminant, and its chromaticity will be a function of random noise; whereas a white surface will map reliably to the chromaticity corresponding to the illuminant spectrum. Hence, combining the two measurements will produce a worse estimate than using the bright region alone. In a simulation study of black-body illuminants, Tominaga *et al.* demonstrated that sensor responses from the brightest intensity regions were most diagnostic in classifying illuminants of different color temperature. We implemented these ideas by generalizing the gray-world model to incorporate weighting by the luminance of each material with the luminance raised to a positive power. The brightness-weighted model in Fig. 4.7 fits the data at least as well as the gray-world model. It is possible that the brightness-weighted model would give a better fit for scenes that contain specular highlights (Lee 1986; Lehman & Palm 2001).

A neural mechanism that integrated over a large spatial area could in principle extract the mean chromaticity. If the outputs of local subunits of such a mechanism were subjected to accelerating nonlinearities before integration, then this mechanism would estimate the illuminant by weighting scene chromaticities as an increasing function of their brightness. The question remains whether such estimates are incorporated by adaptation mechanisms to discount the effect of illuminant changes, since psychophysical measurements indicate that early adaptation mechanisms are extremely local in their spatial properties (MacLeod *et al.* 1992; MacLeod & He 1993; He & MacLeod 1998).

4.4 Role of Global Adaptation to Scene Statistics

Adaptation can account for color constancy if chromatic signals from objects vary by less than a discriminable difference across two illuminants. For the case of a fixed scene and a slowly varying illuminant, Zaidi *et al.* (1997) tested whether adaptation to a variegated scene was sufficient to counter the effect of changes in illuminant spectra. We asked our observers to view a simulated scene, and report if the colors in the scene appeared to change when the effect of an illuminant change was simulated. As shown in Fig. 4.6, the effect of a change in the phase of natural daylight on post-receptoral mechanisms can be simulated by adding a constant to all $L/(L + M)$ chromaticities, and by multiplying all $S/(L + M)$ and $L + M + S$ chromaticities by constants. This enabled us to quantify the tolerance within each post-receptoral mechanism for changes in illumination. Nascimento and Foster (1997) have shown that large-field color changes that keep spatial ratios of cone excitations perfectly constant are perceived as illuminant changes, and are in fact chosen as illuminant changes even over real illuminant changes. Since we were interested in the effect of spatially complex scenes on color constancy, we used random binary and quaternary distributions of squares of uniform size. The binary textures were colored by extremes of each of the $L/(L + M)$, $S/(L + M)$, and $L + M + S$ axes (termed *RG*, *YV*, and *LD* for mnemonic purposes) and the quaternary textures by sums of pairs of binary texture colors (*LDRG*, *RGYV*, and *YVLD*). The space-averaged chromaticity and luminance of all textures was equal to equal-energy white, *W*. The observer adapted to the background for 2 minutes at the initiation of each session and readapted for 2 seconds after each trial (Fig. 4.8). The illuminant on a scene was changed gradually toward and back from a different illuminant as a half-cycle of a sinusoid over a 3 seconds interval. To control for criterion effects, each trial also included another interval in which the illuminant was not altered. The observers indicated the interval in which they perceived a change in the colors of the scene. Thresholds measured for illumination changes in the *R*, *G*, *Y*, *V*, *L*, and *D* color directions on each textured field were compared with thresholds on a uniform achromatic field at *W*.

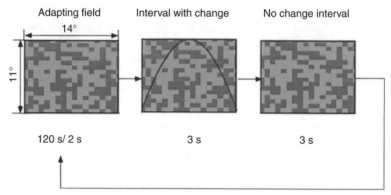

FIG. 4.8 Spatial configuration and temporal sequence of stimuli for global adaptation experiments. The initial adaptation period was 120 s. Each trial consisted of a 2-s period of readaptation, followed by two 3-s intervals, of which one contained a simulated illumination change with a time-course of a half-sinusoid.

Results for two observers are shown in Fig. 4.9. The colors of the background textures are indicated on the abscissa. For each texture class, the threshold for detecting a change in colors as compared with the threshold for detecting a change on the achromatic field is plotted on the ordinate. Separate panels show data for the L, D; R, G; and Y, V directions of simulated illuminant changes. We are interested not in whether there is a small but statistically significant increase in thresholds on the background but whether certain backgrounds functionally mask the effect of illumination changes: the dashed horizontal line at 0.3 identifies the textures that increased the tolerance for an illumination change by at least a factor of 2. The results are systematic and similar for the two observers. Full-field color changes (R, G, Y, V) are less likely to be perceived in the presence of chromatic spatial variations, but thresholds for detection of full-field luminance changes (L, D) are not affected by the presence of spatial variations. Except for one case out of 36, changes toward a chromatic direction are affected only when there is spatial contrast along the same axis. There was no systematic effect of superimposing spatial contrast along a color axis orthogonal to the color direction of the simulated illumination change. The results indicate that the masking effect of spatial contrast is relatively independent within each of the opponent-color mechanisms.

The results show that if the scene contains spatial variations, an observer is less likely to perceive changes in the colors of the scene when the illumination changes than if the scene was spatially uniform at the space-averaged color. The effects of a shift from Sunlight to Skylight on natural scenes can be compared with the experimentally measured thresholds, and shown to be extremely salient. The average shift of signals along the $L/(L + M)$ axis in Fig. 4.6 is 21.3 times the threshold for a similar shift on the W background for observer BS, and 6.4 times for observer KW. Even for the most desensitizing textured background, only 15 per cent of this shift could be tolerated by observer BS, and

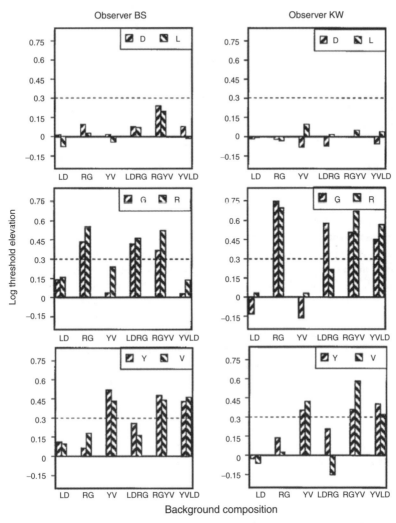

FIG. 4.9 Results for observers BS (left-hand plots) and KW (right-hand plots). The log of the threshold for detecting a change in each color direction minus the log of the baseline threshold for that color direction is plotted against the chromatic content of the background texture (see text). Symbols representing the color direction of the simulated illuminant change are shown in the insets. Dashed horizontal lines are drawn at 0.3 to indicate a doubling of threshold magnitude.

97 per cent by observer KW. The average multiplicative shift along the $S/(L + M)$ axis is 18 times the threshold for a similar shift on the W background for observer BS and nine times for observer KW. On the most desensitizing textured background, BS could tolerate only 19 per cent of the shift, and KW 36 per cent. In general, then, an acute human observer will perceive changes in colors of objects when the illumination shifts over a few seconds between

different phases of natural daylight, despite the fact that the presence of spatial variation will attenuate the perceived magnitudes of the changes.

Objects in the world are almost always seen against variegated backgrounds, but almost all studies of color adaptation have used uniform backgrounds. Using stimuli similar to Fig. 4.8, Zaidi *et al.* (1998) showed that adaptation to a variegated field consists of more than adaptation to the space average, or independently to the constituents, or to any combination thereof. We found that a model for the effects of adapting to variegated fields not only has to take into account different sorts of adaptation at different stages of the visual system, but must also incorporate spatial inhomogeneities in adaptation state across the field and a decision process that involves pooling spatially distributed responses. The model included two classes of spatial locations of neurons. Neurons of one class were constantly exposed to uniformly colored patches in the field, and neurons of the second class were near the edges of color patches. Of those exposed to one color, S versus $L+M$ neurons adapted by multiplicative gain controls determined by the time-integrated level of stimulation, whereas L versus M neurons adapted by a subtraction of a portion of the time-integrated signal (Zaidi *et al.* 1992; Shapiro *et al.* 2001, 2003). On the other hand, neurons that were located near the edges of color patches adapted to temporal modulation of their inputs as a result of eye movements, and this resulted in changes in the shapes of their response functions rather than adaptation to the average stimulation (Zaidi & Shapiro 1993). Global adaptation to a variegated field thus is not determined by the spatial averages that observers use for estimating illuminant color, and has quite different functional benefits as described below.

Adaptation at early stages of the visual system serves to enable good discrimination across a very large domain of lights despite the limited response range of individual neurons. Craik (1938) introduced notions of efficiency into range-resetting, and since then it has been thought to be optimal that when adapted to a certain level, an observer's discrimination should be best at that level. However, this property would be functionally optimal only if it could be assumed that the frequency distribution of stimulation in the near future would have a maximum at or near the adapting level. The situation is quite different when an observer is viewing a spatially variegated field. It has been proposed that, as a result of eye movements, the observer should adapt to the space average (D'Zmura & Lennie 1986; Fairchild & Lennie 1992). However, adapting to the average stimulation alone would not be optimal, because it is unlikely that the highest frequency of future stimuli will occur near the average level. In fact, adaptation to any single level is likely to be grossly suboptimal, and it would be more efficient to adapt the range of sensitivity to the domain of expected stimulation. Zaidi and Shapiro (1993) proposed a model of "response equalization" to account for changes in the response function. This model postulates that the most efficient use of a limited response range is to match the shape of the response function to the expected distribution of inputs, so that on an average, each level of response occurs with equal frequency. If it is assumed that expectations for inputs are set by the recent adaptation history, then the response function should be equated to some function of the cumulative probability distribution of levels in the adapting stimulus. Adaptation to a variegated scene thus is more complex than being a function of the mean level or any other estimate of the illuminant. It is thus not a mechanism that can serve to correct for changes in the illuminant spectrum. On the other hand as the next section shows, range-resetting as a function of the time-integrated signal has specific effects on perceived colors.

4.5 Roles of Local Adaptation and Levels of Reference

The results above show that adaptation to global scene statistics is limited in its effectiveness as a color constancy mechanism. A very large number of studies have shown fairly decent color constancy for single patches of constant reflectance. In a series of experiments Smithson and Zaidi (2004) performed critical tests of whether neural transformations for color constancy of such patches depend on information that is distributed over space, or on information that is spatially localized but distributed over time. In addition, we investigated whether judgments of color appearance under different conditions are well predicted by early adaptation, or whether they reflect higher-level perceptual mechanisms?

In this study we assessed changes in color *appearance* under different illuminants. Our stimulus displays consisted of a square test patch presented on a variegated background of randomly oriented elliptical patches. Examples of these displays are given in Fig. 4.10 (left). Each patch was assigned a reflectance spectrum and rendered under a particular illuminant. We tested a total of 280 simulated materials (Fig. 4.6). Reflectance spectra were chosen from measurements of natural and man-made objects so as to obtain an even coverage of color space. Our background patterns were colored with subsets of 40 reflectance spectra, chosen as described below. Test materials and backgrounds were rendered under either the spectrum of direct sunlight or of zenith skylight. The observer's task was to classify the appearance of sequentially presented test-patches as either red or green in one set of trials, and as either yellow or blue in a second set (Chichilnisky & Wandell 1999). We thus obtained a chromatic locus of test-patches that appeared neither red nor green, and a second locus that appeared neither yellow nor blue. We assume that color boundaries measured under different conditions describe a set of stimuli that generate equivalent signals at the decision stage, hence shifts in the locations of color boundaries provide a measure of the neural transformations performed under different conditions of observing.

In the first experiment, we obtained classification boundaries for conditions in which scenes were rendered under either direct sunlight or zenith skylight. Repeated classifications for each material provided psychometric functions relating stimulus chromaticity to classification-probability i.e. the percentage of times the stimulus is classified as red (versus green), or yellow (versus blue).

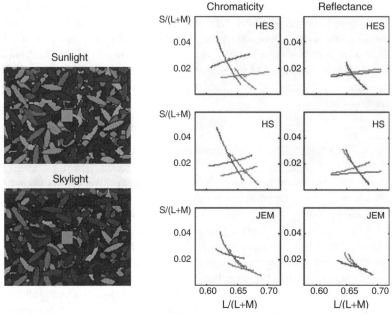

FIG. 4.10 (Left) Examples of stimuli used in color appearance measurements with a global illuminant change on chromatically balanced backgrounds. On each trial, a square test patch was presented on a variegated background of randomly oriented elliptical patches, under skylight or sunlight. (Center) Data for three observers. Panels show traces of classification boundaries in chromaticity space. Red lines show boundaries obtained under sunlight; blue lines show boundaries obtained under skylight. Red and blue open-circles show the corresponding illuminant chromaticities. (Right) Panels show the same boundaries represented in reflectance space (i.e. as if materials were rendered under an equal energy illuminant). (See also Plate 2 at the centre of this book.)

Multiple linear least squares regression was then used to determine the best fitting 3-dimensional polynomial (second- or third-order) relating chromaticity and classification-probability. We assume that the surface in 3-D color space defined by a classification-probability of 0.5 best divides color space into red versus green (or yellow versus blue) and thus represents the classification boundary. The panels of Fig. 4.10 (center) show the lines of intersection of these surfaces with the mean equiluminant plane of the MacLeod–Boynton chromaticity diagram. Traces of classification boundaries are plotted for three observers. Red lines represent boundaries obtained under sunlight illumination; blue lines represent boundaries obtained under skylight illumination. The locations of red/green and yellow/blue boundaries in chromaticity space shift appreciably across illuminants. Panels of Fig. 4.10 (right) show classification boundaries evaluated in reflectance space (i.e. material chromaticities plotted as if rendered under a spectrally uniform illuminant). Classification boundaries obtained under the two illuminant conditions make similar divisions of reflectance space i.e. the grouping of test-materials into color categories is largely unaffected by the illuminant under which they are rendered. This method of demonstrating appearance-based color constancy overcomes many of the shortcomings of conventional methods described by Foster (2003).

A quantitative method to assess the extent of color constancy across an illuminant change is to calculate a color constancy index. These indices typically relate the measured shift in the location of the achromatic point to the shift in the chromaticity of a material of uniform spectral reflectance (Brainard 1998). As illustrated in Fig. 4.6, the effect of an illuminant change on cone-coordinates can be well-summarized by multiplicative scaling, and on opponent signals by multiplicative scaling of the $S/L+M$ opponent signal and translational (additive) scaling of the $L/L+M$ opponent signal. We have defined two color constancy indices, one appropriate for dimensions undergoing multiplicative change (Yang & Shevell 2002), and the other for dimensions undergoing additive change. If b_1 is the coordinate of Illuminant 1, b_2 is the coordinate of Illuminant 2, and a_1 and a_2 are the respective coordinates of the achromatic settings, then the multiplicative constancy index is defined as $C = (\log(a_1/a_2))/(\log(b_1/b_2))$. The value of (a_1/a_2) reveals the scaling factor used by the multiplicative neural transformation; b_1/b_2 quantifies the color conversion imposed by the illuminant change. For perfect constancy $(a_1/a_2) = (b_1/b_2)$ and the index is equal to one. If the co-ordinates of the achromatic settings are not affected by the illuminant, $a_1 = a_2$, and the index is zero. For dimensions undergoing translational scaling, the index is defined as $C = |a_1-a_2|/|b_1-b_2|$. Again, $C = 0$ indicates no constancy, and $C = 1$ indicates perfect constancy. However, since the mapping between chromaticity space and perceptual color space is not known, and is likely to be nonlinear and depend on adaptation state, no constancy index can provide a perceptually accurate measure of how steady a material will appear under an illuminant change.

We derived achromatic points from our data by calculating the point of intersection of the red/green and the blue/yellow classification boundaries. The data showed high levels of constancy, with the averages of the L-, M-, and S-cone constancy indices equal to 0. 87, 0.72, and 0.94, and averages of the $L/(L+M)$ and $S/(L+M)$ constancy indices, equal to 0.87, 0.68, and 0.93 for the three observers.

In the first experiment, the mean chromaticity of the scene could provide a reliable estimate of the cone-coordinates of the illuminant, so good color constancy would be predicted by spatially extended adaptation or alternatively by a high-level mechanism that used the mean to derive an illuminant estimate. In the second experiment, we simulated conditions where the mean chromaticity of the scene does not provide a good estimate of the cone-coordinates of the illuminant. We obtained classification boundaries under four additional conditions. We used sunlight and skylight and red-blue biased, and green-yellow biased sets of reflectances for the background (Fig. 4.11).

Figures 4.12 (left) and (right) show classification boundaries for red-blue and green-yellow biased backgrounds respectively. The red lines represent color boundaries under sunlight and the blue lines represent boundaries under skylight.

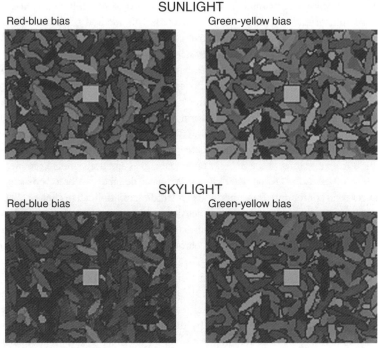

FIG. 4.11 Examples of stimuli used in color appearance measurements with a global illuminant change on chromatically biased backgrounds. The top row shows stimuli rendered under sunlight; the bottom row shows stimuli rendered under skylight. (See also Plate 3 at the centre of this book.)

Again the illuminant has a large effect on the locations of red/green and yellow/blue boundaries in chromaticity space, but the locations of the boundaries in reflectance space are largely unaltered by the illuminant condition. Observers demonstrated high levels of constancy in all conditions. The averages of the $L/(L+M)$ and $S/(L+M)$ constancy indices were 0.87, 0.81, and 0.95 for the three observers.

The results confirm that the color appearance of the test-materials is not set by the mean chromaticity of the global scene. To assess whether performance could be explained by any spatially extended illuminant estimate we performed a critical manipulation. Unknown to the observer, we simulated one illuminant for the test and a different illuminant for the background. Under these conditions, the spatial context provides information only about the background illuminant, so any *global* mechanism would estimate the wrong illuminant for the test, and constancy would be low. In a single trial, the observer has no information about the test-illuminant, since it falls only on a single material and there are no statistical cues to disentangle the material reflectance and the illuminant spectrum. Hence information about the test illuminant is available only by collating information

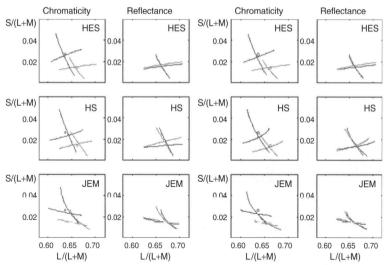

FIG. 4.12 Data for the three observers, with a global illuminant change on
(Left) red-blue biased backgrounds, (Right) green-yellow biased backgrounds.
Panels on the left show traces of classification boundaries in chromaticity space,
obtained under sunlight (red lines) or skylight (blue lines). Open-circles show the
corresponding illuminant chromaticities. Panels on the right show the same boundaries
represented in reflectance space (i.e. as if materials were rendered under an equal
energy illuminant). (See also Plate 4 at the centre of this book.)

over successive trials. We asked whether the classification of test-materials in
the inconsistent illuminant conditions follows that predicted by the background
illuminant, or that predicted by the test illuminant. Again, stimulus displays
comprised a central square test-patch within a variegated background of elliptical
patches. We used the balanced set of background materials, but rather than using
a global illuminant for the whole scene, we either rendered the test-material
under sunlight and the background materials under skylight, or the test-material
under skylight and the background materials under sunlight (Fig. 4.13 (left)).

The dotted lines in Fig. 4.13 (right) show classification boundaries re-plotted
from the first experiment. They are color-coded according to the global illumination used: red for sunlight and blue for skylight. The solid lines show classification
boundaries for the inconsistent illumination conditions, and are color-coded
according to the illuminant falling on the test-patch. So, red lines show performance with sunlight on the test and skylight on the background, and blue lines show
performance with skylight on the test and sunlight on the background. Performance
in the inconsistent illumination conditions is more closely predicted by the illuminant falling on the test-patch than by the illuminant falling on the background. For
observer HS, the blue-yellow boundary was not well-constrained by our data for
the condition with sunlight on the test and skylight on the background.

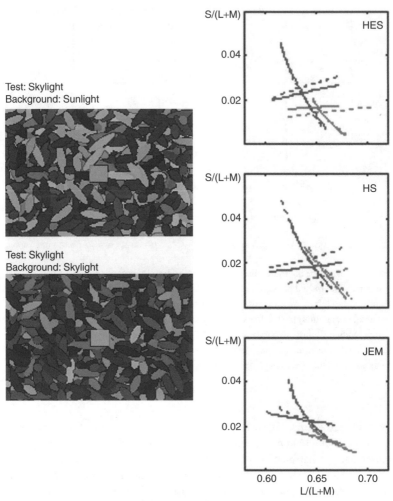

FIG. 4.13 (Left) Examples of stimuli used in color appearance measurements with conflicting illuminants on test and background reflectances. (Right) Data for the three observers. Solid red lines indicate classification boundaries obtained with sunlight illumination on the test, and skylight on the background. Solid blue lines indicate classification boundaries obtained with skylight on the test, and sunlight on the background. Dotted red and blue lines show boundaries obtained with a global illuminant of sunlight or skylight respectively, and are thus color-coded to predict boundary locations based on the test illuminant. Discriminant functions for Observer HS, with sunlight on the test and skylight on the background, were not well-constrained. (See also Plate 5 at the centre of this book.)

We calculated constancy indices for an illuminant change on the test-material only, i.e. a change in the test-illuminant coordinates from b_1 to b_2. In this analysis, a change in the illuminant on the test is not accompanied by a corresponding change in the illuminant on the background, so the spatial context provides no cues to the illuminant change, signalling instead either steady sunlight or skylight. So, if performance were determined by the spatial context, the achromatic coordinates (a_1 and a_2) should be identical, and we should measure constancy indices equal to zero. If however performance were determined by the test illuminant, constancy indices should approach one (or rather the value obtained in the first experiment for a global illuminant change). The averages of the $L/(L+M)$ and $S/(L+M)$ constancy indices were 0.70, 0.45, and 0.82 for the three observers. Constancy indices are in all cases slightly lower than those obtained in the first experiment, but constancy is far from abolished. Observers' performances cannot be explained by any spatially extended process, since the spatial context provided cues to the wrong illuminant. The type of neural mechanism that could perform this temporal collation process could be peripheral or central. A process of spatially localized adaptation, with long time-constants of the order of a few seconds, would converge on the mean chromaticity of the test-materials. Since the mean chromaticity of the test materials was balanced, this would be sufficient to support reasonable constancy.

Early adaptation is not the only neural transformation that could use estimated illuminant cone-coordinates. Later perceptual mechanisms could use these estimates to adjust for color conversions (Adelson & Pentland 1996), without losing information about the illuminant color (Zaidi 1998). For example, Khang & Zaidi (2002) showed that observers were able to identify like versus unlike objects across illuminants, based on perceived similarities between color-shifts of backgrounds and color-shifts of tests. Such non-adaptation mechanisms are particularly salient when the geometrical properties of the scene promote color scission, i.e. separation of the colors of the scene into material colors and the colors of illuminants or transparencies (Hagedorn & D'Zmura 2000).

A different class of transformation mechanism involves the concept of "level of reference" or "anchoring" (Rogers 1941; Helson 1947). Thomas & Jones (1962) showed that matches to a reference color were biased by the distribution of possible matching colors. In its extreme form, if perceived colors in a scene were determined entirely by rank-orders of cone-coordinates, good color constancy would be the result because, as shown in Fig. 4.6, color conversions do not disturb rank-orders of cone-coordinates. This mechanism would not need an estimate for the illuminant but would, like adaptation to the mean, lead to inconstancy if the set of available materials changed.

Our final experiment was designed to determine whether the neural processes that collate information about a temporally extended sample of illuminated spectral reflectances are automatic, or whether they are based on perceptual processes that are selective for information about the test stimuli. We used conflicting illuminants for test and background but now reduced the amount of time observers were exposed to the test-patches to a fraction of the duration of exposure to materials illuminated by the background illuminant. As for all experiments reported here, trial duration was fixed at 1500 ms. But now the test-materials were presented only for 200 ms, after which the display reverted to the background pattern. An automatic adaptation process collates information indiscriminately from test and background. If color constancy is achieved under the test illuminant it must be based on a selective mechanism that collates only the test samples.

The three observers were differently influenced by the reduction in exposure to the test illuminant. For HES, the boundaries obtained with skylight on the test and sunlight on the background were now well-predicted by performance with global sunlight illumination. The red-green boundary obtained with sunlight on the test and skylight on the background was also clearly consistent with the background illuminant, likewise for HS. However, for HS and JEM, the boundaries obtained with skylight on the test and sunlight on the background were well-predicted by the test illuminant. Similarly, the constancy indices indicated that constancy was practically abolished for HES, but remained reasonably high in at least one condition for HS and JEM.

The mixed performance in the final experiment cannot be completely explained by an automatic neural process that acts upon incoming chromatic signals to discount the illuminant. However, in some conditions, observers' judgments were consistent with the hypothesis that the test-materials are illuminated by a different illuminant from the background. In a single trial there is no information about the test illuminant (since this falls only on a single material) so information about the test illuminant can only be obtained by collating information from successive trials. To collate the properties of the test illuminant separately from the properties of the background illuminant requires a process that tracks the chromatic statistics of the task-relevant test-squares. Such a process could be a mechanism of adaptation gated by attention, or it may be a perceptual "level of reference" or "anchoring" (Rogers 1941; Helson 1947) mechanism that segregates test and background presentations. Several cues distinguish test from background. The most obvious is that the test-squares require a judgment while the background ellipses do not. A more subtle cue is highlighted in Forsyth's constancy algorithm (Forsyth 1990). Since the illuminant limits the gamut of spectra reaching the eye, it is possible that (due to the conflicting illuminant) the colors of the test were very unlikely under the background illuminant, and this might provide a cue for the visual system to estimate the illuminant separately for the test-patches.

The majority of experiments on color constancy have focused on the spatial information available in a scene. The primary message from the Smithson and Zaidi (2004) study is that the stability of color appearance is determined mainly by local mechanisms that collate information over time. The color-appearance judgments obtained with conflicting illuminants could be predicted by mechanisms that are either spatially local in extent or that segregate the test from the background. Therefore it is uncertain whether temporal context acts centrally to modify the observer's "adaptation-level" (Helson 1947, 1964), or whether the information reaching the decision-stage is modified automatically by peripheral mechanisms. In certain conditions and for certain observers, the drastic decrease in constancy as a result of reducing exposure to the test is consistent with an adaptation mechanism with a long time constant. However, in other conditions there is little decrease in constancy, indicating the use of a central value that stores contextual information about the stimuli requiring judgment.

4.7 Summary

This paper starts with an example involving lightness identification of 3 D objects across illuminants differing in mean radiance. We show that observers use brightness similarity between materials to perform the lightness identification task, and adaptation serves to make like materials more similar in brightness across illuminants than if luminance is used to judge similarity. The effect of a change in illuminant radiance is to multiply the luminance of all objects in a scene with the same constant, since the luminance of each object is the product of its reflectance and the illuminant radiance. On the other hand, the effect of a change in the spectrum of the illuminant is different for different materials in the field of view since it depends on the spectral reflectance of each material. However, if the effect is calculated in terms of cone-coordinates, then the situation is considerably simplified. Within each cone class, the effect is decently approximated by multiplication by the same constant for all materials. This suggests that if the cone-coordinates of the illuminant can be estimated, then a neural process could invert the effect. We show that when observers are asked to estimate the color of a spotlight, they use a scene statistic that is approximately equal to the mean cone-coordinates of the brightest objects in the scene. Global adaptation to the scene, however, does not use similar statistics, and has limited effectiveness as a color constancy mechanism. On the other hand, spatially local adaptation does play a large role in color constancy. We show that observers can invert the effect of illuminant spectrum changes by collating local information over time. This information seems to be used both in adaptation processes, and in setting levels of reference.

Acknowledgments

The research described in this paper was done in collaboration with Arthur Shapiro, Ben Sachtler, Bill Yoshimi, Branka Spehar, Jeremy DeBonet, Byung-Geun Khang, Hannah Smithson, and Rocco Robillotto. This work was supported by NEI grant EY07556.

References

Adelson, E.H., & Pentland, A.P. (1996). The perception of shading and reflectance. In D. C. Knill, & W. Richards (Eds.), *Perception as Bayesian Inference* (pp. 409–23). Cambridge: Cambridge University Press.

Baylor, D.A., Nunn, B.J., & Schnapf, J.L. (1987). Spectral sensitivity of cones of the monkey Macaca fascicularis. *Journal of Physiology, 390*, 145–60.

Brainard, D.H. (1998). Color constancy in the nearly natural image. 2. Achromatic loci. *Journal of the Optical Society of America A, 15*(2), 307–25.

Brainard, D.H., & Wandell, B.A. (1992). Asymmetric color matching: how color appearance depends on the illuminant. *Journal of the Optical Society of America A, 9*(9), 1433–8.

Brown, R.O. (1994). The world is not gray. *Investigative Ophthalmology & Visual Science, 35*(4), 2165.

Buchsbaum, G. (1980). A spatial processor model for object color perception. *Journal of the Franklin Institute, 310*, 1–26.

Chevreul, M.E. (1839). *De la loi du contraste simultane des couleurs*. Paris: Pitois-Levreault.

Chichilnisky, E.J., & Wandell, B.A. (1999). Trichromatic opponent color classification. *Vision Research, 39*(20), 3444–58.

Chittka, L., Shmida, A., Troje, N., & Menzel, R. (1994). Ultraviolet as a component of flower reflections, and the color perception of Hymenoptera. *Vision Research, 34*(11), 1489–1508.

Craik, K.J.W. (1938). The effect of adaptation on differential brightness discrimination. *Journal of Physiology, 92*, 406–21.

Dannemiller, J.L. (1993). Rank orderings of photoreceptor photon catches from natural objects are nearly illuminant-invariant. *Vision Research, 33*, 131–40.

Derrington, A.M., Krauskopf, J., & Lennie, P. (1984). Chromatic mechanisms in lateral geniculate nucleus of macaque. *Journal of Physiology, 357*, 241–65.

D'Zmura, M., & Lennie, P. (1986). Mechanisms of color constancy. *Journal of the Optical Society of America A, 3*(10), 1662–72.

Evans, R.M. (1974). *The Perception of Color*. New York: Wiley & Sons.

Fairchild, M.D., & Lennie, P. (1992). Chromatic adaptation to natural and incandescent illuminants. *Vision Research, 32*(11), 2077–85.

Forsyth, D. (1990). A novel algorithm for color constancy. *International Journal of Computer Vision, 30*, 5–36.

Foster, D.H. (2003). Does color constancy exist? *Trends in Cognitive Sciences, 7*(10), 439–43.

Foster, D.H., & Nascimento, S.M. (1994). Relational color constancy from invariant cone-excitation ratios. *Proceedings of the Royal Society of London B Biological Sciences, 257*(1349), 115–21.

Golz, J., & MacLeod, D.I. (2002). Influence of scene statistics on color constancy. *Nature, 415*(6872), 637–40.

Hagedorn, J., & D'Zmura, M. (2000). Color appearance of surfaces viewed through fog. *Perception, 29*(10), 1169–84.

Hayhoe, M.M., Benimoff, N.I., & Hood, D.C. (1987). The time-course of multiplicative and subtractive adaptation process. *Vision Research, 27*(11), 1981–96.

He, S., & MacLeod, D.I. (1998). Local nonlinearity in S-cones and their estimated light-collecting apertures. *Vision Research, 38*(7), 1001–6.

Helmholtz, H.v. (1962). *Physiological Optics.* Trans. Vol. 3, J.P.C. Southhall. New York: Dover.

Helson, H. (1938). Fundamental problems in color vision. I. The principle governing changes in hue, saturation, and lightness of non-selective samples in chromatic illumination. *Journal of Experimental Psychology, 23,* 439–76.

Helson, H. (1947). Adaptation-level as frame of reference for prediction of psychophysical data. *Journal of the Optical Society of America, 60,* 1–29.

Helson, H. (1964). *Adaptation-level Theory; An Experimental and Systematic Approach to Behavior.* New York: Harper & Row.

Helson, H., Judd, D.B., & Warren, M.H. (1952). Object-color changes from daylight to incandescent filament illumination. *Illuminating Engineering, 47,* 221–3.

Hering, E. (1964). *Outlines of a Theory of the Light Sense.* Trans. L.M. Hurvich, & D. Jameson. Cambridge, MA: Harvard University Press.

Hiltunen, J. (1996). *Munsell Color Matts (Spectrophotometer Measurements by Hiltunen).* Retrieved September 10, 1999, from http://www.it.lut.fi/ip/research/color/database/ download.html#munsell_spec_matt

Ives, H.E. (1912). The relation between the color of the illuminant and the color of the illuminated object. *Transactions of the Illuminating Engineering Society, 7,* 62–72.

Khang, B.G., & Zaidi, Q. (2002). Cues and strategies for color constancy: perceptual scission, image junctions and transformational color matching. *Vision Research, 42*(2), 211–26.

Khang, B.G., & Zaidi, Q. (2004). Illuminant color perception of spectrally filtered spotlights. *Journal of Vision, 4,* 680–92.

Kingdom, F. (2003). Color brings relief to human vision. *Nature Neuroscience, 6*(6), 641–4.

Koenderink, J.J., & van Doorn, A.J. (1996). Illuminance texture due to surface mesostructure. *Journal of the Optical Society of America A, 13,* 452–63.

Kraft, J.M., & Brainard, D.H. (1999). Mechanisms of color constancy under nearly natural viewing. *Proceedings of the National Academy of Sciences USA, 96*(1), 307–12.

Land, E.H. (1983). Recent advances in retinex theory and some implications for cortical computations: color vision and the natural image. *Proceedings of the National Academy of Sciences USA, 80*(16), 5163–69.

Land, E.H., & McCann, J.J. (1971). Lightness and retinex theory. *Journal of the Optical Society of America, 61,* 1–11.

Lee, H.C. (1986). Method for computing the scene-illuminant chromaticity from specular highlights. *Journal of the Optical Society of America A, 3*(10), 1694–9.

Lehmann, T.M., & Palm, C. (2001). Color line search for illuminant estimation in real-world scenes. *Journal of the Optical Society of America A, 18*(11), 2679–91.

MacLeod, D.I., & Boynton, R.M. (1979). Chromaticity diagram showing cone excitation by stimuli of equal luminance. *Journal of the Optical Society of America, 69*(8), 1183–6.

MacLeod, D.I., & He, S. (1993). Visible flicker from invisible patterns. *Nature, 361*(6409), 256–8.

MacLeod, D.I., Williams, D.R., & Makous, W. (1992). A visual nonlinearity fed by single cones. *Vision Research, 32*(2), 347–63.

Marshall, N.J. (2000). Communication and camouflage with the same 'bright' colors in reef fishes. *Philosophical Transactions of the Royal Society of London B Biological Sciences, 355*(1401), 1243–8.

Nascimento, S.M., Ferreira, F.P., & Foster, D.H. (2002). Statistics of spatial cone-excitation ratios in natural scenes. *Journal of the Optical Society of America A, 19*(8), 1484–90.

Nascimento, S.M., & Foster, D.H. (1997). Detecting natural changes of cone-excitation ratios in simple and complex colored images. *Proceedings of the Royal Society of London B Biological Sciences, 264*(1386), 1395–1402.

Oren, M., & Nayar, S.K. (1995). Generalizations of the Lambertian model and implications for machine vision. *International Journal of Computer Vision, 14*, 227–51.

Robilotto, R., and Zaidi, Q. (2004). Limits of lightness identification for real objects under natural viewing conditions. *Journal of Vision, 4*, 779–97.

Rogers, S. (1941). The anchoring of absolute judgments. *Archives of Psychology Columbia University, 261*, 42.

Sachtler, W.L., & Zaidi, Q. (1992). Chromatic and luminance signals in visual memory. *Journal of the Optical Society of America A, 9*, 877–94.

Shapiro, A., Beere, J., & Zaidi, Q. (2001). Stages of temporal adaptation in the RG color system. *Color Research and Application, 26*, S43–S47.

Shapiro, A., Beere, J., & Zaidi, Q. (2003). Time course of adaptation stages in the S cone color system. *Vision Research, 43*, 1135–47.

Sinha, P., & Adelson, E.H. (1993). Recovering reflectance and illumination in a world of painted polyhedra. *Proceedings of the Fourth International Conference on Computer Vision* (pp. 156–63). Los Alamitos, CA: IEEE Computer Society Press.

Smith, V.C., & Pokorny, J. (1975). Spectral sensitivity of the foveal cone photopigments between 400 and 500 nm. *Vision Research, 15*(2), 161–71.

Smithson, H., & Zaidi, Q. (2004). Color constancy in context: roles of local adaptation and reference levels. *Journal of Vision, 4*, 693–710.

Taylor, A.H., & Kerr, G.P. (1941). The distribution of energy in the visible spectrum of daylight. *Journal of the Optical Society of America, 31*(1), 3–8.

Thomas, D.R., & Jones, C.G. (1962). Stimulus generalization as a function of the frame of reference. *Journal of Experimental Psychology, 64*(1), 77–80.

Tominaga, S., Ebisui, S., & Wandell, B.A. (2001). Scene illuminant classification: brighter is better. *Journal of the Optical Society of America A, 18*(1), 55–64.

Vimal, R.L., Pokorny, J., & Smith, V.C. (1987). Appearance of steadily viewed lights. *Vision Research, 27*(8), 1309–18.

von Kries, J. (1878). Physiology of visual sensations. In D.L. MacAdam (ed.), *Sources of Color Science* (pp. 101–8). Cambridge, MA: MIT Press.

von Kries, J. (1905). Die Gesichtsempfindungen. In W. Nagel (ed.), *Handbuch der Physiologie des Menschen* (Vol. 3) Physiologie der Sinne. Braunschweig: Vieweg und Sohn.

Vrhel, M., Gershon, R., & Iwan, L.S. (1994). Measurement and analysis of object reflectance spectra. *Color Research and Application, 19*, 4–9.

Webster, M.A. (1996). Human color perception and its adaptation. *Network: Computation in Neural Systems, 7*(4), 587–634.

Webster, M.A., Malkoc, G., Bilson, A.C., & Webster, S.M. (2002). Color contrast and contextual influences on color appearance. *Journal of Vision, 2*(6), 505–19.

Webster, M.A., & Mollon, J.D. (1997). Adaptation and the color statistics of natural images. *Vision Research, 37*(23), 3283–98.

Yang, J.N., & Shevell, S.K. (2002). Stereo disparity improves color constancy. *Vision Research, 42*(16), 1979–89.

Zaidi, Q. (1998). Identification of illuminant and object colors: heuristic-based algorithms. *Journal of the Optical Society of America A, 15*(7), 1767–76.

Zaidi, Q. (1999). Color and brightness induction: From Mach bands to 3-D configurations. In K. Gegenfurtner, & L. Sharpe (ed.), *Color Vision: From Genes to Perception*. Cambridge: Cambridge University Press.

Zaidi, Q. (2001). Color constancy in a rough world. *Color Research and Application, 26*(S1), S192–S200.

Zaidi, Q., & Shapiro, A., (1993). Adaptive orthogonalization of opponent-color signals. *Biological Cybernetics, 69*, 415–28.

Zaidi, Q., Shapiro, A., & Hood, D. (1992). The effect of adaptation on the differential sensitivity of the S-cone color system. *Vision Research, 32*, 1297–1318.

Zaidi, Q., Spehar, B., & DeBonet, J. (1997). Color constancy in variegated scenes: role of low-level mechanisms in discounting illumination changes. *Journal of the Optical Society of America A, 14*(10), 2608–21.

Zaidi, Q., Spehar, B., and DeBonet, J. (1998). Adaptation to textured chromatic fields. *Journal of the Optical Society of America A, 15*, 23–32.

Zaidi, Q., Yoshimi, B., Flanigan, N., & Canova, A. (1992). Lateral interactions within color mechanisms in simultaneous induced contrast. *Vision Research, 32*(9), 1695–1707.

Section II

High-Level Vision

5

High-Level Pattern Coding Revealed by Brief Shape Aftcrcffccts

Satoru Suzuki

5.1 Relating Neural Response Properties to Perception of Form Features

Visual form processing is often considered hierarchical in that patterns of illumination on the retina (detected by the rods and cones) are gradually transformed through subcortical and cortical processes into codings of increasingly global and complex patterns[1]. A challenge is to understand what neural codings are used at different processing stages and how they contribute to what people see from moment to moment. On the one hand, detailed neurophysiological research is necessary to understand the variety of responses, interactions and organizations existing in different visual areas of the brain. On the other hand, complementary behavioral research is necessary to infer principles (e.g. computational algorithms) that link the physiological properties and anatomical organizations of visual neurons to the coding of perceived forms.

---

[1] Strictly speaking, the traditional view that the visual form processing is hierarchical is true only with respect to feedforward neural activation. Increasing evidence suggests that consciously perceived patterns are closely associated with feedback (or reentrant) activation of V1 following activation of higher cortical visual areas (e.g. Zipser *et al.* 1996; Dehaene *et al.* 1998; Enns & Di Lollo 2000; Lamme 2001; Pascal-Leone & Walsh 2001).

At the initial stage of cortical visual processing, there is a relatively clear relationship between the variety of neural pattern selectivity and the perceptual features encoded. For example, cells in V1 (the first stage of cortical form processing) have small receptive fields (i.e. each neuron "looks at" a tiny portion of the retina) and are systematically tuned to different orientations and spatial frequencies (e.g. Hubel & Wiesel 1968; De Valois *et al.* 1982). Consistent with these systematic neural tunings, psychophysical studies using patterns designed to stimulate V1 cells (e.g. oriented bars, gratings, and Gabor patches) have revealed repulsive perceptual aftereffects for orientation and spatial frequency (e.g. Gibson & Radner 1937; Blakemore & Sutton 1969; Blakemore *et al.* 1970; Mitchell & Muir 1976; Magnussen & Kurtenbach 1980). Demonstrations of these repulsive aftereffects provided behavioral evidence that perception of orientation and spatial frequency are population coded on the basis of central tendencies of activity[2] of neural units tuned to orientation and spatial-frequency (see Fig. 5.1 for an illustration using tilt aftereffect as an example, and see Section 5.7 for details). The fact that these aftereffects are local (thus indicative of mediation by cells with small receptive fields) and that their tuning properties are similar to those of orientation and spatial-frequency tuned cells in V1, have further supported the idea that perception of local orientation and spatial frequency are population coded in V1 (e.g. Blakemore & Nachmias 1971; Braddick *et al.* 1978; Wenderoth & van der Zwan 1989).

Unfortunately, this clear relationship between organization of neural tuning and coding of perceived features quickly becomes murky as one examines higher cortical visual areas in the ventral visual pathway, V2 → V4 → IT (inferotemporal cortex), thought to mediate form perception (e.g. Ungerleider & Mishkin 1982; Mishkin *et al.* 1983). Though some tunings for orientation and/or spatial-frequency persist in V2, V4, and IT (e.g. Foster *et al.* 1985; Levitt *et al.* 1994; Desimone & Schein 1987; Vogels & Orban 1994), cells in higher visual areas respond preferentially to increasingly complex patterns. Even in V2 (an area adjacent to V1), cells begin to respond to local but complex geometric features such as subjective contours, bent or curved contours, contour intersections, and texture patterns (e.g. Peterhans & von der Heydt 1991; Sheth *et al.* 1996; Leventhal *et al.* 1998; Hegdé & Van Essen 2000). The V4 cells have larger receptive fields

---

[2] Here, it is assumed that perception of form features (presented in isolation or at the focus of attention) are primarily coded by neural population activity on the basis of activation strengths (spike rates) derived from classical receptive fields. It should be noted that recent physiological research has found that (1) neural responses as early as in V1 are influenced by grouping and figure-ground organizations existing well beyond the bounds of classical receptive fields (e.g. Zipser *et al.* 1996; Lamme *et al.* 1999; Nothdurft *et al.* 1999), and (2) some image properties may be coded in V1 as temporal patterns of neural activity (e.g. Ferster & Spruston 1995; Ikegaya *et al.* 2004) providing a means other than activation strengths (i.e. spike rates) to influence downstream neural activity (e.g. Lumer 1998; Fries *et al.* 2001; Reich *et al.* 2001; Suzuki & Grabowecky 2002*b*; Suzuki 2003*b*).

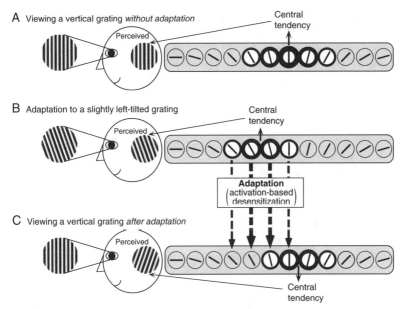

FIG. 5.1 An illustration of how the tilt aftereffect provides behavioral evidence that perceived orientation is coded on the basis of a central tendency of population activity of orientation-tuned cells. The circles with oriented lines represent orientation-tuned cells in the primary visual cortex (V1) with the indicated orientation preferences. A thicker circle indicates stronger neural activation. (A) When a vertical grating is viewed, the vertically tuned cells respond maximally, but cells that are tuned to the neighboring orientations also respond in a graded manner because of their tuning widths. Because the pattern of activation is symmetric about the vertical-tuned cell, the central tendency of the population activity falls at the vertical orientation, and the perceived orientation is vertical (see the grating depicted inside the schematic head of the viewer). (B) When a slightly left-tilted grating is viewed, the central tendency falls at the corresponding orientation (in this case between the preferred orientations of adjacent cells), and a slightly left-tilted orientation is perceived. Importantly, prolonged viewing of this grating results in adaptation (activation-based desensitization which is characteristic of most cortical cells) of the activated cells. (C) When a vertical grating is viewed following this adaptation, the central tendency of population activity shifts to a slightly right-tilted orientation due to the prior desensitization of the cells tuned to left-tilted orientations (dashed arrows). Thus, if perception of orientation is determined by the central tendency of population activity of orientation-tuned cells, the vertical grating should appear slightly tilted to the right; this indeed occurs and the phenomenon is known as the tilt aftereffect.

and respond to combinations and relative positions of curves and angles (e.g. Pasupathy & Connor 1999, 2001), texture patterns (e.g. Gallant *et al.* 1996) and luminance gradients (e.g. Hanazawa & Komatsu 2001). In inferotemporal cortex (IT), cells have very large receptive fields and they respond to a variety of simple and complex geometric patterns with substantial degrees of invariance for position and size (e.g. Desimone, *et al.* 1984; Fujita *et al.* 1992; Logothetis & Sheinberg 1996; Tanaka 1996; Tsunoda *et al.* 2001). Because cells in these higher visual areas respond to a variety of different geometric features with little apparent systematicity (such as the systematic orientation and spatial-frequency tunings in V1), it has been difficult to understand how neural responses in these areas encode perceived features.

5.2 Some Basic Types of Neural Population Coding

At the most general level of conceptualizing neural population coding, per-ceived objects are encoded by overall patterns of distributed neural activity. For example, different classes of common objects (e.g. chairs, houses, bottles, shoes, scissors, and faces) evoke different patterns of neural activity distributed across the temporal visual areas (e.g. Haxby *et al.* 2000, 2001; Tsunoda *et al.* 2001). Objects can then be distinguished on the basis of differences in the gen-eral topography of distributed neural activity, providing virtually unlimited capacity for coding different objects. In this *general-distributed coding*, objects inducing less overlapped neural activities are more readily discriminated (e.g. Abdi *et al.* 2003). General-distributed coding is difficult to crack because one must unravel the principles that relate perceived properties of object features to specific topographies of distributed neural activity.

A subset of distributed coding might include *process-specific coding* where anatomically localized cell assemblies might encode image features that are useful for specific types of processing. Expert object identification (e.g. identification of faces and other objects, such as birds and cars, in which one is an expert), for example, is likely to require encoding of specific feature dimen-sions that are maximally sensitive to identification-relevant image variations (e.g. Young & Yamane 1992; Kobatake *et al.* 1998; Sigala & Logothetis 2002) but minimally sensitive to irrelevant image variations including spurious variations due to changes in illumination, size, orientation, and viewpoint. In contrast, perception of spatial layout, for example, imposes a different (and con-flicting) set of computational demands, requiring viewpoint-dependent encoding of relative positions, sizes and orientations of surfaces and objects to support visually guided action. Human brain imaging (fMRI) results suggest that the processing of objects of expertise preferentially activates the fusiform area (e.g. Kanwisher *et al.* 1997; Gauthier *et al.* 1999, 2000; Gauthier 2000; Rhodes *et al.* 2004), whereas the processing of spatial layouts preferentially activates the parahippocampal area (e.g. Epstein *et al.* 1999, 2003) of the temporal lobe. Whereas any arbitrary categories of objects can be distinguished on the basis of general topographies of distributed neural activity, process-specific codings, utilizing specialized cell assemblies, might have developed to opti-mize discriminability for specific classes of behaviorally-relevant stimuli (see Section 5.6), and to anatomically segregate computationally conflicting processes.

The primary topic of this chapter, *central-tendency coding*, is a special case of process-specific coding. In central-tendency coding, a geometric feature is coded by the central tendency of activity of a population of neural units that are systematically tuned (with overlapped tuning functions) to different values of that feature. For simplicity, discussions in this chapter will be limited to codings of single geometric features (e.g. convexity), though central-tendency codings commonly occur in multi-dimensional feature spaces as most visual neurons are broadly tuned to multiple image features (e.g. V1 cells are simultaneously tuned to orientation, spatial frequency, position, and binocular disparity). The extraction of central tendency might be based on the population activity centroid, vector summation, and/or maximum-likelihood analyses (e.g. Lee *et al.* 1988; Vogels 1990; Young & Yamane 1992; Deneve *et al.* 1999).

Any coding based on patterns of population activity provides resistance against individual (uncorrelated) and global (correlated) fluctuations in neural activity on the basis of averaging and extraction of relative activity. Central-tendency codings in particular can facilitate high-resolution discriminations of the coded features because partially overlapped tuning functions allow interpolations across discretely sampled feature values. For example, in Fig. 5.1(B), the orientation of the grating stimulus is not identical to the preferred orientation of any of the twelve hypothetical orientation-tuned units. However, because each unit has a tuning around its preferred orientation (responding to neighboring orientations in a graded manner), the central tendency can extract the stimulus orientation that falls between the two units, allowing interpolations across discretely sampled orientations. It is thus likely that geometric features that are central-tendency coded in high-level processing are ones for which it is behaviorally important to discriminate their subtle variations.

5.3 Neurophysiological Evidence for Possible High-level Central-tendency Codings of Form Features

In addition to the systematic tunings for local orientation and spatial frequency in V1 and V2 (and to some degree in V4), sub-populations of V2 and V4 cells exhibit tunings for local curvature (Pasupathy & Connor 1999; Hegdé & Van Essen 2000). In V4, however, this "curvature tuning" is complicated by the fact that cells show additional selectivities for sequences of adjacent curves as well as positions of the preferred curves relative to the center of the stimulus pattern (e.g. Pasupathy & Connor 2001). In IT, cells tuned to "similar" geometric patterns tend to be anatomically clustered within "feature columns" (e.g. Fujita *et al.* 1992; Tanaka 1996; G. Wang *et al.* 1996; Y. Wang *et al.* 2000; Tsunoda *et al.* 2001). However, because somewhat arbitrary collections of shapes have been used as stimuli in most studies investigating response properties of IT cells and a single IT cell can exhibit apparently heterogeneous tunings for multiple patterns (e.g. Y. Wang *et al.* 2000), it is not clear which of the large variety of patterns that have been shown to preferentially stimulate individual IT cells indicate central-tendency coded features. There is also evidence that at least some complex patterns (particularly objects with multiple parts) are coded in IT on the basis of part-based distributed patterns of neural activity, in which each sub-cluster of activity appears to represent a part and/or a combination of parts (e.g. Tsunoda *et al.* 2001; Brincat & Connor 2004).

A small set of potentially central-tendency coded features have been reported in IT, however. Face-related features are probably the most well-known example. Neural tunings for variations in global face attributes have been reported, such as roundness of facial outline and amount of hair (Young & Yamane 1992), and facial expression (Hasselmo *et al.* 1989). An optical imaging study also showed that anatomically adjacent regions of IT responded to faces rotated in depth by successive angles (Wang *et al.* 1996). Thus, identity, expression, and 3D orientation of faces appear to be central-tendency coded in IT.

Recently, potential systematic central-tendency codings in IT have also been reported for some non-face features. Kayaert *et al.* (2003, 2004) examined responses of IT cells to various non-accidental geometric features (i.e. features that are preserved across minor viewpoint changes) and to their metric variations, using generalized cones as the stimuli (a set of simple volumes believed by some to be the basic elements of 3D object perception; e.g. Marr 1982; Biederman 1987). They found that some IT cells showed selectivity for specific non-accidental feature "dimensions" such as aspect ratio (overall width and height), curvature, taper (convergence of contours) and convexity, while exhibiting broad tunings for metric variations within the dimensions to which they were sensitive.

5.4 Brief Shape Aftereffects (SAEs) as a "Psycho-anatomical" Tool for Probing High-level Central-tendency Codings of Global Form Features

While neurophysiological studies identify potential central-tendency coded features in terms of systematic neural tunings, complementary behavioral studies are necessary to show that perception of those features is indeed determined by central-tendency coding. Activation-based sensitivity reduction, known as adaptation, is a ubiquitous property of cortical neurons (e.g. for V1 cells, Vautin & Berkeley 1977; Albrecht *et al.* 1984; Hammond *et al.* 1989; Saul & Cynader 1989; Sclar *et al.* 1989; Bonds 1991; Carandini *et al.* 1998; Muller *et al.* 1999; for IT cells, Oram & Perrett 1992; Miller *et al.* 1993*b*; Lueschow *et al.* 1994; Vogels & Orban 1994; Vogels *et al.* 1995). Consequently, a psychophysical signature of central-tendency coding is a "repulsive aftereffect." Roughly speaking, prior exposure (i.e. adaptation) to a feature value (e.g. a left-tilted grating) that is deviated from the test feature value (e.g. a vertical grating) makes the test feature appear distorted in the opposite direction (e.g. it appears right tilted), due to reduction in the relative activity of cells tuned to the adapted value (see Fig. 5.1).

Demonstrations of repulsive aftereffects for local orientation and spatial frequency have confirmed central-tendency codings of local orientation and spatial frequency in V1 (see Fig. 5.1 and Section 5.1). Similar demonstrations of repulsive aftereffects for global geometric features would indicate the existence of central-tendency codings for specific global features. Because neurophysiological results are currently ambiguous as to what global features are central-tendency coded in high-level visual areas, psychophysical demonstrations of global shape aftereffects should be especially helpful in interpreting and potentially guiding neurophysiological research on global shape coding. However, in comparison with the extensive prior research on local orientation and spatial frequency aftereffects, relatively few studies investigated global shape aftereffects (e.g. Regan & Hamstra 1992) prior to Suzuki and colleagues' demonstrations of brief shape aftereffects and recent demonstrations of face-related aftereffects (see Section 5.6). This was primarily due to the difficulty in dissociating global shape aftereffects, indicative of high-level coding of global forms, from local feature aftereffects (the orientation and spatial-frequency aftereffects discussed above, as well as contour-repulsion based figural aftereffects; e.g. Kohler & Wallach 1944; Sagara & Ohyama 1957), indicative of low-level coding of local image features. Isolating high-level aftereffects is difficult because complex shapes are made up of locally oriented contours which necessarily activate low-level processes.

In contrast with conventional methods of measuring aftereffects using prolonged stimuli (e.g. seconds to minutes of adaptation), Suzuki and colleagues noted that rapid sequences of stimuli, that is, (1) brief adaptation and (2) brief test, combined with (3) brief adapt-to-test ISI (inter stimulus interval), could produce robust repulsive aftereffects for global geometric features (see Fig. 5.2).

First, brief adaptors (less than ~150 ms) were found to be effective in producing high-level aftereffects with minimal influences from low-level aftereffects (details follow). This is consistent with the temporal properties of high-level and low-level cells. Inferotemporal (IT) cells in alert monkeys typically adapt to briefly presented stimuli; following a brief exposure to an adaptor stimulus (350–500 ms tested), IT cells reduce their sensitivity to a test stimulus (presented following 300–2000 ms of ISI), especially when the test stimulus is identical or similar to the adaptor stimulus (e.g. Miller *et al.* 1993*b*; Lueschow *et al.* 1994; Vogels & Orban 1994; Vogels *et al.* 1995). In contrast, most V1 cells in alert monkeys do not adapt to briefly presented (up to 500 ms) gratings of preferred orientations (Gur *et al.* 2004; interestingly, V1 cells in anesthetized monkeys adapt rapidly, Muller *et al.* 1999). Furthermore, both behavioral and physiological results indicate that V1 cells adapt slowly over many seconds (e.g. Albrecht *et al.* 1984). Circumventing low-level adaptation by using brief adaptors was particularly important for Suzuki and colleagues to demonstrate aftereffects on relatively simple geometric features consisting of oriented contours. Brief adaptation, however, is not an absolute requirement for generating a high-level aftereffect as evidenced by the fact that face-related aftereffects can be induced by adaptation durations ranging from a second to several minutes (see Rhodes *et al.* this volume).

Second, briefly presenting a test shape (with backward masking) is generally advantageous because it reduces adaptation effects initiated by the test shape,

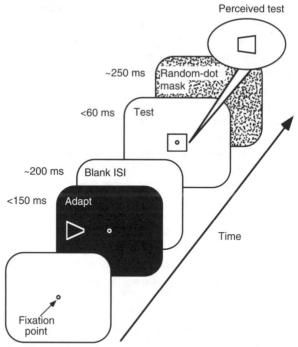

FIG. 5.2 A typical trial sequence used to demonstrate a global shape aftereffect (SAE); a taper aftereffect is shown as an example. The adaptor and test shapes are presented briefly (with an optimum adapt-to-test ISI of ~200 ms) in order to reveal aftereffects due to global-form adaptation unconfounded by low-level local aftereffects (Suzuki 2001). The adaptor display was often presented in reverse contrast (as shown in the figure) to prevent (or substantially reduce) perception of adapt-to-test apparent motion, though apparent motion does not contribute to SAEs (Suzuki & Cavanagh 1998).

and thus increases the sensitivity for detecting aftereffects induced by the adaptor (e.g. Wolfe 1984; Suzuki & Cavanagh 1997). Aftereffects tend to be strengthened when the test stimulus is weakened by reducing its duration, contrast, or presenting it away from the fovea (Suzuki & Cavanagh 1998). Third, in some cases the use of brief adapt-to-test ISI of about 200 ms was crucial to produce aftereffects that were spatially tolerant, that is, to produce aftereffects that diminished only gradually as the position and/or size of the adaptor shape increasingly deviated from the test shape (e.g. Rivest et al. 1998; Suzuki & Cavanagh 1998; Suzuki 2001). Because the sizes of neural receptive fields increase from averaging only 0.3–1° in V1, ~3° in V2, and 1.5–4° in V4 (in parafovea at retinal eccentricities of 2–5° from the fovea), to encompassing large portions of the visual field (a mean of 30° but up to 100°) in IT (e.g. Gross et al. 1972; Desimone & Gross 1979; Dow et al. 1981; Foster et al. 1985;

Desimone & Schein 1987; Gattas *et al.* 1988; Ito *et al.* 1995), aftereffects that show substantial spatial tolerance are likely to be mediated by central-tendency codings in high-level cortical visual areas. Suzuki and colleagues thus called these spatially tolerant aftereffects induced by rapid stimulus sequences, *shape aftereffects* (*SAEs*). The specific types of SAEs found so far suggest that the initial central-tendency coding of local orientation in V1 is elaborated in higher visual areas as central-tendency codings of global skew, taper, curvature, aspect ratio, and convexity (e.g. Suzuki & Cavanagh 1998; Suzuki 1999, 2001, 2003*a*).

For example, a skewed adaptor (e.g. a right-skewed parallelogram) induces an opposite skew on a subsequently flashed symmetric (e.g. rectangular) test shape (Fig. 5.3(A), top). Skew aftereffects are translation tolerant (i.e. occurring when the adaptor and test shapes are presented at completely non-overlapping locations), and they occur even when the adaptor and test shapes have no matching contours (Fig. 5.3(A), bottom), suggesting that skew is central-tendency coded as a global attribute beyond early coding of local orientation. Similarly, a tapered adaptor (e.g. a right pointing triangle) induces an opposite taper (Fig. 5.3(B); also see Fig. 5.2), a curved adaptor induces an opposite curvature (Fig. 5.3(C)), and an elongated adaptor (e.g. a tall ellipse) induces an opposite aspect ratio (Fig. 5.3(D)), on subsequently flashed symmetric test patterns. These aftereffects are translation and scale tolerant (up to 12° of adapt-test separation and 0.3–1.8 in adapt-test linear size ratio; Rivest *et al.* 1998; Suzuki & Cavanagh 1998; Suzuki 2001), suggesting that taper, curvature, and aspect ratio are also central-tendency coded as global attributes. Finally, a convex/concave adaptor (e.g. a diamond/hourglass shape) induces a concave/convex distortion on a subsequently flashed symmetric test pattern (Fig. 5.3(E), top/middle). These convexity aftereffects are scale tolerant (Fig. 5.3(E), bottom), suggesting that convexity is also central-tendency coded as a global attribute. Interestingly, unlike skew, taper, and aspect ratio aftereffects, convexity aftereffects are not translation tolerant, potentially reflecting the fact that the convex–concave distinction for a contour depends on the position of the contour relative to the region of interest. These aftereffects were typically measured using a method of adjustment (having the observer reproduce the appearance of the distorted test shape) or a method of cancellation (nulling the aftereffect using a staircase procedure).

To confirm that a rapid sequence of visual stimulation (Fig. 5.2) uniquely adapted high-level processing without affecting low-level processing, convexity aftereffects induced by convex and concave shapes (Fig. 5.3(E)) were compared with conventional tilt aftereffects induced by oriented gratings (which adapt local-orientation-tuned cells in V1) under closely matched conditions. With prolonged (2600 ms) adaptation, the four patches of oriented gratings locally produced narrowly-tuned tilt aftereffects (Fig. 5.4(A)), which were maximum when the adaptor orientation was ±15° from the test orientation, consistent with the narrow orientation tunings of V1 cells. With brief (134 ms or less) adaptation, however, these gratings produced

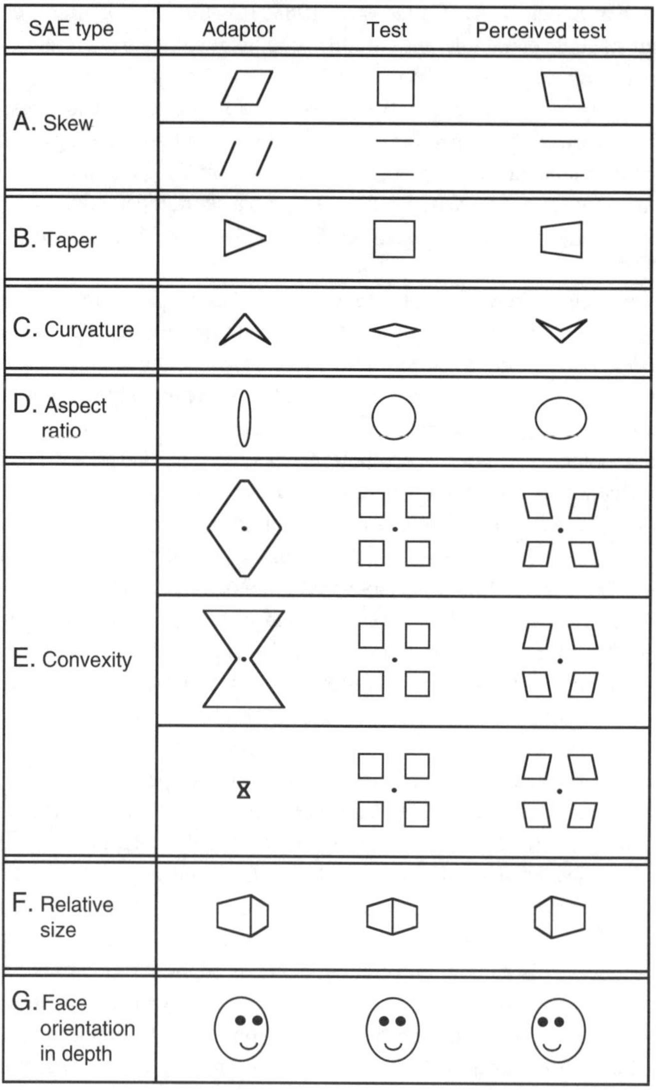

SAE type	Adaptor	Test	Perceived test
A. Skew			
B. Taper			
C. Curvature			
D. Aspect ratio			
E. Convexity			
F. Relative size			
G. Face orientation in depth			

FIG. 5.3 Schematic examples of SAEs demonstrated so far. SAEs are generally translation and scale tolerant. However, in some cases, the magnitude of SAEs can be modulated by the relative position of the adaptor and test shapes (Suzuki & Cavanagh 1998). An array of squares rather than a solid shape was used as the test pattern for measuring convexity aftereffects (E), partly to demonstrate aftereffects acting globally on a grouped array, and partly to facilitate comparisons with local tilt aftereffects (Suzuki 2001).

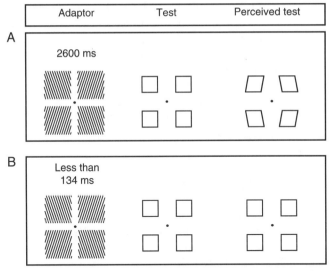

FIG. 5.4 An example of a grating adaptor used in Suzuki (2001) to demonstrate that brief adaptation dissociates global convexity aftereffects from local tilt aftereffects. (A) With prolonged adaptation (2600 ms), the four grating patches locally produce tilt aftereffects, resulting in the overall convex appearance of the four test squares, similar to aftereffects induced by a concave hourglass (see Fig. 3(E), middle). (B) With brief adaptation (less than 134 ms), however, the grating patches produce no aftereffect.

NO aftereffects (Fig. 5.4(B)). In contrast, the convex and concave shapes (Fig. 5.3(E)) produced strong aftereffects with adaptation as brief as 27 ms (undiminished in magnitude relative to 2600 ms adaptation). Control experiments have shown that this dissociation cannot be attributed to differences in spatial frequency contents, or to the possibility that both the convex and concave shapes and the oriented gratings adapted a common orientation-coding mechanism except that briefly presented grating stimuli somehow sub-optimally activated this mechanism (Suzuki 2001).

Parametric investigations have further demonstrated that brief aftereffects induced by the convex and concave shapes were (1) broadly tuned to convexity (maximum when orientations of the side contours were ±30 to ±60° from vertical), (2) indifferent as to the mode of contour definition (e.g. bright lines, high-pass-filtered lines, contours generated by the spatial inhomogeneity of visual sensitivity), (3) already maximum at low contrast energy (saturation within a 3-fold increase in contrast energy beyond detection), (4) strongly modulated by selective attention (see Section 5.5), and (5) relatively size tolerant. As suggested by Suzuki (2001, 2003a), these characteristics of brief convexity aftereffects are paralleled (sometimes even quantitatively) by the response characteristics of high-level pattern-selective neurons, especially in IT. Compared to their low-level counterparts, responses of high-level visual neurons tend to have broader orientation tuning (e.g. Desimone & Schein 1987;

Vogels & Orban 1994; Geisler & Albrecht 1997; McAdams & Maunsell 1999), be relatively indifferent to mode of contour definition (e.g. Sato *et al.* 1980; Rolls & Baylis 1986; Komatsu *et al.* 1992; Ito *et al.* 1994), saturate at lower contrast energy (e.g. Gross *et al.* 1972; Sato *et al.* 1980; Rolls & Baylis 1986; Sclar *et al.* 1990; Cheng *et al.* 1994), be strongly affected by selective attention (when the competing stimuli are presented within the receptive field of a cell; e.g. Luck *et al.* 1997; Chelazzi *et al.* 1998), and be scale tolerant (e.g. Ito *et al.* 1995; Tanaka 1996; Hikosaka 1999). Converging evidence thus suggests that SAEs are indeed mediated by central-tendency codings of global form features, perhaps in IT.

5.5 Attentional Modulations of SAEs

Global pattern processing necessarily pools information from lower-level processes to achieve both complex pattern selectivity and invariance for position and scale (see Riesenhuber & Poggio 2000, for a review). Because of the extensive convergence of neural signals, even small neural modulations that occur in lower-level processing due to attention, contextual factors, and short-term and long-term neural plasticity, can be substantially amplified in high-level processing. For example, though conventional tilt aftereffects (mediated by orientation-tuned cells in V1) are only weakly modulated by attention (Spivey & Spirn 2000), SAEs are strongly modulated by attention (see below). Furthermore, because cells that are tuned to global forms (with position and size tolerance) necessarily have large receptive fields, high-level coding has poor spatial resolution; for example, an IT cell will respond poorly to its preferred shape if other shapes are also present in the vicinity unless the preferred shape is attended (e.g. Miller *et al.* 1993a; Chelazzi *et al.* 1998). Thus, as people live in environments crowded with multiple objects, global form processing must be tightly coupled with attentional selection processes.

Because SAEs selectively probe adaptation of global-form coding mechanisms, they provide a unique means to study how attention modulates incoming signals to influence activations at the level of global-form processing. In neurophysiological research, the degree of attentional selection is often assessed in terms of linear attention weights, that is, how much the input signals from the attended contours are amplified relative to the input signals from the ignored contours in activating a given cell; this way of conceptualizing attention effects at the single-cell level is termed the biased competition model (e.g. Moran & Desimone 1985; Desimone & Duncan 1995; Luck *et al.* 1997; Reynolds *et al.* 1999). Comparable linear attention weights can be behaviorally derived from attentional modulations of SAEs (if one assumes that the magnitude of an SAE is monotonically related to activation of the relevant global-form coding neurons) using a simple formula,

$$w_{attended} - w_{ignored}$$

$$= \frac{[\text{SAE from XY with X attended}] - [\text{SAE from XY with Y attended}]}{[\text{SAE from X alone}] - [\text{SAE from Y alone}]} \times 100\%,$$

where X and Y represent two adaptor shapes, XY represents an adaptor consisting of overlapping X and Y shapes, and $w_{attended}$ and $w_{ignored}$ represent linear attention weights that multiply the input signal when a shape is attended and ignored, respectively; note that although these attention weights are different for the two shapes (e.g. due to differences in their salience), the difference between the attended and ignored weights ($w_{attended} - w_{ignored}$) is the same for each shape under the assumptions of the biased competition model (see Suzuki 2003a for details).

For example, when overlapped hourglass and diamond shapes were used as the adaptor (Suzuki 2001, 2003a), attending to the (convex) diamond produced a concave aftereffect (Fig. 5.5(A)), whereas attending to the (concave) hourglass produced a convex aftereffect (Fig. 5.5(B)); the concave and convex directions of aftereffects were given opposite signs in the equation. The differential attention weights were obtained by expressing this attention-based difference in SAE from the overlapped adaptor as the percentage of the maximum possible difference in SAE from the diamond and hourglass adaptors presented alone. If attention completely suppressed the ignored shape, attending to the diamond or the hourglass in the overlapping adaptor should produce aftereffects identical to those obtained from the diamond or the hourglass adaptor presented alone. This would result in the numerator and denominator of the equation being equal, making the ratio unity (or 100 per cent). Thus, differential attention weights of 100 per cent would indicate complete attentional selection. Psychophysically inferred differential attention weights can be compared with those obtained in neurophysiological studies. Such a comparison is difficult with conventional behavioral measures of selective attention like modulations of response time and accuracy in probe detection tasks.

When different combinations of overlapped shapes were used, the differential attention weights obtained from SAEs were similar. Notably, attentional selection was similar for a combination of opposing shapes (e.g. an hourglass and a diamond that produce opposite convexity aftereffects) and a combination of non-opposing shapes (e.g. an hourglass that produces a convex aftereffect and horizontal lines that produce a vertical-elongation [aspect-ratio] aftereffect). This result ruled out the possibility that attentional selection in SAEs is primarily due to lateral-inhibition-type modulations of population activity within the specific central-tendency coding of the attended feature (e.g. suppression of convex-tuned units when a concave shape is attended). Note, however, that this type of within-coding interaction might still play a role in influencing the course of perceptual multi-stability (see Section 5.8). Interestingly, the differential attention weights derived from the SAE results were ~60 per cent under various conditions (Suzuki 2001, 2003a), comparable to the differential weights achieved at the level of V4 neurons (Reynolds *et al.* 1999). This might suggest that attentional modulations of SAEs are primarily due to modulations of contour processing up to V4.

Because SAEs probe high-level global processing and are sensitive to attentional modulations, SAEs also provide a useful paradigm for studying how attentional selection interacts with various image factors such as salience, scale,

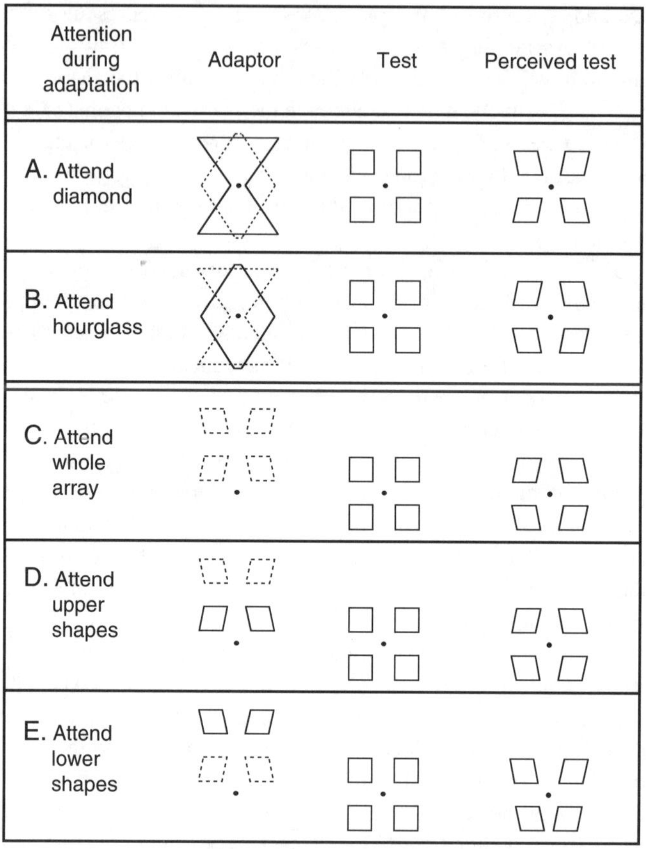

FIG. 5.5 Schematic examples of attentional modulations of SAEs. The attended portion of the adaptor is indicated by dashed contours (for illustration purposes only). When overlapped shapes were used as the adaptor (A and B), the two shapes were given different colors to facilitate attentional selection.

and grouping. For example, it would be beneficial if attention could differentially weight signals regardless of their luminance contrasts; this way, signals from dimmer, but potentially important images, can be selected for higher-level processing as well as signals from salient images. Physiologically, Reynolds and Desimone (2003) have demonstrated that attentional mechanisms can substantially boost the signals from attended low-contrast stimuli against ignored high-contrast stimuli, in controlling responses of V4 neurons. By measuring attentional modulations of SAEs while varying the relative contrasts of the overlapped adaptor shapes, Suzuki (2001) provided psychophysical evidence that the degree of attentional weighting was relatively independent of the salience of the stimuli. In addition, when the overall scale of the overlapped adaptors was varied from 2.3° to 15.8°, the differential attention weights remained largely constant at ~60 per cent, suggesting that the efficiency of attentional selection is relatively scale invariant (Suzuki 2001).

In another SAE study, effects of attending to the whole and parts were assessed by using an adaptor consisting of an array of shapes (Suzuki 1999). For example, a concave array of four parallelograms as the adaptor was flashed in the upper visual field (Fig. 5.5(C–E)). Because the test array was flashed around the fixation point, the bottom row of the adaptor array and the top row of the test array were presented at the same location. Thus, local orientation aftereffects should make the top row of the test array appear tilted outward. To the contrary, when the whole concave adaptor array was attended (attended contours are indicated by dashed lines in Fig. 5.5), the top row of the test array appeared tilted inward and the test array as a whole appeared convex, consistent with a global convexity aftereffect (Fig. 5.5(C)). The result was similar when the top row of the adaptor array was attended (Fig. 5.5(D)), suggesting that when peripheral parts are attended, it is difficult to exclude parts that are closer to the fixation. Interestingly, attending to the bottom row of the adaptor array made the whole test array appear tapered downward (Fig. 5.5(E)), suggesting that attention to parts closer to the fixation can successfully exclude more peripheral parts, and that the selected parts of the adaptor array were processed as having an overall upward taper and the whole test array was processed as a unit. Thus, central-tendency codings of convexity and taper seem to be activated on the basis of the attended portion of an array.

It will be important in future research to gain an integrative understand of attention effects on global-form processing (e.g. studied with SAEs) and those on lower-level processing of luminance, contrast, and local features (e.g. edge orientation). For example, attention results in increased contrast gain and response synchrony in lower-level processes, which might contribute to the increased competitive edge for the attended signals in higher-level processes (Reynolds *et al.* 2000; Fries *et al.* 2001; Cameron *et al.* 2002; Reynolds & Desimone 2003). Future research must specify how signal weighting and synchrony are controlled by feedforward, feedback, and horizontal neural interactions at different stages of processing. Attention effects might also be different for cells with different response properties. For example, while examining attentional modulations of negative afterimages, Suzuki and Grabowecky (2003*b*) found that attentional modulation of brightness adaptation primarily acted on cells that are polarity-independent (responding to patterns whether they are dark or light) rather than cells that are polarity-dependent (responding selectively to dark or light).

5.6   What Global Form Features are Systematically Central-tendency Coded Beyond the Coding of Local Orientation in V1?

The types of SAEs demonstrated so far suggest that the initial central-tendency coding of local orientation in V1 is elaborated into central-tendency codings of global configurations of orientated contours, including skew, taper, curvature, aspect ratio, and convexity (Fig. 5.3(A–E)), perhaps in IT. Others have reported position and scale tolerant aftereffects for various geometric distortions of faces, suggesting high-level central-tendency codings of face-related features. For example, Leopold *et al.* (2001) demonstrated that face-identity aftereffects were undiminished across adapt-to-test retinal separations (implemented as fixation shifts) of up to about half the width of the face (or 6°). Zhao and Chubb (2001) demonstrated that face-distortion aftereffects (originally reported by Webster & MacLin 1999) were still substantial (though reduced in magnitude by half) for adapt-to-test size changes by a factor of two (also see chapters in this volume by Leopold & Bondar, and Rhodes *et al.*). An important question is whether these psychophysically inferred central-tendency coded features represent a fundamental set of high-level image codings, or are merely the tip of the iceberg, and other central-tendency coded features will be uncovered so long as appropriate stimuli are used. Though a definitive answer awaits future research, there are several reasons to believe that these features may be principal.

First, despite the fact that systematic geometric tunings have rarely been reported in IT, there is apparent consistency between the few feature variations for which systematic neural tunings have been found in IT on the one hand, and the set of feature variations for which repulsive aftereffects have been found on the other. For example, neural tunings in IT as well as repulsive aftereffects have been reported for geometric variations in face-related features. In addition, the class of IT cells systematically tuned to variations in aspect ratio (overall height and width), curvature, taper (convergence of contours), and convexity could mediate the SAEs found for aspect ratio, curvature, taper, and convexity (see Sections 5.3 and 5.7).

Second, because high-resolution discriminations of face attributes are crucial for human survival, it is not surprising that face-related features are central-tendency coded; as discussed earlier, central-tendency coding based on overlapped tuning functions allows interpolations between discretely sampled feature values (see Section 5.2 and Fig. 5.1). More generally, if central-tendency coding is an adaptive strategy of the visual system to bestow fast global analyses (rather than part-based analyses) with enhanced perceptual resolution to processing of behaviorally important patterns, it would be beneficial for the visual system to have mechanisms to develop central-tendency codings for behaviorally relevant geometric variations through experience. Brain imaging research using fMRI suggests that coding of objects in which one is an expert (e.g. birds, cars, and artificial creatures such as "greebles") and coding of faces (in which almost everybody is an expert) share the same focal brain region in the fusiform area (e.g. Gauthier *et al.* 1999, 2000; Gauthier 2000). Consistent with this shared-resource idea, there is some evidence that acquired expertise in a non-face category (e.g. cars) can interfere with face processing (e.g. Gauthier *et al.* 2003). Recent fMRI results also suggest that different classes of objects (e.g. faces and other objects of expertise) are processed by relatively non-overlapping sub-populations of cells within the fusiform area (e.g. Rhodes *et al.* 2004).

Single-cell recording studies with monkeys have shown that, with practice, IT cells are capable of developing selectivity for novel complex patterns, such as for paper-clip-like objects made up of wires bent multiple times in different directions (Logothetis *et al.* 1995), schematic fish-like drawings with variations in fin and mouth shapes, schematic faces with variations in eye, nose, and mouth positions (Sigala & Logothetis 2002), a set of complex geometric shapes (Kobatake *et al.* 1998), and for a set of human faces (Young & Yamane 1992). Overall, converging evidence suggests that human fusiform area and monkey IT have the plasticity to develop neural tunings for complex geometric features (including face-related features) that are important for discriminating individuals within a trained class of objects (especially for objects that are structurally similar).

It is not clear, however, whether acquired neural selectivities result in central-tendency codings of the trained features. Indeed, well-practiced discriminations among geometrically distinct objects, not lying along specific geometric continua (e.g. a face versus a chair versus a trumpet), are likely to be based on differences in the general topography of distributed neural activity. Future research should thus examine SAEs in conjunction with pattern learning. If central-tendency codings develop with experience, experts should show repulsive aftereffects for the feature variations in which they are experts. For example, bird experts might show repulsive aftereffects for geometric variations that are crucial for their discrimination of birds. Strong support for this hypothesis would be obtained if a repulsive aftereffect was demonstrated for a trained feature variation for which no aftereffect was observed prior to the training. Such a result would confirm that central-tendency codings generally underlie perception of well-experienced, thus, behaviorally significant, geometric variations.

If central-tendency codings indeed develop with experience, it might be no accident that SAEs have been found for overall skew, taper, curvature, aspect ratio, and convexity. This is because judging 3D orientations of objects is a ubiquitous aspect of daily life, and these features represent a basic set of geometric variations that people routinely experience when flat or moderately curved surfaces are manipulated in depth (most 3D objects can be approximated as being composed of flat or moderately curved surfaces). For example, relative to the fronto-parallel view, a rotation about the vertical axis induces overall tall aspect ratio and laterally pointing taper, both of which increase with greater rotations away from the fronto-parallel view (e.g. from left to right in Fig. 5.6(A)). When an angled intersection of a pair of flat surfaces is rotated about the axis perpendicular to the intersection, an overall curvature is introduced as the surfaces are rotated away from the fronto-parallel view (Fig. 5.6(B)). When the bending angle is changed (while approximately in the fronto-parallel view), the degree of convexity varies. The degree of skew systematically varies as a slanted surface is moved about in space (Fig. 5.6(C)). These 3D-rotation-concomitant geometric distortions occur to flat or moderately curved surfaces of any shape, though the distortions are most evident for symmetric surfaces such as the rectangular surfaces shown in Fig. 5.6.

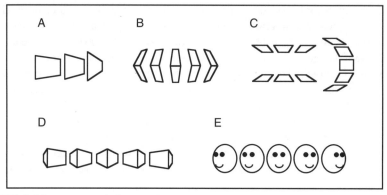

FIG. 5.6 Some geometric features that are systematically distorted when surfaces are rotated in depth. See text for details.

It is thus possible that central-tendency codings of global skew, taper, curvature, aspect ratio, and convexity might be an integral part of the mechanisms that mediate perception of 3D orientations of objects, and small degrees of viewpoint normalization (generating rotated representations to align to a reference viewpoint); for example, approximate 3D rotated views can be generated by applying these 2D geometric distortions via systematically shifting the neural population activities that encode these features. A mechanism like this might mediate 2D-based viewpoint interpolations which are hypothesized to facilitate recognition of objects across different viewpoints (e.g. Ullman 1998). If this is the case, then, repulsive aftereffects should be observed for other image features that also vary systematically as surfaces are rotated in depth. Relative size is an example. As an angled intersection of a pair of flat surfaces is rotated about the axis parallel to the intersection, the visible portion of one surface becomes larger and that of the other surface becomes smaller (Fig. 5.6(D)). Our preliminary results have demonstrated a (translation tolerant) repulsive aftereffect for this feature variation; for example, a flashed polygon showing more of the left surface makes a subsequently flashed symmetric polygon appear to show more of the right surface (see Fig. 5.3(F)).

Our preliminary results have also demonstrated a (translation tolerant) repulsive aftereffect for variations in 3D head orientation, using highly schematic faces (Fig. 5.6(E)); for example, a flashed face looking to the right makes a subsequently flashed forward-looking face appear to be looking to the left (see Fig. 5.3(G)). It is interesting to note that some IT cells show tunings for variations in 3D head orientation (see Section 5.3). Because knowing where a person is looking is of great behavioral significance (and perceived direction of gaze depends in part on perceived head orientation), it may be important to have a dedicated central-tendency coding for head orientation. In fact, Fang and He (2004) have recently reported seemingly object-specific repulsive aftereffects for head orientation as well as for 3D orientations of cars and stick figures, suggesting that the visual system has specialized central-tendency codings of 3D orientation for at least some classes of objects. However, it would not be efficient to have dedicated central-tendency codings for 3D orientation of arbitrary objects. Because objects are composed of surfaces (often large, approximately flat and symmetric surfaces especially for artifacts), the visual system might have instead opted for central-tendency codings of basic geometric distortions that occur when surfaces are rotated and translated in 3D environments.

5.7 Opponent Coding as a Special Case of Central-tendency Coding

It is noteworthy that all of the potentially central-tendency coded global geometric variations discussed so far have two extreme ends and often include a "category boundary" in the middle where perception changes discontinuously (categorically) and where high-resolution discrimination is behaviorally desirable. For example, it is important to be able to quickly determine whether a person has a positive or negative expression (rather than how positive or how negative), whether a person is female or male (rather than how feminine or how masculine), or whether a person is looking to your left or to your right (rather than how far left or how far right). Even for the potential central-tendency codings of skew, taper, curvature, aspect ratio, and convexity, geometrically continuous variations in these features go through a categorical discontinuity at the point of symmetry. Skew, taper, and curvature switch from one direction to the opposite direction when they are varied across the respective null points of symmetry. As aspect ratio is changed continuously through the null point, it changes from elongation along one orientation (e.g. flat) to elongation along the orthogonal orientation (e.g. tall). Convexity switches from convex to concave or vice versa across the null point. Each null point, coinciding with the category boundary, can be considered "the norm" because it lies in the middle of a geometric continuum and represents an "average" of the two extremes.

These considerations suggest that underlying population codings of global geometric features may be based primarily on the relative activities of two opponent populations of cells, one broadly tuned to one side of the norm (e.g. tuned to a flat aspect ratio) and the other broadly tuned to the other side of the norm (e.g. tuned to a tall aspect ratio); the perceived feature value (e.g. the perceived aspect ratio) is determined by the relative activation of the two opponent pools of cells. This is a special case of central-tendency coding, where central tendency is computed on the basis of only two pools of cells broadly tuned to the extreme feature values (Fig. 5.7), rather than on the basis of multiple pools of cells tuned to intermediate feature values (Fig. 5.1). Regan and Hamstra (1992) originally proposed this *opponent-coding* model with respect to coding of aspect ratio. As illustrated in Fig. 5.7(A), the two opponent tuning functions (one broadly tuned to flat aspect ratio and the other broadly tuned to tall aspect ratio) intersect at the norm (neutral aspect ratio) where the slopes are steepest,

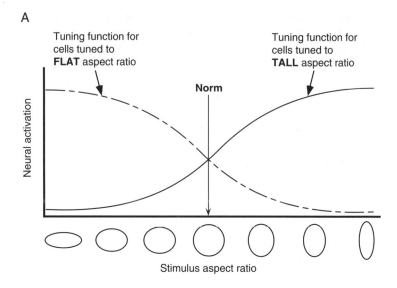

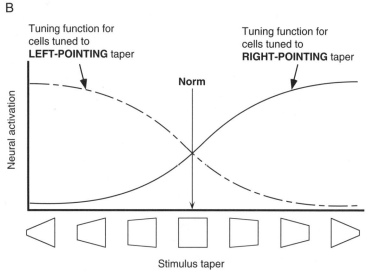

FIG. 5.7 Opponent coding based on two opponent pools of cells broadly tuned to the extreme values of a feature dimension. Two examples are illustrated: (A) opponent coding of aspect ratio (after Regan & Hamstra 1992), and (B) opponent coding of taper. The vertical lines indicate the norms (i.e. neutral aspect ratio, and neutral taper).

such that the relative activation of the opponent-tuned populations changes maximally when the feature value (aspect ratio) is varied near the norm (neutral aspect ratio). This is consistent with the fact that the thresholds for aspect-ratio discriminations are lowest at the neutral aspect ratio (Regan & Hamstra 1992). Regan and Hamstra's opponent-coding model can be applied to coding of other global geometric features; an example is shown in Fig. 5.7(B) for the opponent coding of taper. An opponent coding would be an efficient version of a central-tendency coding especially when the primary perceptual demand is in detecting bi-directional categorical deviations from the norm, with high sensitivity primarily required at the category boundary.

An opponent coding (a central-tendency coding based on two opponent pools of cells) can be distinguished from a *multi-channel coding* (a central-tendency coding based on multiple pools of cells tuned to intermediate feature values) on the basis of the tuning properties of aftereffects. Multi-channel coding predicts repulsive aftereffects with respect to the *relative* feature values of the adaptor and test stimuli. For example, tilt aftereffects are thought to result from the multi-channel coding of local orientation by orientation-tuned cells in V1. As illustrated in Fig. 5.1, adaptation-based desensitization of orientation-tuned cells makes the test orientation appear tilted away from the adaptor orientation. Because there is nothing special about the vertical orientation in the multi-channel coding scheme illustrated in Fig. 5.1, the same repulsive aftereffect is predicted (and occurs) with respect to any test orientation. For example, if the test orientation was 30°, it would appear less than 30° if the adaptor orientation was greater than 30°, and it would appear greater than 30° if the adaptor orientation was less than 30°. Thus, a signature characteristic of multi-channel coding is that when the adaptor feature value (e.g. adaptor orientation) is varied while the test feature value (e.g. test orientation) is fixed, the relevant repulsive aftereffect (e.g. tilt aftereffect) should exhibit an anti-symmetric tuning curve centered at the test feature value (e.g. test orientation).

For example, several tuning curves of tilt aftereffects for different test orientations are illustrated in Fig. 5.8(A) (schematized from Mitchell & Muir 1976 and O'Toole & Wenderoth 1977). Suppose the test orientation is + 45° (the top tuning curve in Fig. 5.8(A)). If the adaptor orientation is identical to the test orientation (+45°), no aftereffect will occur and the test orientation will appear veridical at +45°; this is the node of the tuning curve. If the adaptor orientation is made slightly less than the test orientation (< +45°), the aftereffect will increase the perceived tilt of the test grating, causing the tuning curve to rise above +45°. In contrast, if the adaptor orientation is made slightly greater than the test orientation (> +45°), the aftereffect will decrease the perceived tilt of the test grating, causing the tuning curve to fall below +45°. Because the local orientation tunings of V1 cells are narrow (median orientation bandwidth = 30–40°; Geisler & Albrecht, 1997), these repulsive aftereffects will diminish as the adaptor orientation deviates further from the test orientation, causing the tuning curve to re-converge to +45°; in fact, the tuning curve typically peaks when the adaptor orientation is about ±15° from the test orientation and re-converges when the adaptor orientation is about ±40–60° from the test orientation (e.g. Mitchell & Muir 1976; O'Toole & Wenderoth 1977; Magnussen & Kurtenbach 1980; O'Shea *et al.* 1993).

Under some conditions, this repulsive tilt aftereffect flips to an attractive effect when the adaptor orientation deviates as far as about 50–90° from the test

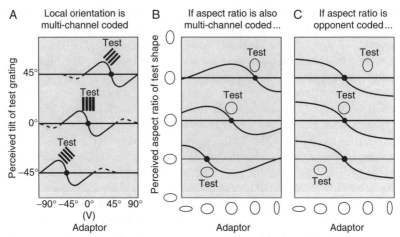

FIG. 5.8 Tuning curves of aftereffects expected from multi-channel coding
(A and B) and from opponent coding (C) when values of the adaptor feature (orientation
or aspect ratio) are varied for fixed values of the test feature. (A) Multi-channel coding
of local orientation generates tuning curves of tilt aftereffect that are anti-symmetric
about the test orientation, with the nodes (indicated by solid circles) occurring at the
test orientations. The dashed portions indicate indirect tilt aftereffects. (B) If aspect
ratio is also multi-channel coded, aspect-ratio aftereffects should produce tuning curves
that are also anti-symmetric about the test aspect ratios (likely with broader tuning
based on previous results). (C) Alternatively, if aspect ratio is opponent coded (see
Fig. 5.7), aspect-ratio aftereffects should be anti-symmetric about the neutral aspect
ratio regardless of the test aspect ratio.

orientation (the dashed portions of the tuning curves shown in Fig. 5.8(A)).
This attractive effect is known as the *indirect* tilt aftereffect. It is typically
smaller in magnitude (e.g. Gibson & Radner 1937; Campbell & Maffei 1971;
O'Shea *et al.* 1993) and less reliable (e.g. Mitchell & Muir 1976) than the repulsive component of tilt aftereffects. Interestingly, the attractive component was
abolished (1) when a square frame was placed around the test grating (e.g.
Wenderoth & van der Zwan 1989), and (2) when an adaptor consisted of multiple gratings with no average tilt (Held & Shattuck 1971; Suzuki 2001; in these
studies, the spatially averaged tilt across the multiple local gratings was the
same as the test orientation [vertical]; see Fig. 5.4 as an example). Such sensitivity to global context (external frame and long-range spatial averaging) suggests
that the attractive component of tilt aftereffects is mediated by a high-level
mechanism involving cells with relatively large receptive fields. In contrast, the
repulsive component of tilt aftereffects is largely unaffected by these manipulations of global context, consistent with its mediation by low-level orientation-
tuned cells with small receptive fields (see Wenderoth & van der Zwan 1989 for a
review of spatial and temporal dissociations between the repulsive and attractive
components of tilt aftereffects). Clifford (in this volume) proposes a dual-process

model of orientation adaptation, in which response-based desensitization contributes to the repulsive component of tilt aftereffects (as described in this chapter; see Fig. 5.1), whereas the adaptive re-scaling of orientation-tuning bandwidths contributes to both the repulsive and attractive components. Regardless of the exact origin of the attractive component of tilt aftereffects, multi-channel coding is clearly associated with its characteristic anti-symmetric tuning curves centered at the test orientation (Fig. 5.8(A)).

If the geometric features revealed by the SAEs are also multi-channel coded by multiple neural units tuned to intermediate feature values, they should also exhibit similar anti-symmetric tuning curves centered at the test feature value. This prediction is illustrated in Fig. 5.8(B) for aspect ratio. If the adaptor aspect ratio is identical to the test aspect ratio, no aftereffects should occur (the node). If the adaptor aspect ratio is made flatter than the test aspect ratio, the after-effect should make the test aspect ratio appear taller than it is, causing the tuning curve to rise above the veridical test aspect ratio. In contrast, if the adaptor aspect ratio is made taller than the test aspect ratio, the aftereffect should make the test aspect ratio appear flatter than it is, causing the tuning curve to fall below the veridical test aspect ratio. Note that the tunings illustrated in Fig. 5.8(B) are broader than in Fig. 5.8(A) because SAEs tend to have broad feature tunings (Suzuki & Rivest 1998; Suzuki 2001).

Qualitatively different tuning curves are expected if aspect ratio is opponent-coded based on the relative activity of the two opponent pools of cells, one broadly tuned to flat aspect ratios and the other broadly tuned to tall aspect ratios (Regan & Hamstra 1992; Suzuki & Rivest 1998; see Fig. 5.7(A)). A neutral adaptor would then adapt the flat and tall pools of cells equally, resulting in no aspect-ratio aftereffect. Thus, unlike in multi-channel coding where the node should follow the test aspect ratio (Fig. 5.8(B)), in opponent coding, the node of the tuning curve should be fixed at the neutral aspect ratio regardless of the test aspect ratio (Fig. 5.8(C)). A flat adaptor would preferentially adapt the flat-tuned pool of cells, making the test aspect ratio appear taller than it is, causing the tuning curve to rise above the veridical test aspect ratio. In contrast, a tall adaptor would preferentially adapt the tall-tuned pool of cells, making the test aspect ratio appear flatter than it is, causing the tuning curve to fall below the veridical test aspect ratio. Thus, if aspect ratio is opponent-coded, all tuning curves should be anti-symmetric about the neutral aspect ratio regardless of the test aspect ratio (Fig. 5.8(C)).

When a series of tuning curves was obtained for aspect ratio aftereffects by orthogonally varying aspect ratios of adaptor and test patterns in one study (Suzuki & Rivest 1998), the shapes of the obtained tuning curves, with their nodes occurring consistently at or near the neutral aspect ratio (Fig. 5.9), were largely consistent with those predicted by opponent coding (Fig. 5.8(C)), and clearly inconsistent with those predicted by multi-channel coding (Fig. 5.8(B)). Recent single-cell results by Kayaert et al. (2004) also support the idea that geometric features such as taper, convexity, and curvature may be opponent-coded in IT in a manner illustrated in Fig. 5.7. First, the IT cells they studied exhibited

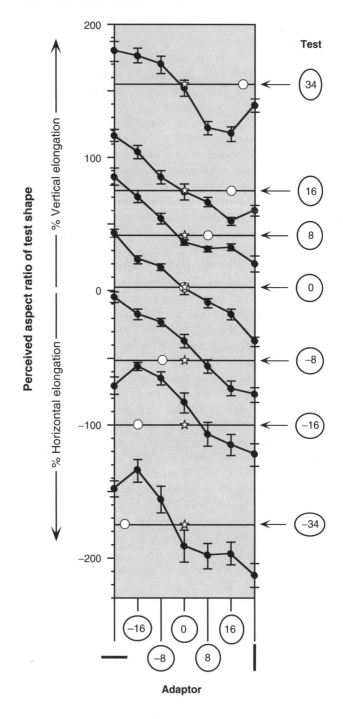

FIG. 5.9 Tuning curves for aspect-ratio aftereffects when the aspect ratios of the adaptor and test shapes were varied orthogonally (data from one observer shown). Aspect ratios were measured as % elongation, ((long axis − short axis)/short axis) × 100%, with positive values indicating vertical elongation and negative values indicating horizontal elongation. The adaptor and test shapes (3.5° in average diameter and presented at 6° eccentricity) were separated by 5°, and were presented in a rapid temporal sequence (see Fig. 5.2); the perceived aspect ratio was measured using a method of adjustment as in Suzuki and Cavanagh (1998). In the figure, the adaptor shapes are illustrated at the bottom and the test shapes on the right (with their % elongations indicated inside). The horizontal line drawn next to each test shape represents its perceived aspect ratio without adaptation (i.e. the baseline); note that the perceived aspect ratio of a briefly flashed (and backward-masked) ellipse tends to be exaggerated (consistent with Suzuki & Cavanagh, 1998). All of the tuning curves obtained for the six test aspect ratios (±8%, ±16%, and ±34% elongations) were more or less anti-symmetric about the neutral (circular) adaptor with baseline crossings (nodes) occurring at or near the neutral adaptor, generally consistent with the opponent-coding hypothesis (see open stars and Fig. 5.8(C) for the predicted baseline crossings), and inconsistent with the multi-channel-coding hypothesis (see open circles and Fig. 5.9(B) for the predicted baseline crossings).

←——————————————————————————————————————

relatively independent tunings for these three geometric features, suggesting that taper, convexity, and curvature are encoded as distinct global dimensions. Second, many of the recorded IT cells responded more strongly to more extreme taper, convexity, and curvature, consistent with the opponent tuning curves illustrated in Fig. 5.7.

There is also evidence that face identity may be partly opponent-coded. Research on identification of caricatured and anti-caricatured faces suggests that faces are encoded in terms of their specific deviations from the norm in the multi-dimensional space defined by face attributes (e.g. Lee *et al.* 2000). Demonstrations of face-specific aftereffects have provided evidence that various face-related dimensions such as simple deformations (e.g. Webster & MacLin 1999), socially relevant dimensions such as face gender, race, expression (e.g. Webster *et al.* 2004), and attractiveness (Rhodes *et al.* 2003) as well as dimensions along which individual faces deviate from the norm (e.g. Leopold *et al.* 2001; Rhodes *et al.* this volume), are represented by a type of central-tendency coding. Significantly, whereas adaptation to a face deviated from the norm caused a distortion on a test face in the opposite direction, adaptation to the norm face caused little distortion (e.g. Webster & MacLin 1999; Leopold *et al.* 2001, also see Leopold and Bondar in this volume). This is similar to aspect ratio aftereffects shown in Fig. 5.8(C) and 5.9 (exhibiting little after-effect from a neutral-aspect-ratio adaptor). As discussed above, this property is consistent with opponent-coding tuning functions such as those shown in Fig. 5.7. In fact, Rhodes *et al.* (this volume) have applied the Regan and Hamstra's opponent coding model to norm-based coding of face-related features.

In distinguishing opponent coding and multi-channel coding, it is notewor-thy that, in the case of a circular dimension such as line orientation (i.e. 180° rotation takes you back to 0° rotation), "opponent-type" aftereffects can be obtained from multi-channel coding. For example, Clifford (this volume) found that following adaptation to a specific orientation, the dots in a random-dot pat-tern appeared to be grouped into the orthogonal orientation. This orthogonal aftereffect is consistent with multi-channel coding of perceived orientation if one assumes that (1) the central tendency is computed as a vector summation along the entire circular dimension of orientation and (2) the orientation-to-vector-direction mapping is such that orthogonal orientations are represented by vectors with opposite directions (see Clifford, this volume, for details). The latter implies an opponent relationship between orthogonal orientations. However, the coding of perceived orientation is still based on central tendency computed over multiple orientation channels with no orientation being uniquely neutral. This is qualitatively different from the opponent coding discussed here (also in Rhodes *et al.* this volume, and Regan & Hamstra 1992; see Fig. 5.7), which is based on two opponent pools of cells and characterized by a special neutral value (e.g. neutral aspect ratio) adaptation which produces no aftereffects.

5.8 Opponent Coding and Perceptual Multi-stability

Indirect support for opponent codings of global skew, taper, curvature, and con-vexity has been found using a rather different experimental paradigm involving the phenomena of perceptual multi-stability. While voluntary attention allows for deliberate selection of behaviorally relevant patterns, the process of pattern selection also sustains meta-stable representations in that visual awareness spontaneously shifts from one object to another or from one image interpreta-tion to another, in the absence of voluntary attention shifts or eye movements (see Attneave 1971; Taylor & Aldridge 1974; and Leopold & Logothetis 1999 for reviews). To study the dynamic process of spontaneous pattern selection involving specific sets of shapes, Suzuki & Grabowecky (2002a) devised stimuli that induced multi-stable binocular rivalry in which the perceived image sponta-neously (and clearly) changed among four shapes.

In binocular rivalry, while the stimulus remains constant, perception changes dramatically due to perturbations in neural responses arising from the conflict-ing signals coming from the two eyes (see Levelt 1965, Blake 1989, and Blake & Logothetis 2002 for reviews). These perturbations could arise from non-linear inhibitory neural interactions coupled with adaptation and stochastic neural noise (e.g. Sugie 1982; Lehky 1988; Blake 1989; Laing & Chow 2002; Kim *et al.* 2005), synchronization and de-synchronization of neural activity (e.g. Lumer 1998; Srinivasan *et al.* 1999; Fries *et al.* 2001; Suzuki & Grabowecky 2002b), and/or from some other yet-to-be specified factors. In conventional binocular rivalry, perception alternates between only two images (one presented to the left eye and the other presented to the right eye). Significantly, in the specific stimulus configurations used by Suzuki and Grabowecky (2002a), perception alternated among four distinct shapes, allowing examinations of transition probabilities (i.e. how visual awareness moves among multiple possible percepts) as well as temporal dynamics (i.e. the duration of each percept) of spontaneous pattern selection.

Note that activities of opponent-tuned pools of cells involved in a specific type of opponent coding (e.g. convex-tuned cells and concave-tuned cells) are likely to be highly interactive. Anatomically, inhibitory connections within IT tend to be short range, limiting strong interactions to primarily within a columnar region (where cells share related pattern selectivity) or across neighboring columns (e.g. Fujita & Fujita 1996; Y. Wang *et al.* 2000). Functionally, mutually inhibitory interactions between opponent-tuned pools of cells would enhance sensitivity for categorical discriminations (e.g. convex versus concave) by facilitating winner-take-all type flipping to one or the other category. If opponent-tuned pools of cells that mediate each opponent coding are indeed anatomically proximal and highly interactive, spontaneous perceptual transitions might be more prevalent between opponent shapes than between non-opponent shapes. Suzuki and Grabowecky (2002a) confirmed this prediction. A perceived image was more likely to change to an opponent shape (as well as to a shape with a similar degree of symmetry). In particular, when they used multistable stimuli in which perception changed among shapes with opposite skew, taper, curvature, and convexity, perceptual transitions were elevated between each pair of opponent shapes. For example, perception was more likely to change from a convex shape to a concave shape or from a left-curved shape to a right-curved shape, and less likely to change from a convex shape to a curved shape. Such phenomena of "perceptual trapping" within a pair of opponent shapes provided indirect support for opponent codings of skew, taper, curvature, and convexity, corroborating the SAE results (also see Leopold 2003; Rubin 2003; Suzuki & Grabowecky 2003a).

5.9 Putting the Codings Together

Ultimately, coding of perceived patterns should be understood on the basis of the overall neural activity throughout the ventral visual pathway (V1 → V2 → V4 → IT). Research on neural pattern tunings and visual aftereffects so far suggests that local orientation and spatial frequency are multi-channel coded in V1 (and up to V4), and certain global configurations of oriented contours such as skew, taper, curvature, aspect ratio, convexity, and relative size, as well as face-specific features, are opponent-coded in IT. Perhaps, any complex geometric features for which a behaviorally significant category boundary lies within a continuum of geometric variations might be opponent-coded in IT. Other object properties that are not conducive to coding in terms of systematic geometric variations around a norm, including highly trained patterns such as English letters and Chinese characters, are probably coded as broadly distributed patterns of activity; the extent of distributed coding might be within IT (e.g. Tsunoda *et al.* 2001), perhaps involving the left inferior temporo-occipital region (Farah 1990), and/or across temporal lobe visual areas (e.g. Haxby *et al.* 2000, 2001), possibly involving lower visual areas such as V4 where there has as yet been no clear evidence of multi-channel or opponent codings of specific geometric features (see Sections 5.1 and 5.3).

As multiple visual areas are activated simultaneously upon viewing almost any visual pattern, a question arises as to how activities in different visual areas contribute to pattern perception. For example, in viewing a vase, local orientations of the luminance-defined contour edges would be multi-channel coded in V1 and V2, local curvatures of those contours and their configurations would be analyzed in V2 and V4, the overall convexity would be opponent-coded in IT, and other image properties such as brightness, color, texture, and 3D part structure (e.g. consisting of a long neck and a bulged base) would be coded (either separately or collectively) as patterns of distributed activity within specific visual areas and/or across multiple relevant areas. It is still largely a mystery as to how all these distributed parallel neural activities result in the rich visual awareness that people experience even in the simple act of appreciating a vase. Nevertheless, if the visual system is designed to adaptively optimize pattern perception for a given task, it is feasible that perception might be dominated by the neural activity involved in the type of coding(s) that maximizes the task performance. In other words, visual awareness might be flexible in "focusing on" whatever coding provides the highest signal-to-noise ratio with respect to the given task (e.g. Ahissar & Hochstein 2002; Paradiso 2002).

It is well-known that almost any perceptual performance (e.g. selecting a target pattern and identifying it) improves with practice, generally with a rapid initial improvement followed by a more gradual long-term improvement (e.g. Newell & Rosenbloom 1981; Heathcote *et al.* 2000). Depending on the task demand, a variety of mechanisms appear to contribute to practice effects, including (1) fine-tuning of the relevant feature detectors and their interactions at different levels of processing, (2) facilitation of attentional selection of task-relevant features while promoting grouping and suppression of irrelevant distractors, and (3) formation of increasingly task-optimized categorical representations (see Suzuki & Goolsby 2003 for a brief review). Practice effects might also optimize specific population codings by adjusting input weightings and decision criteria (e.g. Morgan 1992; Poggio *et al.* 1992). These various optimization processes engage once the observer becomes reasonably comfortable with the task. At the very beginning of performing a task, however, an important process might be to *hone in on the task-optimum coding* (this idea is articulated in the reverse-hierarchy model proposed by Ahissar and Hochstein [e.g. Ahissar & Hochstein 2002; Hochstein & Ahissar 2002], and is also related to the phenomena of abrupt perceptual learning [e.g. Ahissar & Hochstein 1997; Rubin *et al.* 1997]).

For example, suppose the observer discriminates shapes with overall convexity or concavity, and the shapes consist of variously oriented local contour segments. On the one hand, if one were to perform a convex/concave discrimination task while the position and size of the shapes were varied, one's perception should "access" the opponent coding of convexity in IT, which is sensitive to convexity but tolerant for translation and scaling. On the other hand, if one were to perform a fine-grained orientation discrimination task on a particular contour segment at a particular location, one's perception should then access the high-resolution multi-channel coding of local orientation, which is unique to V1 (see Paradiso 2002). If a given task requires a specific geometric coding and the task-optimum coding is selected on the basis of its enhanced activation (e.g. Huk & Heeger 2000), then the initial process of selecting coding might be observed in a brain imaging study in terms of the relatively extensive and rapidly-changing patterns of neural activity at the very beginning of performing the task, quickly converging to localized and stable activity after the rapid initial adjustment period (see Petersen *et al.* 1998 for related results). The process of selecting a task-optimum coding is likely to be especially important when a task is novel. Perhaps poor perceptual learners are those who fail to select the optimum coding for the task; failing at this initial stage would not allow the process of gradual optimization and calibration of the coding to proceed.

5.10 Summary

An ultimate question of visual pattern perception is how neural activity spreads throughout the ventral visual pathway (with concurrent responses to different components and aspects of retinal stimulation) to generate a seemingly coherent and unitary visual awareness of objects and scenes. Extensive research on local aftereffects has linked the systematic organization of neural tunings for orientation and spatial frequency in early cortical visual areas to the central-tendency codings of the perception of those features. Organizations of neural tunings, however, become ambiguous when higher cortical visual areas are examined as cells in those areas integrate a variety of combinations of lower-level signals to achieve increasingly complex and heterogeneous pattern tunings. Indeed, common objects appear to be encoded primarily on the basis of complex and distributed patterns of neural activity. Individual clusters of neural activity might represent parts, combinations of parts, or global aspects of an object. It is largely unclear how these distributed clusters of activity, individually and collectively, map on to different geometric characteristics of an object (e.g. part shape, part structure, global geometry).

Recent demonstrations of global-shape aftereffects suggest that at least some well-learned global geometric attributes are central-tendency coded in high-level visual areas, perhaps because central-tendency codings afford fast and fine-tuned discriminations along the coded dimensions. For example, shape aftereffects (SAEs) using brief stimulus sequences have revealed central-tendency codings for a set of global geometric features, including skew, taper, curvature, aspect ratio, convexity, relative size, and face orientation in depth (Fig. 5.3).

The fact that these geometric features correspond to those that are systematically distorted when surfaces are rotated in depth (Fig. 5.6) suggests that central-tendency codings of these features might be an integral part of the mechanisms that mediate pictorial-cue-based extraction of 3D surface orientation and viewpoint normalization. Other researchers have demonstrated aftereffects for face-specific features, revealing central-tendency codings of face-related attributes. Interestingly, while low-level central-tendency codings of local orientation and spatial frequency are mediated by cells tuned to multiple intermediate feature values (e.g. Fig. 5.1)–multi-channel coding (perhaps, optimized for fine-grained analyses of local details), the tuning properties of global aftereffects suggest that each high-level central-tendency coding is mediated primarily by two opponent pools of cells broadly tuned to opposite feature directions across a norm (e.g. Fig. 5.7)–opponent coding (perhaps, optimized for norm-based categorical discriminations of complex patterns).

It is likely that different types of codings, such as general-purpose codings by distributed patterns of neural activity, specialized codings including central-tendency codings (e.g. multi-channel coding and opponent coding), as well as temporal codings based on the precise dynamics of neural firing (e.g. Ferster & Spruston 1995; Mechler *et al.* 1998; Sugase *et al.* 1999; Ikegaya *et al.* 2004), modify and/or develop adaptively with experience. A challenge is to specify what types of interactions among stimuli, perceptual demands, and preexisting neural circuits lead to developments of different codings, and how those codings are anatomically and physiologically organized within and across different areas of the brain. An equally challenging task is to understand how different codings, spread across the ventral visual pathway, selectively and/or interactively contribute to the rich perceptual experience of visual objects and scenes.

Acknowledgements

I would like to thank Marcia Grabowecky for her invaluable comments on early versions of the manuscript. This work was supported by a National Institutes of Health grant EY014110.

References

Abdi, H., Jiang, F., O'Toole, A.J., & Haxby, J. (2003). Pattern-based analyses for brain imaging data: applications to face processing. *Abstracts of the Psychonomic Society*, 8, 26.

Ahissar, M., & Hochstein, S. (1997). Task difficulty and the specificity of perceptual learning. *Nature*, *387*, 401–6.

Ahissar, M., & Hochstein, S. (2002). The role of attention in learning simple visual tasks. In M. Fahle, & T. Poggio (ed.), *Perceptual Learning* (pp. 253–72). Cambridge, MA: MIT Press.

Albrecht, D.G., Farrar, S.B., & Hamilton, D.B. (1984). Spatial contrast adaptation characteristics of neurons recorded in the cat's visual cortex. *Journal of Physiology*, *347*, 713–39.

Attneave, F. (1971). Multistability in perception. *Scientific American, 225*, 63–71.

Biedermen, I. (1987). Recognition by components: a theory of human image understanding. *Psychological Review, 94*, 115–47.

Blake, R. (1989). A neural theory of binocular rivalry. *Psychological Review, 96*, 145–167.

Blake, R., & Logothetis, N.K. (2002). Visual competition. *Nature Neuroscience, 3*, 1–11.

Blakemore, C, & Nachmias, J. (1971). The orientational specificity of two visual after-effects. *Journal of Physiology, 213*, 157–74.

Blakemore, C., Nachmias, J., & Sutton, P. (1970). The perceived spatial frequency shift: Evidence for frequency selective neurons in the human brain. *Journal of Physiology, 210*, 727–50.

Blakemore, C., & Sutton, P. (1969). Size adaptation: A new aftereffect. *Science, 166*, 245–7.

Bonds, A.B. (1991). Temporal dynamics of contrast gain in single cells of the cat striate cortex. *Visual Neuroscience, 6*, 239–55.

Braddick, O., Campbell, F.W., & Atkinson, J. (1978). Channels in vision: Basic aspects. In R. Held, H.W. Leibowitz, & L.-H. Teuber (ed.), *Handbook of Sensory Physiology: Vol. 8. Perception* (pp. 3–38). Berlin: Springer-Verlag.

Brincat, S.L., & Connor, C.E. (2004). Underlying principles of visual shape selectivity in posterior inferotemporal cortex. *Nature Neuroscience, 8*(7), 880–6.

Cameron, E.L., Tai, J.C., & Carrasco, M. (2002). Covert attention affects the psychometric function of contrast sensitivity. *Vision Research, 42*, 949–67.

Campbell, F. W., & Maffei, L. (1971). The tilt after-effect: a fresh look. *Vision Research, 11*, 833–40.

Carandini, M., Movshon, J.A., & Ferster, D. (1998). Pattern adaptation and cross-orientation interactions in the primary visual cortex. *Neuropharmacology, 37*, 501–11.

Chelazzi, L., Duncan, J., Miller, E. K., & Desimone, R. (1998). Responses of neurons in inferior temporal cortex during memory-guided visual search. *Journal of Neurophysiology, 80*(6), 2918–40.

Cheng, K., Hasegawa, T., Saleem, K.S., & Tanaka, K. (1994). Comparison of neural sensitivity for stimulus speed, length, and contrast in the prestriate visual cortical areas V4 and MT of the macaque monkey. *Journal of Neurophysiology, 71*(6), 2269–80.

De Valois, R.L., Albrecht, D.G., & Thorell, L.G. (1982). Spatial frequency selectivity of cells in macaque visual cortex. *Vision Research, 22*, 545–59.

Dehaene, S., Naccache, L., Le Clec'H, G., Koechlin, E., Mueller, M., Dahaene-Lambertz, G. *et al.* (1998). Imaging unconscious semantic priming. *Nature, 395*, 597–600.

Deneve, S., Latham, P.E., & Pouget, A. (1999). Reading population codes: a neural implementation of ideal observers. *Nature Neuroscience, 2*(8), 740–45.

Desimone, R., Albright, T.D., Gross, C.G., & Bruce, C. (1984). Stimulus-selective properties of inferior temporal neurons in the macaque. *Journal of Neuroscience, 8*, 2051–62.

Desimone, R., & Duncan, J. (1995). Neural mechanisms of selective visual attention. *Annual Review of Neuroscience, 18*, 193–222.

Desimone, R., & Gross, C.G. (1979). Visual areas in the temporal cortex of the macaque. *Brain Research, 178*, 363–80.

Desimone, R., & Schein, S.J. (1987). Visual properties of neurons in area V4 of the macaque: sensitivity to stimulus form. *Journal of Neurophysiology, 57*(3), 835–68.

Dow, B.M., Snyder, A.Z., Vautin, R.G., & Bauer, R. (1981). Magnification factor and receptive field size in foveal striate cortex of the monkey. *Experimental Brain Research, 44*, 213–28.

Enns, J.T., & Di Lollo, V. (2000). What's new in visual masking? *Trends in Cognitive Sciences*, *4*(9), 345–52.

Epstein, R., Graham, K.S., & Downing, P.E. (2003). View-point specific scene representations in human parahippocampal cortex. *Neuron*, *37*, 865–76.

Epstein, R., Harris, A., Stanley, D., & Kanwisher, N. (1999). The parahippocampal place area: recognition, navigation, or encoding? *Neuron*, *23*, 115–25.

Fang, F., & He, S. (2004). Viewer-centered object representations in human visual system revealed by viewpoint aftereffect. *Abstracts of the Vision Sciences Society*, *4*, 71.

Farah, M.J. (1990). *Visual Agnosia: Disorders of Object Vision and What They Tell Us About Normal Vision*. Cambridge, MA: MIT Press.

Ferster, D. & Spruston, N. (1995). Cracking the neuronal code. *Science*, *270*, 756–7.

Foster, K.H., Gaska, J.P., Nagler, M., & Polen, D.A. (1985). Spatial and temporal frequency selectivity of neurons in visual cortical areas V1 and V2 of the macaque monkey. *Journal of Physiology*, *365*, 331–68.

Fries, P., Reynolds, J.H., Rorie, A.E., & Desimone, R. (2001). Modulation of oscillatory neural synchronization by selective visual attention. *Science*, *291*, 1560–63.

Fujita, I., & Fujita, T. (1996). Intrinsic connections in the macaque inferior temporal cortex. *Journal of Computational Neurology*, *368*, 467–86.

Fujita, I., Tanaka, K., Ito, M., & Cheng, K. (1992). Columns for visual features of objects in monkey inferotemporal cortex. *Nature*, *360*, 343–6.

Gallant, J.L., Connor, C.E., Rakshit, S., Lewis, J.W., & Van Essen, D.C. (1996). Neural responses to polar, hyperbolic, and cartesian gratings in area V4 of the macaque monkey. *Journal of Neurophysiology*, *76*(4), 2718–39.

Gattass, R., Sousa, A.P.B., & Gross, C.G. (1988). Visuotopic organization and extent of V3 and V4 of the macaque. *Journal of Neuroscience,* *8*(6), 1831–45.

Gauthier, I. (2000). What constrains the organization of the ventral temporal cortex? *Trends in Cognitive Sciences*, *4*(1), 1–2.

Gauthier, I., Curran, T., Curby, K.M., & Collins, D. (2003). Perceptual interference supports a non-modular account of face processing. *Nature Neuroscience*, *6*(4), 428–32.

Gauthier, I., Skudlarski, P., Gore, J.C., & Anderson, A.W. (2000). Expertise for cars and birds recruits brain areas involved in face recognition. *Nature Neuroscience*, *3*(2), 191–7.

Gauthier, I., Tarr, M.J., Anderson, A.W., Skudlarski, P., & Gore, J.C. (1999). Activation of the middle fusiform 'face area' increases with expertise in recognizing novel objects. *Nature Neuroscience*, *2*(6), 568–73.

Geisler, W.S., & Albrecht, D.G. (1997). Visual cortex neurons in monkey and cats: Detection, discrimination, and identification. *Visual Neuroscience*, *14*, 897–919.

Gibson, J.J., & Radner, M. (1937). Adaptation, aftereffect and contrast in the perception of tilted lines. *Journal of Experimental Psychology*, *20*, 453–67.

Gross, C.G., Rocha-Miranda, C.E., & Bender, D.B. (1972). Visual properties of neurons in inferotemporal cortex of the macaque. *Journal of Neurophysiology*, *35*, 96–111.

Gur, M., Kagan, I., & Snodderly, M.D. (2004). Lack of short-term adaptation in V1 cells of the alert monkey. *Abstracts of the Vision Sciences Society*, *4*, 255.

Hammond, P., Pomfrett, C.J.D., & Ahmed, B. (1989). Neural motion after-effects in the cat's striate cortex: orientation selectivity. *Vision Research*, *29*(12), 1671–83.

Hanazawa, A., & Komatsu, H. (2001). Influence of the direction of elemental luminance gradients on the responses of V4 cells to textured surfaces. *Journal of Neuroscience*, *21*(12), 4490–7.

Hasselmo, M.E., Rolls, E.T., & Baylis, G.C. (1989). The role of expression and identity in the face-selective responses of neurons in the temporal visual cortex of the monkey. *Behavioral Brain Research*, *32*, 203–18.

Haxby, J.V., Gobbini, M.I., Furey, M.L., Ishai, A., Schouten, J.L., & Pietrini, P. (2001). Distributed and overlapping representations of faces and objects in ventral visual cortex. *Science*, *293*, 2425–30.

Haxby, J.V., Ishai, A., Chao, L.L., Ungerleider, L.G., & Martin, A. (2000). Object-form topology in the ventral temporal lobe. *Trends in Cognitive Sciences*, *4*(1), 3–4.

Heathcote, A., Brown, S., & Mewhort, D.J.K. (2000). The power law repealed: the case for an exponential law of practice. *Psychonomic Bulletin & Review*, *7*, 185–207.

Hegdé, J., & Van Essen, D.C. (2000). Selectivity for complex shapes in primate visual area V2. *Journal of Neuroscience*, *20*, RC61.

Held, R., & Shattuck, S.R. (1971). Color- and edge-sensitive channels in the human visual system: tuning for orientation. *Science*, *174*, 314–16.

Hikosaka, K. (1999). Tolerances of responses to visual patterns in neurons of the posterior inferotemporal cortex in the macaque against changing stimulus size and orientation, and deleting patterns. *Behavioral Brain Research*, *100*, 67–76.

Hochstein, S., & Ahissar, M. (2002). View from the top: hierarchies and reverse hierarchies in the visual system. *Neuron*, *36*, 791–804.

Hubel, D.H., & Wiesel, T.N. (1968). Receptive fields and functional architecture of monkey striate cortex. *Journal of Physiology*, *195*, 215–43.

Huk, A.C., & Heeger, D.J. (2000). Task-related modulation of visual cortex. *Journal of Neurophysiology*, *83*, 3525–36.

Ikegaya, Y., Aaron, G., Cossart, R., Aronov, D., Lampl, I., Ferster, D. *et al.* (2004). Synfire chains and cortical songs: temporal modules of cortical activity. *Science*, *304*, 559–64.

Ito, M., Fujita, I., Tamura, H., & Tanaka, K. (1994). Processing of contrast polarity of visual images in inferotemporal cortex of the macaque monkey. *Cerebral Cortex*, *5*, 499–508.

Ito, M., Tamura, H., Fujita, I., & Tanaka, K. (1995). Size and position invariance of neuronal responses in monkey inferotemporal cortex. *Journal of Neurophysiology*, *73*(1), 218–26.

Kanwisher, N.G., McDermott, J., & Chun, M.M. (1997). The fusiform face area: a module in human extrastriate cortex specialized for face perception. *Journal of Neuroscience*, *17*, 4301–11.

Kayaert, G., Op de Beeck, H., Biederman, I., & Vogels, R. (2004). Shape dimension-dependent coding of macaque IT neurons. *Abstracts of the Vision Sciences Society*, *4*, 70.

Kayaert, G., Biederman, I., & Vogels, R. (2003). Shape tuning in macaque inferior temporal cortex. *Journal of Neuroscience*, *23*(7), 3016–27.

Kim, Y.-J., Grabowecky, M., & Suzuki, S. (2005). Stochastic resonance in binocular rivalry. Submitted.

Kobatake, E., Wang, G., & Tanaka, K. (1998). Effects of shape-discrimination training on the selectivity of inferotemporal cells in adult monkeys. *Journal of Neurophysiology*, *80*, 324–30.

Kohler, W., & Wallach, H. (1944). Figural aftereffects: an investigation of visual processes. *Proceedings of the American Philosophical Society*, *88*, 269–357.

Komatsu, H., Ideura, Y., Kaji, S., & Yamane, S. (1992). Color selectivity of neurons in the inferior temporal cortex of the awake macaque monkey. *Journal of Neuroscience*, *12*(2), 408–24.

Lamme, V.A.F. (2001). Blindsight: the role of feedforward and feedback corticocortical connections. *Acta Psychologica*, *107*, 209–228.

Lamme, V.A.F., Rodriguez-Rodriguez, V., & Spekreijse, H. (1999). Separate processing dynamics for texture elements, boundaries and surfaces in primary visual cortex of the macaque monkey. *Cerebral Cortex*, *9*, 406–413.

Lee, C., Rohrer, W.H., & Sparks, D.L. (1988). Population coding of saccadic eye movements by neurons in the superior colliculus. *Nature*, *332*, 357–60.

Lee, K., Byatt, G., & Rhodes, G. (2000). Caricature effects, distinctiveness, and identification: testing the face-space framework. *Psychological Science*, *11*(5), 379–85.

Lehky, S.R. (1988). An astable multivibrator model of binocular rivalry. *Perception*, *17*, 215–28.

Leopold, D.A. (2003). Visual perception: shaping what we see. *Current Biology*, *13*, R10–R12.

Leopold, D.A., & Logothetis, N.K. (1999). Multistable phenomena: changing views in perception. *Trends in Cognitive Sciences*, *3*, 254–64.

Leopold, D.A., O'Toole, A.J., Vetter, T., & Blanz, V. (2001). Prototype-referenced shape encoding revealed by high-level after-effects. *Nature Neuroscience*, *4*(1), 89–94.

Levelt, W.J.M. (1965). *On Binocular Rivalry*. Soesterberg, The Netherlands: Institute for Perception RVO-TNO.

Leventhal, A.G., Wang, Y., Schmolesky, M.T., & Zhou, Y. (1998). Neural correlates of boundary perception. *Visual Neuroscience*, *15*, 1107–18.

Levitt, J.B., Kiper, D.C., & Movshon, J.A. (1994). Receptive fields and functional architecture of macaque V2. *Journal of Neurophysiology*, *71*(6), 2517–42.

Laing, C.R., & Chow, C.C. (2002). A spiking neuron model for binocular rivalry. *Journal of Computational Neuroscience*, *12*, 39–53.

Logothetis, N.K., Pauls, J., & Poggio, T. (1995). Shape representation in the inferior temporal cortex of monkeys. *Current Biology*, *5*, 552–63.

Logothetis, N.K., & Sheinberg, D.L. (1996). Visual object recognition. *Annual Review of Neuroscience*, *19*, 577–621.

Luck, S.J., Chelazzi, L., Hillyard, S., & Desimone, R. (1997). Neural mechanisms of spatial selective attention in areas V1, V2, and V4 of macaque visual cortex. *Journal of Neurophysiology*, *77*, 24–42.

Lueschow, A., Miller, E.K., & Desimone, R. (1994). Inferior temporal mechanisms for invariant object recognition. *Cerebral Cortex*, *5*, 523–31.

Lumer, E.D. (1998). A neural model of binocular integration and rivalry based on the coordination of action-potential timing in primary visual cortex. *Cerebral Cortex*, *8*, 553–61.

Magnussen, S., & Kurtenbach, W. (1980). Linear summation of tilt illusion and tilt aftereffect. *Vision Research*, *20*, 39–42.

Marr, D. (1982). *Vision*. San Francisco: Freeman.

McAdams, C.J., & Maunsell, J.H.R. (1999). Effects of attention on orientation-tuning functions of single neurons in macaque cortical area V4. *Journal of Neuroscicence*, *19*(1), 431–41.

Mechler, F., Victor, J.D., Purpura, K.P., & Shapley, R. (1998). Robust temporal coding of contrast by V1 neurons for transient but not for steady-state stimuli. *Journal of Neuroscience*, *18*(16), 6583–98.

Miller, E.K., Gochin, P.M., & Gross, C.G. (1993a). Suppression of visual responses of neurons in inferior temporal cortex of the awake macaque monkey by addition of a second stimulus. *Brain Research*, *616*, 25–9.

Miller, E.K., Li, L, & Desimone, R. (1993b). Activity of neurons in anterior inferior temporal cortex during a short-term memory task. *Journal of Neuroscience, 13*(4), 1460–78.

Mishkin, M., Ungerleider, L.G., & Macko, K.A. (1983). Object vision and spatial vision: two central pathways. *Trends in Neurosciences, 6*, 414–17.

Mitchel, D.E. & Muir, D.W. (1976). Does the tilt after-effect occur in the oblique meridian? *Vision Research, 16*, 609–13.

Moran, J., & Desimone, R. (1985). Selective attention gates visual processing in extrastriate cortex. *Science, 229*, 782–4.

Morgan, M.J. (1992). Hyperacuity of those in the know. *Current Biology, 2*(9), 481–2.

Muller, J.R., Metha, A.B., Krauskopf, J., & Lennie, P. (1999). Rapid adaptation in visual cortex to the structure of images. *Science, 285*, 1405–8.

Newell, A., & Rosenbloom, P.S. (1981). Mechanisms of skill acquisition and the power law of practice. In J.R. Anderson (ed.), *Cognitive Skills and Their Acquisition* (pp. 1–55). Hillsdale, NJ: Erlbaum.

Nothdurft, H-C., Gallant, J.L., & Van Essen, D.C. (1999). Response modulation by texture surround in primate area V1: Correlates of "popout" under anesthesia. *Visual Neuroscience, 16*, 15–34.

O'Shea, R.P., Wilson, R.G., & Duckett, A. (1993). The effects of contrast reversal on the direct, indirect, and interocularly-transferred tilt aftereffect. *New Zealand Journal of Psychology, 22*(2), 94–100.

O'Toole, B., & Wenderoth, P. (1977). The tilt illusion: Repulsion and attraction effects in the oblique meridian. *Vision Research, 17*(3), 367–74.

Oram, M.W., & Perrett, D.I. (1992). Time course of neural responses discriminating different views of the face and head. *Journal of Neurophysiology, 68*(1), 70–84.

Paradiso, M.A. (2002). Perceptual and neuronal correspondence in primary visual cortex. *Current Opinion in Neurobiology, 12*, 155–161.

Pascal-Leone, A., & Walsh, V. (2001). Fast backprojections from the motion to the primary visual area necessary for visual awareness. *Science, 292*, 510–21.

Pasupathy, A., & Connor, C.E. (1999). Responses to contour features in macaque area V4. *Journal of Neurophysiology, 82*, 2490–502.

Pasupathy, A., & Connor, C.E. (2001). Shape representation in area V4: position-specific tuning for boundary conformation. *Journal of Neurophysiology, 86*, 2505–19.

Peterhans, E., & von der Heydt, R. (1991). Subjective contours—bridging the gap between psychophysics and physiology. *Trends in Neurosciences, 14*, 112–9.

Petersen, S.E., van Mier, H., Fiez, J. A., & Raichle, M.E. (1998). The effects of practice on the functional anatomy of task performance. *Proceedings of the National Academy of Sciences USA, 95*, 853–60.

Poggio, T., Fahle, M., & Edelman, S. (1992). Fast perceptual learning in visual hyperacuity. *Science, 256*, 1018–21.

Regan, D., & Hamstra, S.J. (1992). Shape discrimination and the judgment of perfect symmetry: dissociation of shape from size. *Vision Research, 32*, 1845–64.

Reich, D.S., Mechler, F., & Victor, J.D. (2001). Temporal coding of contrast in primary visual cortex: when, what, and why. *Journal of Neurophysiology, 85*, 1039–50.

Reynolds, J.H., Chelazzi, L., & Desimone, R. (1999). Competitive mechanisms subserve attention in macaque areas V2 and V4. *Journal of Neuroscience, 19*(5), 1736–53.

Reynolds, J.H., & Desimone, R. (2003). Interacting roles of attention and visual salience in V4. *Neuron, 37*, 853–63.

Reynolds, J.H., Pasternak, T., & Desimone, R. (2000). Attention increases sensitivity of V4 neurons. *Neuron, 26,* 703–14.

Rhodes, G., Byatt, G., Michie, P.T., & Puce, A. (2004). Is the fusiform face area specialized for faces, individuation, or expert individuation? *Journal of Cognitive Neuroscience, 16*(2), 189–203.

Rhodes, G., Jeffery, L., Watson T.L., Clifford C.W.G., & Nakayama K. (2003). Fitting the mind to the world: face adaptation and attractiveness aftereffects. *Psychological Science, 14*(6), 558–66.

Riesenhuber, M., & Poggio, T. (2000). Models of object recognition. *Nature Neuroscience, 3,* 1199–204.

Rivest, J., Intriligator, J., Suzuki, S., & Warner, J. (1998). A shape distortion effect that is size invariant. *Investigative Ophthalmology & Visual Science (Suppl.), 39*(4), S853.

Rolls, E.T. & Baylis, G.C. (1986). Size and contrast have only small effects on the responses to faces of neurons in the cortex of the superior temporal sulcus of the monkey. *Experimental Brain Research, 65,* 38–48.

Rubin, N. (2003). Binocular rivalry and perceptual multi-stability. *Trends in Neurosciences, 26*(6), 289–91.

Rubin, N., Nakayama, K., & Shapley, R. (1997). Abrupt learning and retinal size specificity in illusory-contour perception. *Current Biology, 7,* 461–7.

Sagara, M., & Ohyama, T. (1957). Experimental studies of figural aftereffects in Japan. *Psychological Bulletin, 54,* 327–38.

Sato, T., Kawamura, T., & Iwai, E. (1980). Responsiveness of inferotemporal single units to visual pattern stimuli in monkeys performing discrimination. *Experimental Brain Research, 38,* 313–19.

Saul, A.B., & Cynader, M.S. (1989). Adaptation in single units in visual cortex: The tuning of aftereffects in the spatial domain. *Visual Neuroscience, 2,* 593–607.

Sclar, G., Lennie, P., & DePriest, D.D. (1989). Contrast adaptation in striate cortex of macaque. *Vision Research, 29*(7), 747–55.

Sclar, G., Maunsell, J.H.R., & Lennie, P. (1990). Coding of image contrast in central visual pathways of the macaque monkey. *Vision Research, 30*(1), 1–10.

Sheth, B.R., Sharma, J., Rao, S.C., & Sur, M. (1996). Orientation maps of subjective contours in visual cortex. *Science, 274,* 2110–5.

Sigala, N., & Logothetis, N.K. (2002). Visual categorization shapes feature selectivity in the primate temporal cortex. *Nature, 415,* 318–20.

Spivey, M.J., & Spirn, M.J. (2000). Selective visual attention modulates the direct tilt aftereffect. *Perception & Psychophysics, 62*(8), 1525–33.

Srinivasan, R., Russell, D.P., Edelman, G.M., & Tononi, G. (1999). Increased synchronization of neuromagnetic responses during conscious perception. *Journal of Neuroscience, 19*(13), 5435–48.

Sugase, Y., Yamane, S., Ueno, S., & Kawano, K. (1999). Global and fine information coded by single neurons in the temporal visual cortex. *Nature, 400,* 869–73.

Sugie, N. (1982). Neural models of brightness perception and retinal rivalry in binocular vision. *Biological Cybernetics, 43,* 13–21.

Suzuki, S. (1999). Influences of contexts on a non-retinotopic skew-contrast effect. *Investigative Ophthalmology & Visual Science (Suppl.), 40*(4), S812.

Suzuki, S. (2001). Attention-dependent brief adaptation to contour orientation: a high-level aftereffect for convexity? *Vision Research, 41*(28), 3883–902.

Suzuki, S. (2003a). Attentional selection of overlapped shapes: a study using brief shape aftereffects. *Vision Research, 43*, 549–61.

Suzuki, S. (2003b). The high and low of visual awareness. *Neuron, 39*, 883–84.

Suzuki, S., & Cavanagh, P. (1997). Focused attention distorts visual space: an attentional repulsion effect. *Journal of Experimental Psychology: Human Perception and Performance, 23*, 443–63.

Suzuki, S., & Cavanagh, P. (1998). A shape-contrast effect for briefly presented stimuli. *Journal of Experimental Psychology: Human Perception and Performance, 24*(5), 1315–41.

Suzuki, S., & Goolsby, B.A. (2003). Sequential priming is not constrained by the shape of long-term learning curves. *Perception & Psychophysics, 65*(4), 632–48.

Suzuki, S., & Grabowecky, M. (2002a). Evidence for perceptual "trapping" and adaptation in multistable binocular rivalry. *Neuron, 36*, 143–57.

Suzuki, S., & Grabowecky, M. (2002b). Overlapping features can be parsed on the basis of rapid temporal cues that produce stable emergent percepts. *Vision Research, 42*, 2669–92.

Suzuki, S., & Grabowecky, M. (2003a). Response: Binocular rivalry and perceptual multi-stability. *Trends in Neurosciences, 26*(6), 287–9.

Suzuki, S., & Grabowecky, M. (2003b). Attention during adaptation weakens negative afterimages. *Journal of Experimental Psychology: Human Perception and Performance, 29*(4), 793–807.

Suzuki, S., & Rivest, J. (1998). Interactions among "aspect-ratio channels." *Investigative Ophthalmology & Visual Science (Suppl.), 39*(4), S855.

Tanaka, K. (1996). Inferotemporal cortex and object vision. *Annual Review of Neuroscience, 19*, 109–39.

Taylor, M.M., & Aldridge, K.D. (1974). Stochastic processes in reversing figure perception. *Perception & Psychophysics, 16*(1), 9–27.

Tsunoda, K., Yamane, Y., Nishizaki, M., & Tanifuji, M. (2001). Complex objects are represented in macaque inferotemporal cortex by the combination of feature columns. *Nature Neuroscience, 4*(8), 832–8.

Ullman, S. (1998). Three-dimensional object recognition based on the combination of views. *Cognition, 67*, 21–44.

Ungerleider, L.G., & Mishkin, M. (1982). Two cortical visual systems. In D.J. Ingle, M.A. Goodale, & R.J.W. Mansfield (ed.), *Analysis of Visual Behavior* (pp. 549–86). Cambridge, MA: MIT Press.

Vautin, R.G., & Berkley, M.A. (1977). Responses of single cells in cat visual cortex to prolonged stimulus movement: Neural correlates of visual aftereffects. *Journal of Physiology, 40*(5), 1051–65.

Vogels, R. (1990). Population coding of stimulus orientation by striate cortical cells. *Biological Cybernetics, 64*, 25–31.

Vogels, R., & Orban, G.A. (1994). Activity of inferior temporal neurons during orientation discrimination with successively presented gratings. *Journal of Neurophysiology, 71*(4), 1428–51.

Vogels, R., Sary, G., & Orban, G.A. (1995). How task-related are the responses of inferior temporal neurons? *Visual Neuroscience, 12*, 207–14.

Wang, G., Tanaka, K., & Tanifuji, M. (1996). Optical imaging of functional organization in the monkey inferotemporal cortex. *Science, 272*, 1665–8.

Wang, Y., Fujita, I., & Maruyama, Y. (2000). Neuronal mechanisms of selectivity for object features revealed by blocking inhibition in inferotemporal cortex. *Nature Neuroscience, 3*(8), 807–13.

Webster, M., Kaping, D., Mizokami, Y., & Dumahel, P. (2004). Adaptation to natural face categories. *Nature*, *428*, 558–61.

Webster, M., & MacLin, O.H. (1999). Figural after-effects in the perception of faces. *Psychonomic Bulletin & Review*, *6*(4), 647–53.

Wenderoth, P., & van der Zwan, R. (1989). The effects of exposure duration and surrounding frames on direct and indirect tilt aftereffects and illusions. *Perception & Psychophysics*, *46*(4), 338–44.

Wolfe, J.M. (1984). Short test flashes produce large tilt aftereffects. *Vision Research*, *24*(12), 1959–64.

Young, M.P., & Yamane, S. (1992). Sparse population coding of faces in the inferotemporal cortex. *Science*, *256*, 1327–31.

Zhao, L., & Chubb, C. (2001). The size-tuning of the face-distortion after-effect. *Vision Research*, *41*, 2979–94.

Zipser, K., Lamme, V.A.F., & Shiller, P.H. (1996). Contextual modulation in primary visual cortex. *Journal of Neuroscience*, *16*(22), 7376–89.

6

fMRI Adaptation: A Tool for Studying Visual Representations in the Primate Brain

ZOE KOURTZI AND KALANIT GRILL-SPECTOR

6.1 Adaptation and Short-term Brain Plasticity in High-level Object Areas

One of the most fundamental properties of the brain that clearly distinguishes it from artificially constructed computational devices is its ability to continuously update its functional properties based on prior experience. This property, also termed brain "plasticity" is manifested on many levels of organization and at many time scales. In recent years, clear demonstrations of experience-dependent modifications of brain activity in the human visual cortex have been established. Fairly long-term changes (on the order of days) were observed after subjects learned to recognize unfamiliar shapes (Gauthier *et al.* 1999), or when trained to recognize subliminally-presented visual objects (Grill-Spector *et al.* 2000) and even single presentations of objects (van Turennout *et al.* 2000). Experience-dependent changes are not only evident on long range time scales lasting days, but also in short time scales in the order of seconds.

A particularly robust phenomenon is repetition-suppression, or adaptation, in which repeated presentation of the same visual stimulus leads to a consistent and gradual reduction in activation within seconds of the occurrence of the first image presentation. This phenomenon was termed fMR-adaptation (fMR-A) (Grill-Spector *et al.* 1999; Grill-Spector & Malach 2001), and is also referred to as repetition-suppression or repetition-priming (Buckner & Koutstaal 1998; Koutstaal *et al.* 2001; Vuilleumier *et al.* 2002). Similar stimulus-specific repetition-suppression (or mnemonic filtering) has been found in physiological recordings in macaque inferotemporal (IT) cortex (Miller *et al.* 1991, 1993).

Visual adaptation is an ubiquitous phenomenon that has been implicated in many perceptual processes, such as contrast and color adaptation (Hadjikhani *et al.* 1998; Engel & Furmanski 2001), as well as tilt (Graham 1972; see Clifford, this volume) and motion aftereffects (Clifford, this volume; Tootell *et al.* 1995; Culham *et al.* 2000; Huk *et al.* 2001). However, much less is known about the neural correlates of the adaptation phenomenon in high-level visual areas.

6.2 What is the Source of the Activity Reduction?

Although of fundamental importance, the neural mechanisms underlying fMRI adaptation are not fully understood. Several mechanisms have been proposed to account for adaptation, such as habituation and priming.

Adaptation may be a manifestation of the basic phenomenon of habituation, in which the system suppresses temporally repetitive stimuli. The behavioral correlate of prolonged habituation is typically reduced sensitivity of the observer for test stimuli which have similar properties as the adapting stimulus. This kind of adaptation has revealed orientation selectivity (Graham 1972), direction selectivity (Tootell *et al.* 1995; Culham *et al.* 2000; Huk *et al.* 2001), and color opponent mechanisms (Bradley *et al.* 1988; Webster & Mollon 1994).

Some researchers (Schacter and Buckner 1998) have suggested that fMRI adaptation may correspond to the behavioral phenomenon of visual priming in which the performance of the subject improves with repeated presentations of a stimulus. Behaviorally, visual priming reflects improved performance both in faster reaction times and in higher accuracy. In contrast to habituation, visual priming can be manifested after a single exposure to a stimulus (i.e., the "prime"), and is preserved in time scales ranging from seconds to even a year (Cave 1997). However, it is rather counterintuitive that a reduced cortical response would be correlated with improved performance. Two theories on the mechanisms underlying priming have been proposed: priming of selective neurons and inhibition of non-selective neurons.

The first approach proposes that the initial processing of the input may leave a trace or prime on selective neurons that are specifically involved in processing the objects that are presented. As a consequence, less neural processing is required in order to generate a response to the repeated presentation of the same object. This reduced neural processing could be manifested in a shorter neural duty cycle; that is, neurons fire robustly, but for a shorter period of time. Indeed physiological studies in the macaque (Ringo 1996) indicate that early visual responses are not affected by image repetition, and suppression occurs only at later times (beginning 200 ms after stimulus onset). Further data suggest that repetition suppression occurs for excitatory but not inhibitory neurons (Sobotka & Ringo 1994) and is stronger for neurons that respond more vigorously to the first stimulus presentation, suggesting that neurons that are selective to the stimulus are adapted more strongly than non-selective neurons (Miller *et al.* 1993). Importantly, both the mechanism of priming by shortening the duty cycle of selective neurons and habituation by suppressing responses to temporally repetitive stimuli suggest that the selective neurons involved in the initial processing of the stimulus are the ones that are suppressed. It is still an open question whether habituation after prolonged exposure and priming of selective neurons after a single exposure reflect different mechanisms that operate at different time scales or rather different expressions of a single underlying mechanism.

A different model for improved visual processing which underlies priming has been suggested by Li *et al.* (1993) and has been considered by others (e.g. Wiggs & Martin 1998; Henson & Rugg 2003). This model suggests that improved visual processing by priming occurs by inhibition of non-selective neurons which are initially activated, whereas the selective neurons remain unchanged and are not suppressed. Thus, image repetition generates a more efficient and sparser representation of the visual stimulus across the cortex. This hypothesis suggests that fMRI adaptation reflects the suppression of the irrelevant (non-selective) neurons rather than more efficient processing of the repeated visual stimulus by the selective neurons. However, it is unclear why a sparser representation across the cortex as suggested by this model would predict faster visual processing (which is the behavioral signature of priming). Furthermore, there is no evidence from Li *et al.*'s experiments or other studies that the selective neurons are not suppressed and that the non-selective neurons are suppressed. On the contrary, most of the data suggest that the suppression is highly specific. Finally, evidence from neuroimaging studies suggests that regions that are selective for objects and particular object categories (such as faces) are the same regions that show fMRI adaptation (Grill-Spector *et al.* 1999; Avidan *et al.* 2002*a,b*).

To sum up, while there are yet many unknowns for the neural mechanisms underlying fMRI adaptation, results from both single unit studies and imaging studies suggest that this phenomenon reflects the suppression of neurons involved in the processing of the stimulus, that this suppression is stimulus specific. Thus, fMRI adaptation can be used as an important experimental tool to tag specific neural populations.

6.3 fMRI Adaptation: A Tool for Investigating Properties of Neural Populations in Sub-voxel Resolution

One of the limitations of conventional fMRI paradigms that rely on the subtraction of activation between different stimulus types is that they average across neural populations that may respond homogeneously across stimulus changes or may be differentially tuned to different stimulus attributes. Thus, in most cases, it is impossible to infer the properties of the underlying imaged neural populations. fMRI adaptation paradigms have been recently employed to study the properties of neuronal populations beyond this limited spatial resolution of fMRI. These paradigms capitalize on the reduction of neural responses for stimuli that have been presented for prolonged time or repeatedly (Lisberger & Movshon 1999; Mueller *et al.* 1999). A change in a specific stimulus dimension that elicits increased responses (i.e. rebound of activity) identifies neural populations that are sensitive to the modified stimulus attributes (Fig. 6.1). The fMRI adaptation paradigms have been used in both monkey and human fMRI studies as a sensitive tool that allows us to investigate (a) the sensitivity of the neural populations and (b) the invariance of their responses within the imaged voxels. Adaptation across a change between two stimuli provides evidence for a common neural representation invariant to that change, while recovery from adaptation suggests neural representations sensitive to specific stimulus properties.

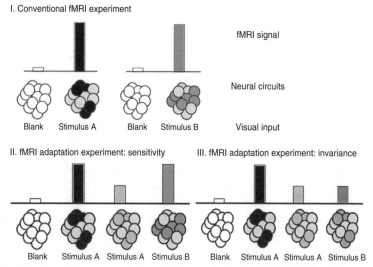

FIG. 6.1 Conventional versus Adaptation fMRI paradigms: (I) Conventional imaging experiment: fMRI responses to two stimulus conditions A and B are compared to each other. If different neural subpopulations in the measured voxel encode the two stimuli, it is possible that the strength of the BOLD signal will be the same under these two conditions. Therefore, this conventional imaging experiment may fail to characterize the properties of these neural populations. (II) Adaptation experiment: stimulus A is shown for a prolonged time or repeatedly resulting in adaptation of the BOLD signal. If different neural subpopulations encode stimuli A and B then after presentation of stimulus B the signal shows a rebound; that is release from adaptation. (III) If the same neural subpopulations encode stimuli A and B, then the responses for stimulus B remain adapted after adaptation to stimulus A.

6.4 fMRI Adaptation for the Study of Neuronal Sensitivity

Recent imaging studies tested whether the neural populations in the early visual areas are tuned to visual features, e.g. orientation, color, direction of motion (Tootell *et al.* 1998; Engel & Furmanski 2001; Huk & Heeger 2001; Tolias *et al.* 2001). For example, after prolonged exposure to the adapting motion direction, observers were tested with the same stimulus in the same or in an orthogonal motion direction. Decreased fMRI responses were observed in MT when the test stimuli were at the same motion direction as the adapting stimulus. However, recovery from this adaptation effect was observed for stimuli presented at an orthogonal direction. These studies suggest that the neural populations in MT are tuned to the direction of motion. Similarly, recent studies have shown stronger adaptation in MT/MST for coherently than for transparently moving plaid stimuli. These findings provide evidence that fMRI adaptation responses are linked to the activity of pattern-motion rather than component-motion cells in MT/MST (Huk & Heeger 2002). Thus, these studies provide evidence that the fMRI signal can reveal neural sensitivity consistent with the sensitivity established by neurophysiological methods.

Recently, combined monkey (Fig. 6.2) and human (Fig. 6.3) fMRI studies showed that coherent shape perception involves early (retinotopic) and higher (occipitotemporal) visual areas that may integrate local elements to global shapes at different spatial scales (Kourtzi *et al.* 2003*b*). fMRI responses across visual areas to collinear contours versus random patterns were tested. The collinear patterns consisted of a number of similarly oriented elements embedded into a background of randomly oriented elements, while the random patterns consisted of a field of randomly oriented elements. The collinear patterns yield the perception of a global figure in a randomly textured background and are thought to emerge from a segmentation process relying on the integration of the similarly oriented line-segments into global configurations (Kovacs & Julesz 1993, 1994; Hess & Field 1999, for review). In the fMRI adaptation paradigm used, stimulus sensitivity was deduced by changes in the course of adaptation to a pattern of randomly oriented elements. Adaptation was observed when the adapting random pattern was followed by an identical test pattern. Recovery from adaptation (rebound) was observed in early visual areas measured in the monkey (V1, V2/V3), and in both retinotopic and higher occipitotemporal regions in the human measurements, when the adapting random pattern was followed by a different random or a collinear pattern. More importantly, this rebound effect was stronger for collinear than random patterns. Thus, in contrast to traditional approaches, sensitivity to collinear shapes was shown not only in higher visual areas that are implicated in shape processing, but also in early visual areas where sensitivity depended on the signal (collinear elements) -to- noise (random background elements) ratio within the receptive field.

Further human fMRI studies (Altmann *et al.* 2003) showed decreased detection performance and fMRI activations when misalignment of the contour elements disturbed the perceptual coherence of the contours. However, grouping

I. Stimuli

A Random Patterns   B Collinear Patterns

II. Regions of interest in the monkey brain

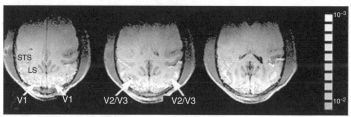

III. fMRI adaptation

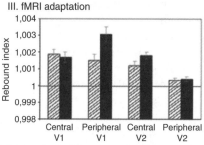

FIG. 6.2 Monkey fMRI study on collinear shapes (Kourtzi *et al.* 2003). (I) Stimuli
rendered by oriented line segments: (A) Random Pattern used as the adapting stimulus and
(B) Collinear Pattern used as the test stimulus. (II) Localization of the visual areas in the monkey
brain. Three consecutive slices (posterior to anterior) from one subject showing the visual areas
(V1, V2/V3) that were selected as regions of interest for the analysis of the adaptation experiment. These regions responded significantly more strongly to a full field rotating polar stimulus
than blank stimulation periods. Significance charts indicate the results of t-tests. The arrows point
to the activated visual areas, the borders of which were identified based on anatomical criteria.
Major sulci are labeled: LS: Lunate Sulcus, and STS: superior temporal sulcus. (III) fMRI
Adaptation results: An fMRI rebound index (percent signal change in each condition/percent
signal change in the Identical (adapted) Random Pattern condition) is plotted. A ratio of 1 (horizontal line) indicates adaptation, whereas a ratio higher than 1 indicates recovery from adaptation
compared to the minimum responses (adapted fMRI responses) in the Identical condition. This
rebound index is plotted for the responses to the Random-to-Collinear Pattern (solid bars) and to
the Different Random Pattern (striped bars) conditions across visual areas. The error bars indicate
standard errors on the percent signal change averaged across scans and subjects. Collinearity
effects were observed in peripheral V1 and central V2, but not in central V1, where only a small
number of collinear elements was within the small size receptive fields, and peripheral V2, where
the number of random background elements within the receptive field was possibly larger than
the number of collinear elements. These fMRI adaptation results suggest that early visual areas
contribute to the integration of local elements to global shapes based on the signal (collinear
elements) -to- noise ratio (random background elements) within their receptive field.

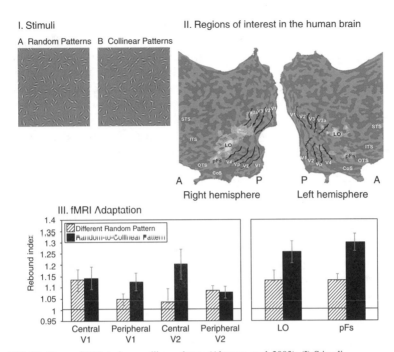

FIG. 6.3 Human fMRI study on collinear shapes (Altmann *et al.* 2003). (I) Stimuli
rendered by Gabors. Examples of (A) the random patterns and (B) the collinear patterns used as
stimuli. (II) Localization of the visual areas in the human brain. Functional activation maps for
one subject showing the early retinotopic regions and the LOC (lateral occipital complex).
The functional activations are superimposed on flattened cortical surfaces of the right and left
hemispheres. The sulci are coded in darker gray than the gyri and the Anterior-Posterior
orientation is noted by A and P. Major sulci are labeled: STS: superior temporal sulcus, ITS:
inferior temporal sulcus, OTS: occipitotemporal sulcus, CoS: collateral sulcus. The borders
(shown by lines) of the early visual regions (V1, V2, VP, V3, V3a, V4v) were defined with
standard retinotopic techniques. The LOC was defined as the set of all contiguous voxels in
the ventral occipitotemporal cortex that were activated more strongly ($p < 10^{-4}$) by intact than
by scrambled images of objects. The posterior (LO) and anterior regions (pFs) of the LOC were
identified based on anatomical criteria. (III) fMRI Adaptation results: An fMRI rebound index
(percent signal change in each condition/percent signal change in the Identical (adapted)
Random Pattern condition) reported for the Random-to-Collinear Pattern (solid black bars) and
the Different Random Pattern (striped bars) conditions across visual areas. A ratio of 1
(horizontal line) indicates adaptation. This rebound index is shown for central and peripheral
subregions of V1 and V2, posterior (LO) and anterior (pFs) subregions of the LOC. The error
bars indicate standard errors on the percent signal change averaged across scans and subjects.
Similar to the monkey fMRI adaptation study, collinearity effects were observed in peripheral
V1 and central V2 consistent with the signal (collinear elements) -to- noise (random background
elements) ratio within their receptive field. Interestingly, the collinearity effects in the LOC,
where the large receptive fields encode the whole stimulus that consisted of more background
than collinear elements, suggest that neural populations in the LOC encode the perceived global
shape rather than local configurations.

of the misaligned contour elements by disparity resulted in increased performance and fMRI activations, suggesting that similar neural mechanisms may
underlie grouping of local elements to global shapes by different visual features
(orientation or disparity). These studies provide additional evidence for the role
of early perceptual organization processes and their interactions with higher
stages of visual analysis in unified visual perception. Taken together, these findings provide evidence for common mechanisms in the human and non-human
primate brain that are involved in coherent shape perception and bridge the gap
between previous monkey electrophysiological and human fMRI findings on
the neural processing of shapes.

Furthermore, recent human fMRI studies have used adaptation to test the
sensitivity of the responses of neural populations in the Lateral Occipital Complex
(LOC), a region in the lateral occipital cortex extending anteriorly in the temporal
cortex, that has been shown to be involved in shape processing (Kanwisher
et al. 1996; Malach *et al.* 1995). Here, fMRI adaptation was used to test
whether the LOC is involved in the processing of object shape independent of
low level image features that define the shape (Fig. 6.4; Kourtzi & Kanwisher
2001). An event-related fMRI adaptation paradigm was employed, in which a
pair of consecutively-presented stimuli was presented in each trial that lasted
for 3 seconds. These studies showed adaptation in the LOC when the perceived
shape was identical but the image contours differed (because occluding bars
occurred in front of the shape in one stimulus and behind the shape in the other).
In contrast, recovery from adaptation was observed when the contours were identical but the perceived shapes were different (because of a figure-ground reversal).

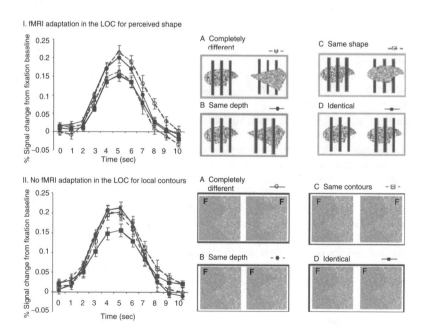

Consistent with these results, adaptation was also shown for grayscale images and line drawings of the same objects (Kourtzi & Kanwisher 2000) but not for objects that differed in their 3D structure (i.e. convex versus concave) (Kourtzi *et al.* 2003*a*). These results suggest that neural populations in the LOC may not represent simple image features, such as contours, but represent higher-level shape information and 3D objects independent of image cues (i.e. shading and line contours).

6.5 fMRI Adaptation for the Study of Neuronal Invariances

Understanding the representation of objects in the brain is crucial for understanding how object recognition occurs efficiently and rapidly. One of the biggest challenges of the object recognition system is dealing with the variability in the appearance of objects without losing acuity in discriminating between objects that are similar. Theories of object recognition differ most critically in their prediction about the nature of the representation of objects. Some theories (Biederman 1987) suggest a 3D object-centered representation, while other theories posit that multiple 2D views of an object span its representation (Poggio & Edelman 1990; Ullman 1996; Edelman & Duvdevani-Bar 1997).

Using fMRI adaptation we investigated (Grill-Spector *et al.* 1999) the invariant properties of object representations using a variety of objects (animals, man-made objects, faces), formats (gray-level photos, sketches, and line drawings), and transformations (size, position, rotation around the vertical, and illumination). To test invariance we measured the extent of fMRI adaptation in the LOC when objects were viewed undergoing only one transformation at a time, and keeping the others constant. We found that different kinds of image transformations produce different levels of adaptation within the LOC (which includes object selective regions LO and the fusiform gyrus, Fig. 6.5). Adaptation in the fusiform was found to be largely invariant to size and position, but not invariant

FIG. 6.4 Shape Processing in the human LOC (Kourtzi & Kanwisher 2001). Data averaged across 10 subjects showing fMRI adaptation effects in the LOC, that is decreased responses (% signal change from fixation baseline) for identical images of objects (compared to the responses for different objects in a trial). (I) Adaptation is shown for images that have the same perceived shape but different contours due to occlusion. That is, decreased fMRI responses were observed for the Same Shape compared to the Completely Different condition. (II) In contrast, no adaptation is shown for images that when rendered stereoscopically have the same contours but different perceived shape due to figure ground reversal (F indicates the shape perceived as the figure in front of the background for each image). That is, increased fMRI responses were observed for the Same Contours compared to the Identical condition. These fMRI adaptation results suggest that neural populations in the LOC encode the perceived shape of objects rather than their local contours.

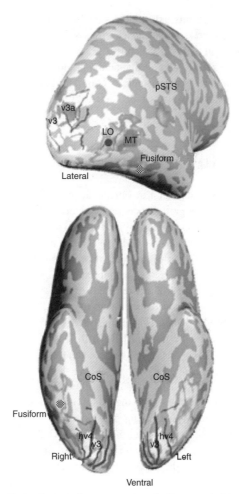

FIG. 6.5 Regions that activate to faces more strongly than novel objects, houses, cars, and scenes with $p < 10^{-4}$ at the voxel level. Lines indicate visual meridians: blue: horizontal visual meridian; red: upper visual meridian; green: lower visual meridian. Location of MT is indicated in blue. Three main regions show higher activation for faces compared to controls: a region in the fusiform gyrus, a region in LO, and a region in the posterior STS. (See also Plate 6 at the centre of this book.)

to the direction of illumination and rotation around the vertical axis. Figure 6.6(A) shows the data obtained for faces; similar results were found for cars (Fig. 6.6(B)) and animals (Grill-Spector *et al.* 1999). This suggests that the representation of objects and faces at least in the level of the fusiform is view-based rather than object-based. In contrast, LO did not show size or position invariance, although it was adapted by presentation of identical images (Fig. 6.6).

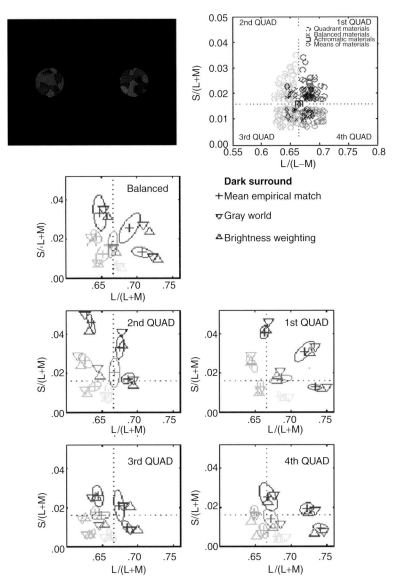

PLATE 1 (Top left) Red spotlight cast on green-yellow materials on the left and the same red spotlight on gray materials on the right. Observers were asked to estimate the color of the spotlight moving on chromatic materials and to match it by adjusting the color of the spotlight moving on gray materials. (Top right) MacLeod–Boynton chromaticities (under equal energy light) of the 240 materials used, which consisted of 6 sets of 40 materials, 4 sets of chromatic materials from each quadrant, one set of balanced chromatic materials, one set of achromatic materials. Colored diamonds indicate mean of each quadrant's materials, while the square and the gray diamond at the intersection of the horizontal and vertical dotted lines represent both the achromatic materials and the mean of the balanced chromatic materials. (Bottom) Mean chromaticities of the match spotlights (+), and predictions from a gray-world model (△) and a model that gives greater weight to the brighter materials (▽). The results are color-coded to correspond roughly to the appearance of the spotlight on the achromatic materials. (see also Chapter 4, Fig. 4.7.)

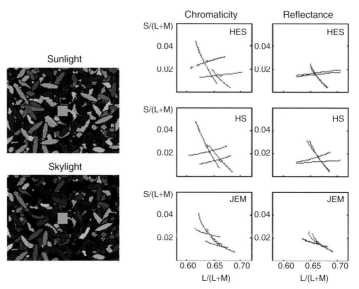

PLATE 2 (Left) Examples of stimuli used in color appearance measurements with a global illuminant change on chromatically balanced backgrounds. On each trial, a square test patch was presented on a variegated background of randomly oriented elliptical patches, under skylight or sunlight. (Center) Data for three observers. Panels show traces of classification boundaries in chromaticity space. Red lines show boundaries obtained under sunlight; blue lines show boundaries obtained under skylight. Red and blue open-circles show the corresponding illuminant chromaticities. (Right) Panels show the same boundaries represented in reflectance space (i.e. as if materials were rendered under an equal energy illuminant). (See also Chapter 4, Fig. 4.10.)

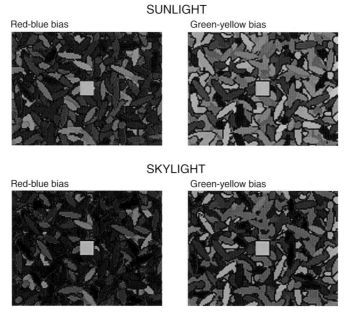

PLATE 3 Examples of stimuli used in color appearance measurements with a global illuminant change on chromatically biased backgrounds. The top row shows stimuli rendered under sunlight; the bottom row shows stimuli rendered under skylight. (See also Chapter 4, Fig. 4.11.)

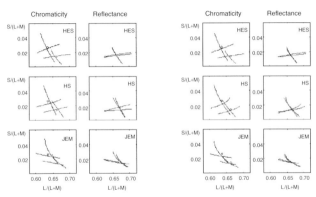

PLATE 4 Data for the three observers, with a global illuminant change on
(Left) red-blue biased backrounds, (Right) green-yellow biased backrounds. Panels
on the left show traces of classification boundaries in chromaticity space, obtained
under sunlight (red lines) or sky light (blue lines). Open-circles show the
corresponding illuminant chromaticities. Panels on the right show the same boundaries
represented in reflectance space (i.e. as if materials were rendered under an equal
energy illuminant). (See also Chapter 4, Fig. 4.12.)

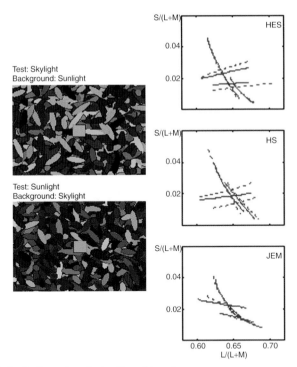

PLATE 5 (Left) Examples of stimuli used in color appearance measurements with
conflicting illuminants on test and background reflectances. (Right) Data for the three
observers. Solid red lines indicate classification boundaries obtained with sunlight
illumination on the test, and skylight on the background. Solid blue lines indicate
classification boundaries obtained with skylight on the test, and sunlight on the
background. Dotted red and blue lines show boundaries obtained with a global
illuminant of sunlight or skylight respectively, and are thus color-coded to predict
boundary locations based on the test illuminant. Discriminant functions for
Observer HS, with sunlight on the test and skylight on the background, were not
well-constrained. (See also Chapter 4, Fig. 4.13.)

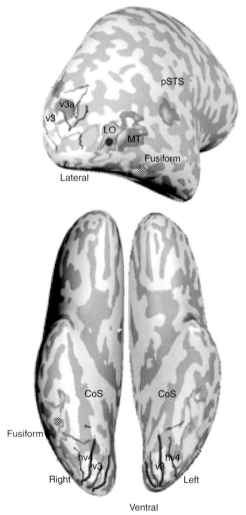

PLATE 6 Regions that activate to faces more strongly than novel objects, houses, cars, and scenes with $p < 10^{-4}$ at the voxel level. Lines indicate visual meridians: blue: horizontal visual meridian; red: upper visual meridian; green: lower visual meridian. Location of MT is indicated in blue. Three main regions show higher activation for faces compared to controls: a region in the fusiform gyrus, a region in LO, and a region in the posterior STS. (See also Chapter 6, Fig. 6.5.)

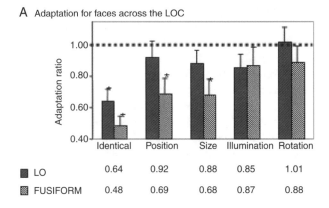

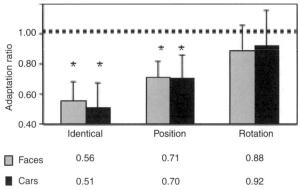

FIG. 6.6 Adaptation ratios across object transformations calculated relative to the non-adapting block of gray-level photographs of different individuals (or objects) taken under the same viewing conditions: adaptation ratio = % signal (condition)/% signal (different). A ratio of 1 indicates no adaptation because the activation is the same as for the non-adapting stimulus. A ratio less than one indicates adaptation. Asterisks indicate significant adaptation compared to the non-adapting condition. Error bars indicate SEM. Identical: repetitions of the same individual taken under the same viewing conditions. Position: same individual in different positions displaced 6 degrees around fixation. Size: same individual in different sizes (size changes were 3 fold). Illumination: same individual illuminated from 5 different directions. Rotation: same individual in different rotation around the vertical axis ranging from $-90°:90°$.

(A) Adaptation ratios for faces across object transformations in LO and fusiform regions of interest averaged across 14 subjects.

(B) Adaptation ratios for faces and cars in the fusiform gyrus averaged across 9 subjects.

The fact that the more posterior subdivision of the LOC (LO) was sensitive to size and position changes is consistent with macaque studies suggesting a progression of areas in the IT cortex, from TEO or PIT that retains some degree of retinotopy to TE or AIT in which the representations are more invariant (Ito *et al.* 1995; Gross *et al.* 1972). These neuronal invariances to changes in size and position should be contrasted with the high degree of shape selectivity in LOC revealed by the relative lack of adaptation in the blocks where objects from the same basic category (i.e. cars or faces) were presented under identical viewing conditions. Furthermore, the differential profile of adaptation within LOC sub-regions is also incompatible with a global, non-specific arousal being the source of fMRI adaptation.

6.6 Interpretation of fMRI Adaptation Results

Two points should be considered while interpreting the results of fMRI adaptation. First, the level of adaptation can be measured relative to a minimum of activation corresponding to the adapting state (Figs. 6.2 and 6.3 – rebound index = % signal in a condition/% signal in adapted condition) or a maximum of activation, corresponding to a non-adapted state (Fig. 6.6) – adaptation ratio = % signal in a condition/% signal in non-adapted state. In our experiments, the non-adapted state consisted of conditions in which different exemplars within an object category were presented. However, we cannot rule out the possibility that some adaptation did occur even in these presumably "non-adapting" epochs. For example, if there were common features among the different object exemplars used in the non-adapting conditions, these may have adapted neurons specifically tuned to such repeating features. Thus, conclusions that can be derived from adaptation studies refer only to the *relative* effects exerted by one set of images compared to another. Second, the adaptation effect reflects the overall changes in activity of a very large neuronal population; consequently, it may mask opposite effects that may occur within a smaller neuronal population intermixed within the larger population. For example, one could envision that a small subset of neurons in LOC is invariant to face viewpoint, and shows strong adaptation when faces are rotated; however, this adaptation is masked by a larger, viewpoint sensitive neuronal population – leading to the impression of overall viewpoint-sensitivity. Single-cell recordings are useful in providing additional information about the nature of view dependent representations and about the percentage of cells manifesting view dependent or invariant properties.

Keeping these cautionary points in mind, one can still make educated hypotheses regarding the representation of objects in high order object areas. Using conventional BOLD imaging, previous fMRI studies reported a similar fMRI signal for different face viewpoints (Kanwisher *et al.* 1997) implying viewpoint-invariant representation of faces in the fusiform gyrus. However, conventional methods cannot distinguish between voxels containing viewpoint-invariant neurons and voxels containing a mixture of neuronal populations tuned to specific ranges of views. The use of fMRI adaptation enabled us to demonstrate that the representation of faces and objects within the fusiform gyrus is actually sensitive to rotation of these objects (faces and cars). This indicates that the representation of a face, at least at the level of the majority of fusiform neurons, is not viewpoint-invariant, arguing against a full 3D object-centered representation as proposed by some theories.

One surprising result was that viewing the same object under different directions of illumination resulted in substantial recovery from adaptation. Several models suggest that extraction of illumination could be done by lower visual areas (Lekhy & Sejnowski 1988). Our results suggest that sensitivity to the direction of illumination is retained even in higher levels of the visual hierarchy. While size and position changes are probably compensated for in the level of the fusiform, illumination is not. These results are in line with the reported sensitivity of IT neurons to stimulus shading (Ito *et al.* 1994) and results from some psychophysical experiments (Tarr *et al.* 1998).

6.7 Summary

In summary, fMRI adaptation has been recently used as a tool for the study of visual representations. This paradigm capitalizes on the logic that repeated or prolonged presentation of the same stimulus results in decreased responses compared to the presentation of different stimuli. Used in conjunction with imaging techniques, adaptation is a powerful tool for studying the properties of networks of neurons in the human and non-human primate brain. Also, fMRI adaptation allows us to investigate the sensitivity and invariance of the responses of neural populations within the imaged voxels. This is not possible with conventional fMRI paradigms that rely on the subtraction of activation between different stimulus types since they average across neural populations that may respond similarly across stimulus changes or may be differentially tuned to different stimulus attributes. Thus, this paradigm goes beyond the limited spatial resolution of conventional fMRI paradigms and allows us to test the nature of visual representations at a higher resolution in the primate brain. We summarize studies using fMRI adaptation to test for selective responses to different types of stimuli and investigate the invariant properties of visual representations across early and higher visual areas. Although adaptation is a property of neural responses, the relationship between the adaptation of the BOLD signal and neuronal activity is currently not known. Simultaneous recordings of the BOLD signal and electrophysiological activity during adaptation are likely to provide further insights about the relationship between BOLD and neuronal adaptation.

References

Altmann, C.F., Bulthoff, H.H., & Kourtzi, Z. (2003). Perceptual organization of local elements into global shapes in the human visual cortex. *Currrent Biology, 13*(4), 342–9.

Avidan, G., Harel, M., Hendler, T., Ben-Bashat, D., Zohary, E., & Malach, R. (2002a). Contrast sensitivity in human visual areas and its relationship to object recognition. *Journal of Neurophysiology*, *87*, 3102–16.

Avidan, G., Hasson, U., Hendler, T., Zohary, E., & Malach, R. (2002b). Analysis of the neuronal selectivity underlying low fMRI signals. *Currrent Biology*, *12*, 964–72.

Bradley, A., Switkes, E., & De Valois, K. (1988). Orientation and spatial frequency selectivity of adaptation to color and luminance gratings. *Vision Research*, *28*, 841–56.

Biederman, I. (1987). Recognition-by-components: a theory of human image understanding. *Psychological Review*, *94*, 115–47.

Buckner. R.L., & Koutstaal, W. (1998). Functional neuroimaging studies of encoding, priming, and explicit memory retrieval. *Proceedings of the National Academy of Sciences of the U S A*, *95*, 891–8.

Cave, C.B. (1997). Very long-lasting priming in picture naming. *Psychological Science*, *8*, 322–5.

Culham, J.C., Verstraten, F.A., Ashida, H., & Cavanagh, P. (2000). Independent aftereffects of attention and motion. *Neuron*, *28*, 607–15.

Edelman, S., & Duvdevani-Bar, S. (1997). A model of visual recognition and categorization. *Philosophical Transactions of the Royal Society of London, Series B Biological Sciences*, *352*, 1191–202.

Engel, S.A., & Furmanski, C.S. (2001). Selective adaptation to color contrast in human primary visual cortex. *Journal of Neuroscience*, *21*, 3949–54.

Gauthier, I., Tarr, M.J., Anderson, A.W., Skudlarski, P., & Gore, J.C. (1999). Activation of the middle fusiform 'face area' increases with expertise in recognizing novel objects. *Nature Neuroscience*, *2*, 568–73.

Graham, N. (1972). Spatial frequency channels in the human visual system: effects of luminance and pattern drift. *Vision Research*, *12,* 53–68.

Grill-Spector, K., & Malach, R. (2001). fMR-adaptation: a tool for studying the functional properties of human cortical neurons. *Acta Psychologica (Amst)*, *107*, 293–321.

Grill-Spector, K., Kushnir, T., Hendler, T., & Malach, R. (2000). The dynamics of object-selective activation correlate with recognition performance in humans. *Nature Neuroscience*, *3*, 837–43.

Grill-Spector, K., Kushnir, T., Edelman, S., Avidan, G., Itzchak, Y., & Malach, R. (1999). Differential processing of objects under various viewing conditions in the human lateral occipital complex. *Neuron*, *24*, 187–203.

Gross, C.G., Rocha, M.C., & Bender, D.B. (1972). Visual properties of neurons in inferotemporal cortex of the Macaque. *Journal of Neurophysiology*, *35*, 96–111.

Hadjikhani, N., Liu, A.K., Dale, A.M., Cavanagh, P., & Tootell, R.B. (1998). Retinotopy and color sensitivity in human visual cortical area V8. *Nature Neuroscience*, *1*, 235–41.

Henson, R.N., & Rugg, M.D. (2003). Neural response suppression, haemodynamic repetition effects, and behavioural priming. *Neuropsychologia*, 41, 263–70.

Hess, R., & Field, D. (1999). Integration of contours: new insights. *Trends in Cognitive Sciences*, *3*(12), 480–6.

Huk, A.C., & Heeger, D.J. (2002). Pattern-motion responses in human visual cortex. *Nature Neuroscience*, *5*, 72–5.

Huk, A.C., Ress, D., & Heeger, D.J. (2001). Neuronal basis of the motion aftereffect reconsidered. *Neuron*, *32*, 161–72.

Ito, M., Fujita, I., Tamura, H., & Tanaka, K. (1994). Processing of contrast polarity of visual images in inferotemporal cortex of the macaque monkey. *Cerebral Cortex, 4*, 499–508.

Ito, M., Tamura, H., Fujita, I., & Tanaka, K. (1995). Size and position invariance of neuronal responses in monkey inferotemporal cortex. *Journal of Neurophysiology, 73*, 218–26.

Kanwisher, N., Chun, M.M., McDermott, J., & Ledden, P.J. (1996). Functional imaging of human visual recognition. *Brain Research Cognitive Brain Research, 5*, 55–67.

Kanwisher, N., McDermott, J., & Chun, M.M. (1997). The fusiform face area: a module in human extrastriate cortex specialized for face perception. *Journal of Neuroscience, 17*, 4302–11.

Koutstaal, W., Wagner, A.D., Rotte, M., Maril, A., Buckner, R.L., & Schacter, D.L. (2001). Perceptual specificity in visual object priming: functional magnetic resonance imaging evidence for a laterality difference in fusiform cortex. *Neuropsychologia, 39*, 184–99.

Kourtzi, Z., & Kanwisher, N. (2000). Cortical regions involved in perceiving object shape. *Journal of Neuroscience, 20*, 3310–8.

Kourtzi, Z., & Kanwisher, N. (2001). Representation of perceived object shape by the human lateral occipital complex. *Science, 293*, 1506–9.

Kourtzi, Z., Erb, M., Grodd, W., & Bulthoff, H.H. (2003a). Representation of the perceived 3-D object shape in the human lateral occipital complex. *Cerebral Cortex, 13*(9), 911–20.

Kourtzi, Z., Tolias, A.S., Altmann, C.F., Augath, M., & Logothetis, N.K. (2003b). Integration of local features into global shapes: monkey and human FMRI studies. *Neuron, 37*(2), 333–46.

Kovacs, I., & Julesz, B. (1993). A closed curve is much more than an incomplete one: effect of closure in figure-ground segmentation. *Proceedings of the National Academy of Sciences of the U S A, 90*(16), 7495–7.

Kovacs, I., & Julesz, B. (1994). Perceptual sensitivity maps within globally defined visual shapes. *Nature, 370*(6491), 644–6.

Lekhy, S.R., & Sejnowski, T.J. (1990). Neural network model of visual cortex determining surface curvature from images of shaded surfaces. *Proceedings of the Royal Society of London, Series B [Biol], 240*, 251–78.

Li, L., Miller, E.K., & Desimone, R. (1993). The representation of stimulus familiarity in anterior inferior temporal cortex. *Journal of Neurophysiology, 69*, 1918–29.

Lisberger, S.G., & Movshon, J.A. (1999). Visual motion analysis for pursuit eye movements in area MT of macaque monkeys. *Journal of Neuroscience, 19*, 2224–46.

Malach, R., Reppas, J.B., Benson, R.B., Kwong, K.K., Jiang, H., & Kennedy, W.A., (1995). Object-related activity revealed by functional magnetic resonance imaging in human occipital cortex. *Proceedings of the National Academy of Sciences of the U S A, 92*(18), 8135–9.

Miller, E.K., Li, L., & Desimone, R. (1991). A neural mechanism for working and recognition memory in inferior temporal cortex. *Science, 254*, 1377–9.

Miller, E.K., Li, L., & Desimone, R. (1993). Activity of neurons in anterior inferior temporal cortex during a short-term memory task. *Journal of Neuroscience, 13*, 1460–78.

Mueller, J.R., Metha, A.B., Krauskopf, J., & Lennie, P. (1999). Rapid adaptation in visual cortex to the structure of images. *Science, 285*, 1405–8.

Poggio, T., & Edelman, S. (1990). A network that learns to recognize three-dimensional objects. *Nature, 343,* 263–6.

Ringo, J.L. (1996). Stimulus specific adaptation in inferior temporal and medial temporal cortex of the monkey. *Behavioral Brain Research, 76,* 191–7.

Schacter, D.L., & Buckner, R.L. (1998). Priming and the brain. *Neuron, 20,* 185–95.

Sobotka, S., & Ringo, J.L. (1994). Stimulus specific adaptation in excited but not in inhibited cells in inferotemporal cortex of macaque. *Brain Research, 646,* 95–9.

Tarr, M.J., Kersten, D., & Bulthoff, H.H. (1998). Why the visual recognition system might encode the effects of illumination. *Vision Research, 38,* 2259–76.

Tolias, A.S., Smirnakis, S.M., Augath, M.A., Trinath, T., & Logothetis, N.K. (2001). Motion processing in the macaque: revisited with functional magnetic resonance imaging. *Journal of Neuroscience, 21*(21), 8594–601.

Tootell, R.B., Hadjikhani, N.K., Vanduffel, W., Liu, A.K., Mendola, J.D., Sereno, M.I., et al. (1998). Functional analysis of primary visual cortex (V1) in humans. *Proceedings of the National Academy of Sciences of the U S A, 95*(3), 811–7.

Tootell, R.B., Reppas, J.B., Dale, A.M., Look, R.B., Sereno, M.I., Malach, R., Brady, T.J., & Rosen, B.R. (1995). Visual motion aftereffect in human cortical area MT revealed by functional magnetic resonance imaging. *Nature, 375,* 139–41.

Ullman, S. (1996). *High Level Vision.* Cambridge: MIT Press.

van Turennout, M., Ellmore, T., & Martin, A. (2000). Long-lasting cortical plasticity in the object naming system. *Nature Neuroscience, 3,* 1329–34.

Vuilleumier, P., Henson, R.N., Driver, J., & Dolan, R.J. (2002). Multiple levels of visual object constancy revealed by event-related fMRI of repetition priming. *Nature Neuroscience, 5,* 491–9.

Webster, M., & Mollon, J. (1994). The influence of contrast adaptation on color appearance. *Vision Research, 34,* 1993–2020.

Wiggs, C.L., & Martin, A. (1998). Properties and mechanisms of perceptual priming. *Current Opinion in Neurobiology, 8,* 227–33.

7

Adaptation to Complex Visual Patterns in Humans and Monkeys

DAVID A. LEOPOLD AND IGOR BONDAR

Seldom do we question the veracity of our percepts. Our brain, it seems, is remarkably skilled at transforming optical images on the retina into accurate and meaningful objects and scenes in our mind. On occasions, however, perception deviates from the true structure of the world, and by studying such instances we are able to gain insight into the processes underlying normal vision. Starting with a somewhat trivial example, consider the percept that follows exposure to intense light, perhaps from sunlight reflected off the rippled surface of a lake. For a few seconds, the visual surroundings appear strewn with ghostly purplish spots that jump from object to object with each shift of one's gaze. Perception is clearly mistaken in that these spots are not really there. Fortunately, experience teaches us that these potentially alarming apparitions, which are similar in nature to the afterimages that can be generated and studied in the laboratory (Craik 1940), eventually subside and normal vision (usually) returns. In this example, abnormally high light intensity has led to temporary disruption of photoreceptor function in the retina. The brain itself may thus be forgiven for the perceptual inaccuracy, since tainted information was clearly passed on to it from its primary sensory organ.

In contrast to afterimages, the equally famous after*effects* are widely thought to be a product of the visual cortex. They also involve temporary misperceptions following exposure to an adapting visual stimulus. However, aftereffects generally do not appear as new structures painted upon the world, but rather as distortions of existing visual patterns. Their diversity and range of complexity suggest an origin deep within the neural circuits underlying perceptual organization, which is the process by which the 2-D spatiotemporal optical pattern on the retina is reinterpreted into perceptually meaningful quantities, such as objects and their 3-D spatial relationships. For the uninitiated, the impact of adaptation on perception can be surprising. After one gazes at a waterfall, a stationary pattern can appear to drift upwards (Wohlgemuth 1911). After one stares at a curved line, a straight one can appear to bend in the opposite direction (Gibson 1933). And, unlike afterimages, aftereffects cannot be primarily retinal in origin, since adaptation through one eye results in distortions of a test stimulus viewed through the other.

It is interesting, and perhaps no coincidence, that the diversity of aftereffects, for motion direction, color, orientation and spatial frequency, and many other stimulus attributes, closely mirrors the physiological response selectivity in the visual system. As a tool for studying visual processing in the brain, adaptation is effective at isolating and distorting single attributes within a pattern (e.g. motion), while leaving others untainted (e.g. color). For this reason, aftereffects have been famously termed the "psychologist's microelectrode" (Frisby 1979), though, as we will see, their role may be best described as complementary to single-unit studies. Interestingly, despite centuries of study (Wade 1999) and a number of recent electrophysiological (Maffei *et al.* 1973; Movshon & Lennie 1979; Carandini *et al.* 1998, 2000; Kohn & Movshon 2004) and neuroimaging (Tootell *et al.* 1995; Culham *et al.* 1999; Taylor *et al.* 2000; Huk *et al.* 2001; Tolias *et al.* 2001) investigations, the cortical mechanisms of aftereffects remain mysterious. As discussed in detail below, this is probably because aftereffects, like most perceptual phenomena, are not the product of a single visual area or processing stage. In fact, a number of findings suggest that our intuition about the generation and expression of aftereffects, which usually hinges on the balance of activity among feature selective sensory neurons, may be somewhat off the mark. Indeed, even the simple retina-based explanation of after*images* provided above is likely to be a gross oversimplification of their perceptual determinants (Wade 1978; Shimojo *et al.* 2001; Suzuki & Grabowecky 2003). One difficulty that emerges in formalizing any theory of adaptation is that aftereffects are expressed in perceptual, rather than physical quantities, and that perception can be simultaneously shaped by contributions from all over the brain, none of which are particularly well-understood.

Given that we have only a vague notion of their neural basis, what can aftereffects teach us about the brain function? Ironically, they may be most instructive precisely because their origin *cannot* be easily localized. Unlike single-unit or even imaging experiments, aftereffects provide a glimpse at distributed systems in the brain as they are functionally coupled in normal vision. In the present article, we explore aftereffects from a particular point of view, namely, with regard to the complexity of the stimuli that generate them. We first ask, given the hierarchical structure of the visual system, and the many types of stimuli for which adaptation is effective, does stimulus complexity affect the expression of the well-studied tilt aftereffect (TAE)? If aftereffects are a product of selective sensory neurons, complex stimuli might be expected to elicit very different effects, reflecting their processing at higher processing stages in the visual hierarchy. We then focus on aftereffects generated by adaptation to faces, which have recently shed new light on the brain mechanisms of both aftereffects and face processing. We show in humans and monkeys that such aftereffects are best explained if the brain takes an unseen, average face as a *norm* or reference point during adaptation. Finally, we reflect on the generality of norm-based encoding in the brain, not just for faces but for a wide range of stimuli, and speculate how such a scheme might emerge and contribute to our normal vision.

7.1 Aftereffects to Simple and Complex Stimuli

Although it is common to speak of simple and complex aftereffects, it is more meaningful to instead apply these terms to the stimuli that generate the aftereffects. Traditionally, adapting stimuli have been impoverished, usually consisting of a single prominent attribute, such as orientation or direction of motion. Recently, a number of aftereffects have been reported that use more complex adapting patterns, such as geometric shapes (Petersik *et al.* 1984; Suzuki 2001; Fang *et al.* 2004), spatiotemporal sequences (Arnold & Anstis 1993; van der Smagt *et al.* 1999), and natural images (Webster & MacLin 1999; Leopold *et al.* 2001). The expression of these aftereffects often cannot be predicted based on local adaptation to the component parts of the stimuli, and this has been taken as evidence for the selective activation of high-level selective neurons. In contrast, aftereffects elicited by adaptation to simpler stimuli are usually considered to arise from earlier cortical sites, such as the primary visual cortex (V1). However, given the paucity of direct physiological data on this point, are these assumptions really sound? As mentioned previously, adaptation with virtually any stimulus will influence neurons at early, intermediate, and late stages of visual processing, all of which will have the potential to contribute to the percept in one way or another.

Thus before proceeding on to a survey of more complex aftereffects, let us begin by examining whether simple aftereffects are indeed likely to be the product of feature selective circuitry in earliest cortical processing stages. We focus on the tilt aftereffect (TAE) (Gibson & Radner 1937), which refers to the slightly rotated perception of a bar or grating that follows adaptation to a different orientation. After staring for half a minute at a small grating patch oriented 15° to the right of the vertical, a subsequently viewed vertical grating patch will appear as if it were rotated 1–2° leftward. Adaptation to one portion in the visual field will cause an aftereffect only in the direct vicinity of the adapting location. This highly reproducible, localized, repulsive effect serves to demonstrate the principle of adaptation in psychology textbooks, and is embraced by neuroscientists because of its apparently direct connection to orientation-selective neurons in the primary visual cortex, area V1 (Hubel & Wiesel 1968). Models of the TAE typically invoke the fatigue of a subset of V1 neurons during the adaptation period, which creates a subsequent imbalance in the cortical analysis of local orientation. According to this view, temporary biasing of orientation processing is applied early, in the primary visual cortex, and then passed along to higher "perceptual" centers in a manner somewhat analogous to the purplish spots described above (Coltheart 1971). But it may be seen as somewhat surprising that there is a widespread acceptance of this view, given the lack of direct physiological data to support it. Single unit studies from the primary visual cortex have generally observed orientation-selective suppression following extended periods of adaptation (Movshon & Lennie 1979; Carandini *et al.* 1998). But these observations, while consistent with a role of V1 in adaptational aftereffects, do not provide a strong test for the hypothesis that the TAE is a product of the primary visual cortex. Thus the question remains open. As we now examine more thoroughly the family of aftereffects involving orientation, we will see how surprisingly difficult it is for any feature-based model of aftereffect generation to accommodate all instances of the TAE. Even simple aftereffects, it appears, are not so simple.

7.1.1 The Tilt Aftereffect and Norms

The original characterization of the TAE came from the seminal work of Gibson and Radner (1937). A few years before, Gibson had reported that extended inspection of curved line segments would cause them ever so slowly to lose their apparent curvature. He also found that subsequently viewed straight lines then appeared to bend in the opposite direction (Gibson 1933). Upon finding similar effects in the domain of orientation, Gibson and Radner decided to investigate this tilt aftereffect systematically. Using vertical lines as test stimuli, they discovered that the magnitude and direction of perceived rotation changed according to the orientation of the adapting stimulus. A small tilt in the adapting stimulus caused the test to appear rotated *away* from the adapting orientation, while a larger one was drawn *towards* it. Gibson and Radner termed the repulsive and attractive effects as the *direct* and *indirect* effects respectively.

The existence of direct and indirect effects poses problems for simple V1-based models of the TAE, and some psychophysical evidence suggested that indirect effects invoke altogether different cortical mechanisms than the direct effects (Wenderoth & Johnstone 1988; van der Zwan & Wenderoth 1995). Unlike the direct effects, indirect effects are unreliable (Koehler *et al.* 1944), and sensitive to the presence of visual orientation context, such as a frame, surrounding the stimulus (Wenderoth & Johnstone 1988). They also appear to act upon the global representation of orientation, and therefore do not require the strict matching in the stimulus size, position, and spatial frequency content between the adapting and test stimuli that is characteristic of direct effects (Wenderoth & van der Zwan 1989; Wenderoth & Smith 1999). Despite these obstacles, some models have successfully incorporated both components into a single, comprehensive model of the TAE (Bednar & Mukkulainen 2000; Clifford *et al.* 2000).

Gibson and Radner, in trying to understand the nature of the aftereffects that they observed with tilt and curvature, postulated the existence of implicit *norms* to serve as references for the visual system in generating a percept. According to their ideas, an aftereffect was not simply the product of an adapting and test pattern, but was also critically dependent on a third, implicitly represented stimulus. The size and direction of a perceptual aftereffect was first and foremost a function of the difference between the adapting pattern and an internal norm. For orientation, the cardinal directions (horizontal and vertical) served this function, while for curvature a straight line was the reference point.

While these were landmark notions, they are generally no longer accepted because they cannot account for some simple observations. Koehler and Wallach (Koehler *et al.* 1944), for example, showed that adaptation to a horizontal line created an aftereffect for oblique lines (Koehler *et al.* 1994, Figure 60), which would not be predicted if horizontal were a special norm orientation. Later studies provided additional examples to further weaken norm-based accounts of adaptation (Morant & Harris 1965; Mitchell & Muir 1976). It thus became gradually apparent that a simple norm-based theory could not account for all cases of the TAE, and the theory of norms faded away into the history of psychophysics. It is important to consider, however, that the limitations on a theory should not necessarily lead to its complete rejection. Interestingly, since that time, norm-based theories of perception have reemerged in a completely different context, in the study of face recognition (Rhodes *et al.* 1987), where the concept of norms was originally closely tied to that of category prototypes (e.g. Posner *et al.* 1968). Given their role in adaptation, as well as face recognition, it is perhaps not altogether surprising that norms are at the center of the discussion of face aftereffects, as discussed later.

7.1.2 What Makes an Aftereffect Simple?

A number of demonstrations reveal that vastly different stimuli can give rise to similar aftereffects. Consider, for example, the TAE elicited by adaptation to the stimulus in Fig. 7.1(A), based on the work of Joung and van der Zwan (Joung *et al.* 2000). If the reader inspects the upper pattern for a period and then shifts his or her gaze to the lower one, it will appear to tilt to the right although it is in fact vertical. Joung and colleagues found that such stimuli, whose orientation is defined only by the axis of symmetry, produce surprisingly ordinary tilt aftereffects, similar in direction and magnitude to that encountered with luminance contours (Joung *et al.* 2000; Joung & Latimer 2003). This similarity even extends to both direct and indirect components. In considering the neural mechanisms underlying the aftereffect, the receptive field size and structure of neurons in V1 would suggest that they cannot be sensitive to the orientation of the adapting and test patterns, which is defined only at a global level.

Analogous demonstrations exist for other types of simple aftereffects, such as the spatial frequency shift (Blakemore & Sutton 1969), which has also been speculated to reflect local adaptation in the primary visual cortex. While this

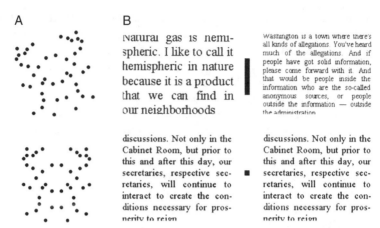

FIG. 7.1 Two derivatives of well-known "low-level" aftereffects whose appearance cannot be easily accounted for by low-level mechanisms alone. (A) Axis of symmetry tilt aftereffect. When the upper pattern is examined for half a minute before shifting one's gaze to the lower pattern (adapted from Joung *et al.* 2000), the lower pattern appears to lean to the right. This tilt aftereffect shares many properties in common with the well known illusion following adaptation to a luminance bar or grating. (B) If one restricts one's gaze to the vertical bar between the text in the upper half of the figure, and then moves the eyes to the lower square, the text on the right appears as a larger font than that on the left. These aftereffects, while bearing marked similarities to their low-level counterparts, are thought to require global, rather than local feature-based processing, and are therefore thought to depend upon higher-level mechanisms as well.

aftereffect is usually demonstrated with simple gratings, adaptation to a variety of more complex textures produces similar perceptual distortions (Durgin 2001; McKay 1964). The stimulus in Fig. 7.1(B), for example, based on a demonstration by Anstis (1974), shows that higher-level stimulus attributes can also be affected by such adaptation. In this case, prolonged inspection of the upper text patches gives rise to systematic changes in the perceived font size of the lower text blocks. While some of this effect can be accounted for by general, spatial frequency-selective adaptation, recent experiments have shown that a significant portion of texture aftereffects occurs independent of spatial frequency content (Durgin & Huk 1997), apparently acting on the representation of the texture itself (in the case of Fig. 7.1(B), text).

Thus it seems unwise to assign aftereffects to brain areas based upon the complexity of the adapting pattern. The common phenomenology of the TAE with vastly different stimuli suggests instead that a more general mechanism is at work, even if it is currently beyond our grasp.

This is further emphasized by examining adaptation to subjective contours, which have been studied both in terms of their cortical representations as well as their ability to generate aftereffects. Tilt aftereffects following such adaptation, to stimuli like those shown in Fig. 7.2(A), for instance (adapted from

A

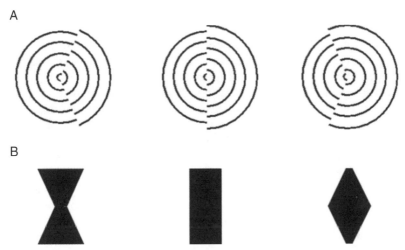

B

FIG. 7.2 Three examples of stimuli giving rise to "high-level" adaptational aftereffects. In each case, adaptation to the stimulus on the left, followed by brief presentation of the stimulus in the middle, produces a percept in the direction of the stimulus on the right. (A) Illusory or "subjective" contours produce by and large normal tilt aftereffects (adapted from Paradiso *et al.* 1989). (B) Aftereffects to simple concave and convex patterns such as this (adapted from Suzuki 2001) recently raised the possibility of opponent mechanisms governing the perception of simple shapes.

Paradiso *et al.* 1989), closely resemble those obtained with luminance contours (Smith & Over 1975; Paradiso *et al.* 1989). This generalization also holds for both direct and indirect components (van der Zwan & Wenderoth 1995), despite the very different physical nature of the real and subjective contours. This is perhaps unsurprising given the robustness of the TAE to contours defined by different attributes, including color, texture, motion, and binocular disparity (Cavanagh 1989). However, it does further weaken the argument that the TAE is a product of activity in area V1, where subjective contours generally fail to activate orientation-selective neurons (von der Heydt & Peterhans 1989). Interestingly, neurons in neighboring area V2 do respond reliably to such patterns. Thus, while orientation analysis in V1 is clearly an important step in early visual analysis, the often-made assumption that the same machinery is at the core of the TAE may need to be reconsidered.

7.1.3 Aftereffects of Shape

We next consider shape aftereffects, of which surprisingly few examples have been reported. It is interesting that despite extensive knowledge about the physiology of the visual cortex, and the associated aftereffects to simple patterns, our ability to predict the form of an aftereffect to an arbitrary shape is almost nonexistent. If nothing else, this underscores our poor understanding of their neural basis. In general, aftereffects for shapes are more difficult to demonstrate than those for simpler stimuli. It was recognized shortly after Gibson's original studies that certain two- and three-dimensional shapes can give rise to figural aftereffects (Koehler & Wallach 1944; Koehler & Emery 1947; Regan & Hamstra 1992). Yet, in the following decades, while scores of reports investigated aftereffects of orientation, motion, and color, relatively few focused on simple or complex shapes. A series of recent studies from Suzuki and colleagues has drawn new interest to this potentially important topic. The authors observed that even a brief presentation of an "adapting" line or shape can strongly and reliably influence the appearance of a subsequently shown pattern (Suzuki & Cavanagh 1998; Suzuki 2001; see also Suzuki, this volume). In one experiment, Suzuki adapted to and tested with stimuli such as those shown in Fig. 7.2(B), and found that particular pairs of shapes, say a convex and a concave one, were complementary for the formation of aftereffects. Based on this, he argued that shape perception may rely on "opponent" processing, analogous to the representation of color in the early visual system. It is interesting to reflect that while the stimuli and paradigm differ markedly from Gibson's, many of the results and conclusions are reminiscent of the original experiments with adaptation to line curvature (Gibson 1933).

Shape aftereffects are generally more robust to changes in size and even position between the adapting and test stimuli than aftereffects with simple stimuli (Suzuki 2001). This observation has led to speculation that shape aftereffects reflect selective adaptation of neurons beyond the earliest cortical areas, perhaps in the inferotemporal cortex where shape-selective responses show similar invariant properties (Ito et al. 1995). But, in light of the previously identified dangers in assigning a perceptual effect to a given brain area, we might first ask whether the contribution from earlier areas is also measurable. One approach that Suzuki introduced to potentially disentangle this web of early and late contributions uses adaptation *duration* as an additional experimental variable. He found that by severely reducing the adaptation time he was able to eliminate aftereffects related to internal oriented texture, but that the same conditions had little effect on aftereffects generated by the outline contour. The latter effects were robust to changes in size and position, and therefore may have tied more directly to later stages of visual representation. Although the real basis of this dissociation remains a matter of speculation, the results suggest that early and late contributions to a perceptual aftereffect can be, in some cases, evaluated separately. They also highlight adaptation duration as a potentially important variable for teasing apart low- and high-level contributions to perceptual aftereffects.

In summary, despite the venerable history of adaptation, the many uses of aftereffects for probing visual function are still being discovered. Adaptation with complex stimuli is beginning to provide new insights into the brain's processing mechanism and the encoding of shapes and objects. At the same time, we have to remember that aftereffects with simple stimuli are likely to involve more than the selective exhaustion of tuned V1 neurons. We now turn to faces, a natural stimulus category to which our brains should be even more accustomed. Face recognition is in some ways the pinnacle of our visual performance. In faces, we are able to capitalize on miniscule structural differences to distinguish between individuals, despite enormous variation in the images reaching the eye due to changes in viewing angle, illumination, and facial expression. Faces are of great social value, providing information not only about identity, but also about the disposition and even intentions of others. Yet none of these qualities makes strong predictions about the degree to which face perception might be susceptible to adaptation, which is discussed in the next section.

7.2 Adaptation to Faces

How might prolonged exposure to one face affect the perception of subsequently viewed faces? As with each of the stimuli discussed above, a face first impacts cortical neurons in area V1. Though it is important to point out that "first", in this case, refers more to the conceptual than temporal order of activation since, after the initial presentation transient, the stimulus is available to adapt all levels of processing simultaneously. Theoretically, the image of a face should activate a subpopulation of V1 neurons based upon its constellation of low-level, localized features. At (conceptually) later stages of processing, such as the inferotemporal cortex, higher order aspects of the same image activate face-selective neurons (Perrett et al. 1982). For faces and other patterns, the low-level details of the stimuli are often disregarded in this area, in favor of overall, holistic structure (Sary et al. 1993; Ito et al. 1995). While most of the available data on face-selective neurons comes from the monkey, recent evidence suggests that similar neural responses are present in the human brain as well (Kreiman et al. 2000). Imaging reveals that the cortex of both monkeys and humans displays widespread, selective activation in response to faces (Kanwisher et al. 1997; Haxby et al. 2000). There is thus good evidence that adaptation to a face simultaneously activates diverse specific and many more unspecific neurons at many levels of cortical processing.

Bringing faces into the domain of stimuli that can be investigated by adaptation, an influential experiment by Webster and MacLin (1999) first demonstrated that faces, like other stimuli, can robustly generate and express figural aftereffects. They showed that adapting to a grotesquely distorted face caused subsequently viewed normal faces to appear distorted in the opposite manner, an effect that transferred between faces of different identity. Face aftereffects, like those of geometrical shapes, were later shown to be robust to changes in the relative position (Leopold et al. 2001), size (Zhao & Chubb 2001), and angular orientation (Watson & Clifford 2003) of the adapting and test stimuli. Yet unlike other complex patterns, faces possess a number of "special" dimensions, such as identity and expression, for which our perception appears finely tuned. Recent experiments have shown that even such high-level, socially relevant stimulus properties can be isolated and studied using adaptation. The subtle physical differences that define facial identity, for example, can be probed using adaptation (Leopold *et al.* 2001; Rhodes *et al.*, this volume), as described in detail in the next section. In addition, gender, ethnicity, expression (Webster *et al.* 2004), and even attractiveness (Rhodes *et al.* 2003) can be independently isolated to a surprising degree using adaptation.

Next, we briefly describe a study demonstrating that individual *identity* is a dimension of face analysis that can be selectively adapted and probed with a perceptual aftereffect. We then show that the expression of this aftereffect, which is one of the most specialized forms of adaptation known to date, is very similar for a rhesus monkey looking at human faces. These studies set the stage for electrophysiological investigations of face encoding in the monkey that are currently underway (Leopold 2003).

7.2.1 Face Identity Aftereffect

The physical difference between the faces of two individuals is often remarkably subtle, amounting to slight differences in the shape or configuration of the same basic features. Yet we are readily able to recognize thousands of different faces, sometimes based on these structural differences alone. We developed an adaptation paradigm to investigate how the brain might accomplish this task. We started with the models of face recognition that postulate the brain's decoding of individual faces to be based on the natural statistics of a large number of faces. The average face, in particular, has often been a particularly important statistic, serving as a norm for interpreting facial structure (Rhodes & Tremewan 1994). Note that the norms in face recognition, just as those postulated much earlier by Gibson for the perception of lines, are thought to be represented *implicitly* in the visual processing apparatus. As such, they can be used to decode the sensory input and, when faced with adaptation, determine the magnitude and duration of a perceptual aftereffect. Norm-based models have previously been used to account for several features of face recognition, most notably the tolerance of recognition to caricaturization (Valentine & Bruce 1986; Rhodes *et al.* 1987). In such models, it is the *difference* of a face from the average that informs the recognition system about the identity of the individual[1]. It is interesting now to reflect on the fact that norm-based models have had a prominent theoretical role, quite independently, both in the study of simple aftereffects and in the coding of face identity. In retrospect, this common denominator might be seen to predict that norms would play a central role in aftereffects involving face identity, and that is indeed what we found.

---

[1] The terminology here can be confusing. The average face is sometimes referred to as the "prototype". This term comes from the literature on categorization, since the average face might be seen to be the prototype for the category of faces. It is also referred to as the "norm" because of its putative role as an implicit reference.

We tested adaptation to face identity using realistic human faces as the adapting and test stimuli (Leopold *et al.* 2001). We designed our stimuli to occupy particular positions within an abstract *face space* (Valentine 1991), where single faces are considered as points or vectors in a high-dimensional space centered on the average face (see Fig. 7.3(A)). The stimuli consisted of morphs of scanned, realistic faces available from the Max Planck Face Database (http://www.kyb.tuebingen.de/~faces). Vetter and colleagues previously developed the computational methods to generate realistic faces at arbitrary points within this space (Vetter & Troje 1997; Blanz *et al.* 1999).

Using these stimuli, we asked whether adaptation could be so precise as to leave an identity-specific trace in the visual system. The methods and some of the results have been previously described in detail (Leopold *et al.* 2001), but we will give a brief overview here. Subjects were first trained and then tested on their ability to discriminate between four different faces at several levels of identity strength (i.e. distance from the center in face space). We first measured the basic sensitivity to this variable without any adaptation (Fig. 7.3(B,C)). Next, we repeated the measurements, but in this case, each test pattern was preceded by an adapting stimulus, which was an anti-face[2] in some cases, and the average face in others. The anti-face adapting stimuli in some cases lay along the *same* trajectory as the test ("anti-face same" condition), and in some cases along *different* trajectories ("anti-face different" condition). Based on pilot studies, and on the previous observation that short test stimuli give rise to strong adaptational aftereffects (Wolfe 1984), we used an adaptation duration of 5000 ms and a test duration of 200 ms.

Sensitivity following adaptation is shown in the black curves in Fig. 7.4, for the anti-face same (Fig. 7.4(A)), anti-face different (Fig. 7.4(B)), and average face (Fig. 7.4(C)) adaptation conditions. These data show that face perception is biased toward correctly identifying the test face following adaptation to an anti-face lying on the same trajectory as the test face, but is biased in the opposite direction (and hence performance is disrupted) when the faces were on different trajectories. Subjects reported that in the latter case, faces appeared as "hybrids", with recognizable features from both the trajectories involved. This requirement that the adapting and test stimuli be on the same trajectory for facilitation demonstrates that anti-face adaptation is specific for the subtle physical differences that make each individual face unique.

The misperception of identity was also reflected in the mean response times, shown in Fig. 7.5. Additional experiments showed that the identity-specific effects were robust to stimulus translations of at least six degrees on the retina,

---

[2] *Anti-faces* refer to faces morphed onto the other side of the mean for each of the four test faces. Anti-faces appear just as normal faces with a unique identity. In the context of the face space, there is an "opposite" relationship between a face and its anti-face. Psychophysical work has shown that the morphing between a face and its anti-face involves a perceptual discontinuity in identity upon passing the average stimulus (Blanz *et al.* 2000).

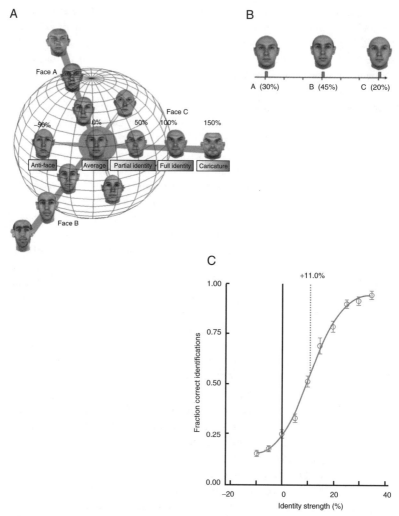

FIG. 7.3 Sensitivity to face identity in the context of a multidimensional face space. (A) Norm-based face space, showing the relative positions of different degrees of caricaturization for three different individuals' identity trajectories. (B) Sensitivity was tested with multiple 200 ms presentations at different identity strengths. Subjects were required to indicate the identity of the face following each presentation by pressing one of four buttons on a choice box. (C) The resulting psychometric function showed that roughly 30% identity strength was sufficient for subjects to approach 100% performance (N = 7). The dotted line (11.0%) corresponds to threshold in identification performance, based on the inflection point of the best fitting probit function (gray line). Chance performance corresponds to a fraction of 0.25 correct identification.

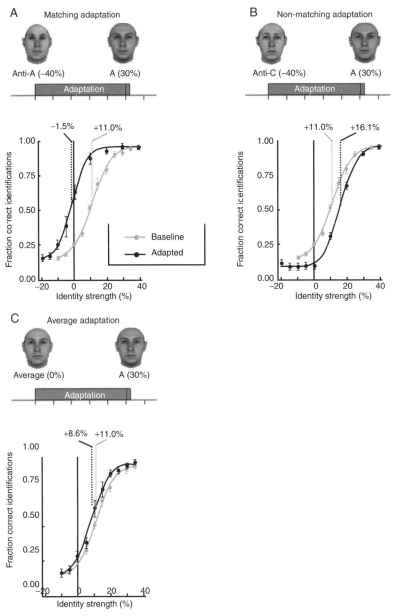

FIG. 7.4 Effects of adaptation to one face on perception of another. The effect of adaptation was highly dependent on the relative positions of the adapting and test faces in the multidimensional face space. (A) When the adapting face was on the same identity trajectory but on the opposite side of the average face, perception was biased in the direction of the test face, which was thus correctly identified at values quite close to the average face. (B) In contrast, when the adapting and test faces were on different trajectories, performance was impaired since perception was biased in a different direction. (C) Following adaptation to the average face (i.e. the center of face space), there was a small but statistically significant improvement in performance. Dotted vertical lines show the identification thresholds for the baseline and adapted conditions.

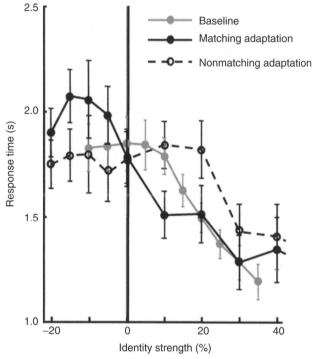

FIG. 7.5 Reaction time as a function of identity strength.

suggesting that their origin cannot be a constellation of low-level, localized after-effects. And, similar to the results of Webster and MacLin (1999), the aftereffect was expressed for inverted as well as upright faces (Leopold 2001). This suggests that the face aftereffect, while highly specific for face identity, involves mechanisms that are distinct from those responsible for the profound and selective disruption of faces following inversion (Yin 1969; Rhodes & Tremewan 1994; Kanwisher *et al.* 1998).

In summary, these results demonstrate that adaptation can precisely bias the perception of face identity toward or away from a particular individual, with results that are consistent with norm-based models of face recognition. We next explore the generality of this observation by testing whether a non-human primate, confronted with the same adapting and test stimuli, experiences similar perceptual aftereffects.

7.2.2 Human Face Aftereffect in the Monkey

The motivation for testing a monkey under identical conditions to the human was two-fold. First, we wanted to explore generality of the effect between these two species, which have similar visual faculties but markedly different cognitive capabilities. Perceptual aftereffects have been previously demonstrated in animals (Roberts 1984) including old world monkeys (Scott & Powell 1963). Monkeys, like humans, are highly sensitive to the facial identity and expressions of their conspecifics (Pascalis *et al.* 2000), and appear to have a similar network of areas involved in the analysis of faces (Kanwisher *et al.* 1997; Logothetis *et al.* 1999; Haxby *et al.* 2000; Tsao *et al.* 2003). Nonetheless, given the profound sensitivity to subtle structural and social nuances that characterize face recognition, it is possible that face-processing modules are species-specific. The other (and primary) motivation is our ongoing exploration of face representations with microelectrode recordings in trained monkeys (Leopold *et al.* 2003). We have been recording the activity of face-responsive neurons in the inferotemporal cortex of monkeys. Neurons were evaluated in their responses to faces at several points along an identity trajectory, both with and without anti-face adaptation. During the testing, one monkey was trained to report the identity of the test faces just as had been done by the humans. It is the psychophysical performance of this animal that we report here.

The fitted curves in Fig. 7.6 show the monkey's recognition of human faces as a function of identity strength (black line), as compared to the performance of the seven individual humans from Fig. 7.3(C). For the monkey, as for the humans, data were pooled over all four identity trajectories. The similarity between the monkey and human data is striking, with the monkey showing only a slightly lower sensitivity to face identity. This may reflect small behavioral fluctuations typical of animal studies, or it may reflect a true difference in the recognition of human faces. It is perhaps interesting to point out that the monkey's performance with human faces was most comparable to the human performance on the same faces when they were inverted (Leopold *et al.* 2001). Thus these data do not provide a definitive answer regarding the absolute sensitivity of human face processing in the monkey, but they do indicate that monkeys are able to see and interpret faces of diminished identity in a manner that is comparable to humans. We next tested the more interesting question of how adaptation affects the monkey's percept.

The data in Fig. 7.7 show that the perceptual effects of adaptation were very similar for the monkey and humans. This can be best seen by comparing Fig. 7.7(A) with Fig. 7.4(A), and Fig. 7.7(B) with Fig. 7.4(B), respectively. This observation might be taken as evidence that a face processing module, whose operation covers both human and monkey faces, is evolutionarily conserved between the two species from a common ancestor. An alternative interpretation might be that the aftereffect has relatively little to do with faces *per se*, but instead represents a general mechanism for analyzing complex visual patterns, and that the monkey's adeptness with human faces represents an experience-dependent specialization. It is difficult to differentiate between these two possibilities in the current study, given the magnitude of training for both humans and the monkey that may have gradually shaped the manner in which the adapting and test faces were processed.

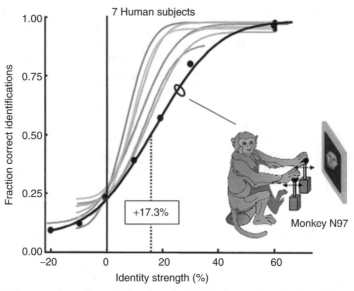

FIG. 7.6 Comparison of sensitivity of monkey N97 to human face identity with that of 7 human subjects during the same task. The monkey's overall performance was slightly worse than the humans', with the identity threshold (dotted line) roughly 6% higher (17.3% versus 11.0% mean for 7 humans) and near-perfect performance requiring roughly 50% identity strength. MONKEY TRAINING: The training regimen consisted of reward-based operant conditioning, where a drop of apple juice was received for correct answers. Like the human subjects, the monkey was trained to identify the four faces, first at high and then at lower identity levels. Instead of responding with a button box, the animal used two bi-directional levers to signal which of the faces was recognized, and received a juice reward. Training for the baseline and adaptation tasks required approximately three and two months, respectively. The training period was deemed complete when the monkey would perform above 95% on full-identity trials. Note that the monkey was required to provide a response with each presentation, and we therefore took necessary precautions in the reward schedule to encourage good performance. First, rather than rewarding automatically with each correct response, we employed a probabilistic schedule, where each correct response led to a probability of reward, generally between 0.4 and 0.8. Second, while incorrect responses were generally not rewarded, an exception was made for very low identity strengths (≤10%), which were rewarded randomly – encouraging the monkey to "guess" when recognition was difficult or impossible.

7.3 Internal References for Visual Processing

Based on the face identity aftereffect, as well as the handful of classical and more recent aftereffects for orientation and faces referenced above, we thus conclude that norms, which are seldom included in modern descriptions of vision, may indeed serve an important function in shaping our percept. The paradigm

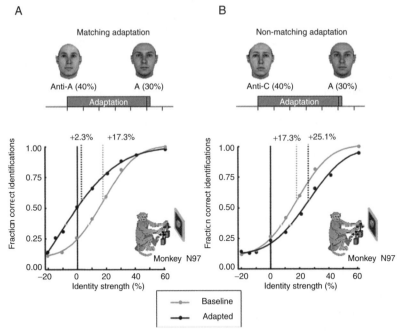

FIG. 7.7 Effects of adaptation on human face perception in one monkey. The psycho-physical paradigm, including the stimuli, was identical to that used with the humans with one exception – the adapting stimulus was shown for 4 seconds rather than 5 seconds. (A) Following adaptation to an anti-face, performance with test stimuli lying on the same trajectory is improved since perception is biased in that direction. (B) Performance with test stimuli lying on different trajectories declines because the perception is biased in a different direction. These results closely mirror those found in human subjects.

of adaptation seems particularly suited for tapping into such stored internal quantities, since they may not be directly measurable with electrophysiological or neuroimaging techniques. Such perceptual assays, while providing a healthy complement to physical measurements of brain function, blur the distinction somewhat between implicit and explicit neural representations.

In this vein, one might object to an unnecessary level of abstraction put forth here, invoking an unseen, internal stimulus representation to guide visual processing. Would not simple, antagonistic (or opponent) connectivity between neurons with dissimilar preferred features be sufficient to explain the same data? We would argue that the answer is both yes and no. Yes because it is likely that the aftereffect is, ultimately, a product of highly refined neural connectivity. But, no because a simple, mechanistic explanation of a neural circuit, making no reference to a norm stimulus, bypasses the essence of the experimental results and is therefore incomplete.

Consider the face identity aftereffect. In face space, our experiments revealed that only faces on opposite sides of the average face are, in fact, "opponent". This was shown by the specificity of adaptation between a particular anti-face and its corresponding original face. Other pairs of equally dissimilar faces do not possess this quality (see Rhodes *et al.*, this volume). If we consider a neural model of this opponency that involves antagonistic connectivity between neurons responding to a face and its anti-face, one must explain how exactly that pattern of connectivity came to be. To account for this specificity, one must invoke the average face as having a special role in the genesis of any such anatomical or physiological specificity, even if the details of this process are unknown. This conclusion is bolstered by recent neurophysiological findings from the monkey inferotemporal cortex (IT), which find that the average face occupies a privileged position in the tuning of face-selective neurons (Leopold *et al.* 2003) . Using the set of faces from the experiments described above, as well as an additional set that was controlled for its low-level stimulus properties, we found that neurons in anterior IT were tuned to face identity in a unique and unexpected way. Namely, responsive units very often fired *less* spikes for the average face than for faces of higher identity strength. This was often the case even when the cells were responsive to several different face identities, in which case the average face typically elicited the smallest response of all the faces shown. Thus, while more work needs to be done on this issue, these results suggest that face-selective responses might best be described not in terms of the physical quantities of a stimulus, but rather in the *deviation* of that stimulus from the stored average or norm.

These results question, how might such a face gain this special status to serve as the "decoder" for incoming faces? One property of norm-based encoding schemes is that they are well-suited to adapt themselves over time to the statistics of their environment. This point is particularly relevant for our perception of individuals, where the "diet" of faces might ultimately determine, over time, the structure of the norm (Webster & MacLin 1999; Rhodes *et al.* 2003). These ideas resonate closely with work from Purves and colleagues, who have recently championed the more general notion that our perceptual mechanisms are fine-tuned for the visual statistics of the environment (Purves & Lotto 2003). In a series of experiments, they endeavored to measure scene statistics directly, and have used these measurements to offer explanations for a host of simple visual illusions, including those of orientation (Nundy 2000; Howe & Purves 2002). The shaping of visual processing, and thus perception, according to such statistics bears some equivalence to the implicit storage of norms, and is also ultimately expressed as connectivity between visually responsive neurons. And their results, like those reported here, emphasize that our sensory processing is finely tuned to solve precisely the visual problems that we are most likely to encounter.

7.4 Summary

We examined the properties of diverse visual aftereffects, including the face identity aftereffect and several others previously reported in the literature.

We first compared with the studies of the tilt aftereffect that used simple and complex adapting patterns, and found that the perceptual effects were remarkably similar despite the fact that the stimuli were likely to activate different cortical areas. This led us to conclude that simple models of the tilt aftereffect based on connectivity between orientation selective neurons in V1 are likely to be incorrect or incomplete. We then described the expression of the face identity aftereffect in humans and a rhesus monkey. In both cases, adaptation resulted in consistent and precise misperception in facial identity, according to the relative positions of the adapting stimulus and the average face in a norm-centered face space. Preliminary electrophysiological studies suggest that the norm face plays a particularly important role with regard to the tuning of the neurons to face stimuli. In light of these results, we conclude that visual adaptation provides a means to gauge aspects of visual processing that are currently intractable with other techniques. The host of aftereffects to complex stimuli that have surfaced in the last few years questions many of the standard assumptions about the generation and expression of aftereffects, both simple and complex. And the classical concept of norm-based coding, which has seldom been invoked in recent decades, may in fact hold great value for understanding how the brain senses and interprets the structure of visual patterns.

Acknowledgments

Thanks to Drs. Christof Koch, Alexander Maier, and Melanie Wilke, and to Kai-Markus Mueller and Evgeniy Bart for their comments on the manuscript. The face images were collected by Drs. N. Troje, T. Vetter and others in the laboratory of Prof. H. Bülthoff, and the experiments were performed in the laboratory of Prof. N. Logothetis at the Max Planck Institute for Biological Cybernetics. The morphed stimuli were produced by Drs. T. Vetter and V. Blanz, who contributed to the human psychophysics described here, along with Dr. A. O'Toole. Thanks to J. Werner for technical assistance. This work was supported by the Max Planck Society.

References

Anstis, S.M. (1974). Size adaptation to visual texture and print: evidence for spatial frequency analysis. *American Journal of Psychology, 87*, 261–7.

Arnold, K., & Anstis, S.M. (1993). Properties of the visual channels that underlie adaptation to gradual change of luminance. *Vision Research, 33*, 47–54.

Bednar, J.A., & Mukkulainen, R. (2000). Tilt aftereffects in a self-organizing model of the primary visual cortex. *Neural Computation, 12*, 1721–40.

Blakemore, C., & Sutton, P. (1969). Size adaptation: a new aftereffect. *Science, 166*, 245–7.

Blanz, V., O'Toole, A.J., & Vetter, T. (2000). On the other side of the mean: the perception of dissimilarity in human faces. *Perception, 29*(8), 885–91.

Blanz, V., & Vetter, T. (1999). A morphable model for the synthesis of 3d faces. *Symposium on Interactive 3D Gaphics – Proceedings of SIGGRAPH'99* (pp. 187–94). New York: ACM Press.

Carandini, M. (2000). Visual cortex: fatigue and adaptation. *Current Biology, 10,* R605–R607.

Carandini, M., Movshon, A.J., & Ferster, D. (1998). Pattern adaptation and cross-orientation interactions in the primary visual cortex. *Neuropharmacology, 37,* 501–11.

Cavanagh, P. (1989). Multiple analyses of orientation in the visual system. In D. Lam, & C. Gilbert (ed.), *Neural Mechanisms of Visual Perception* (pp. 261–80). Woodlands, TX: Portfolio Publishing.

Clifford, C.W.G., Wenderoth, P., & Spehar, B. (2000). A functional angle on some after-effects in cortical vision. *Proceedings of the Royal Society of London - Series B: Biological Sciences, 267,* 1705–10.

Coltheart, M. (1971). Visual feature-analyzers and aftereffects of tilt and curvature. *Psychological Review, 78,* 114–21.

Craik, K.J.W. (1940). Origin of visual afterimages. *Nature, 145,* 512.

Culham, J.C., Dukelow, S.P., Vilis, T., Hassard, F.A., Gati, J.S., Menon, R.S. *et al.* (1999). Recovery of fMRI activation in motion area MT following storage of the motion aftereffect. *Journal of Neurophysiology, 81*(1), 388–93.

Durgin, F.H. (2001). Texture contrast aftereffects are monocular; texture density aftereffects are binocular. *Vision Research, 41,* 2619–30.

Durgin, F.H., & Huk, A.C. (1997). Texture density aftereffects in the perception of artificial and natural textures. *Vision Research, 37,* 3273–82.

Fang, F., & He, S. (2004). Stabilized structure from motion without disparity induced disparity adaptation. *Current Biology, 14,* 247–51.

Frisby, J.P. (1979). *Seeing: Illusion, Brain and Mind.* Oxford, England: Oxford University Press.

Gibson, J.J. (1933). Adaptation, after-effect and contrast in the perception of curved lines. *Journal of Experimental Psychology, 16,* 1–31.

Gibson, J.J., & Radner, M. (1937). Adaptation, after-effect, and contrast in the perception of tilted lines.i.quantitative studies. *Journal of Experimental Psychology, 20,* 453–67.

Haxby, J.V., Hoffman, E.A., & Gobbini, M.I. (2000). The distributed human neural system for face perception. *Trends in Cognitive Sciences, 4,* 223–33.

Howe, C.Q., & Purves, D. (2002). Range image statistics can explain the anomalous perception of length. *Proceedings of the National Academy of Sciences of the United States of America, 99,* 13184–8.

Hubel, D.H., & Wiesel, T.N. (1968). Receptive fields and functional architecture of monkey striate cortex. *Journal of Physiology, 195,* 215–43.

Huk, A.C., Ress, D., & Heeger, D.J. (2001). Neuronal basis of the motion aftereffect reconsidered. *Neuron, 32,* 161–72.

Ito, M., Tamura, H., Fujita, I., & Tanaka, K. (1995). Size and position invariance of neuronal responses in monkey inferotemporal cortex. *Journal of Neurophysiology, 73,* 218–26.

Joung, W., & Latimer, C. (2003). Tilt aftereffects generated by symmetrical dot patterns with two or four axes of symmetry. *Spatial Vision, 16,* 155–82.

Joung, W., van der Zwan, R., & Latimer, C. (2000). Tilt aftereffects generated by bilaterally symmetrical patterns. *Spatial Vision, 13,* 107–28.

Kanwisher, N., McDermott, J., & Chun, M.M. (1997). The fusiform face area: A module in human extrastriate cortex specialized for face perception. *Journal of Neuroscience, 17,* 4302–11.

Kanwisher, N., Tong, F., & Nakayama, K. (1998). The effect of face inversion on the human fusiform face area. *Cognition, 68*(1), B1–11.

Koehler, W., & Emery, D.A. (1947). Figural after-effects in the third dimension of visual space. *American Journal of Psychology*, *60*, 159–201.

Koehler, W., & Wallach, H. (1944). Figural after-effects: an investigation of visual processes. *Proceedings of the American Philosophical Society*, *88*, 269–357.

Kohn, A., & Movshon, J.A. (2004). Adaptation changes the direction tuning of macaque MT neurons. *Nature Neuroscience*, *7(7)*, 764–72.

Kreiman, G., Koch, C., & Fried, I. (2000). Category-specific visual responses in the human medial temporal lobe. *Nature Neuroscience*, *3*, 946–53.

Leopold, D.A., Bondar, I.V., Giese, M.A., & Logothetis, N.K. (2003). Prototype-referenced encoding of faces in the monkey inferotemporal cortex. Society for Neuroscience Abstracts, Program No. 590.7.

Leopold, D.A., O'Toole, A.J., Vetter, T., & Blanz, V. (2001). Prototype-referenced shape encoding revealed by high-level aftereffects. *Nature Neuroscience*, *4*, 89–94.

Logothetis, N.K., Guggenberger, H., Peled, S., & Pauls, J. (1999). Functional imaging of the monkey brain. *Nature Neuroscience*, *2*, 555–62.

Maffei, L., Fiorentini, A., & Bisti, S. (1973). Neural correlate of perceptual adaptation to gratings. *Science*, *182*, 1036–8.

McKay, D.M. (1964). Central adaptation in mechanisms of form vision. *Nature*, *203*, 993–4.

Mitchell, D.E., & Muir, D.W. (1976). Does the tilt aftereffect occur in the oblique meridian? *Vision Research*, *16*, 609–13.

Morant, R.B., & Harris, J.R. (1965). Two different aftereffects of exposure to visual tilts. *American Journal of Psychology*, *78*, 218–26.

Movshon, J.A., & Lennie, P. (1979). Pattern-selective adaptation in visual cortical neurons. *Nature*, *278*, 850–2.

Nundy, S., Lotto, B., Coppola, D., Shimpi, A., & Purves, D. (2000). Why are angles misperceived? *Proceedings of the National Academy of Sciences of the United States of America*, *97*, 5592–7.

Paradiso, M.A., Shimojo, S., & Nakayama, K. (1989). Subjective contours, tilt aftereffects, and visual cortical organization. *Vision Research*, *29(9)*, 1205–13.

Pascalis, O., Petit, O., Kim, J.H., & Campbell, R. (2000). Picture perception in primates: the case of face perception. In J. Fagot (ed.), *Picture Perception in Animals* (pp. 263–94). East Sussex, UK: Psychology Press Ltd.

Perrett, D.I., Rolls, E.T., & Caan, W. (1982). Visual neurones responsive to faces in the monkey temporal cortex. *Experimental Brain Research*, *47*, 329–42.

Petersik, J.T., Shepard, A., & Malsch, R. (1984). A three-dimensional motion aftereffect produced by prolonged adaptation to a rotation simulation. *Perception*, *13*, 489–97.

Posner, M.I., & Keele, S.W. (1968). On the genesis of abstract ideas. *Journal of Experimental Psychology*, *77*, 353–63.

Purves, D., & Lotto, R.B. (2003). *Why We See What We Do: An Empirical Theory of Vision*. Sunderland, MA: Sinauer Associates, Inc.

Regan, D., & Hamstra, S.J. (1992). Shape discrimination and the judgement of perfect symmetry: dissociation of shape from size . *Vision Research*, *32*, 1845–64.

Rhodes, G., Jeffery, L., Watson, T.L., Clifford, C.W.G., & Nakayama, K. (2003). Fitting the mind to the world: face adaptation and attractiveness aftereffects. *Psychological Science*, *14*, 558–66.

Rhodes, G., Brennan, S., & Carey, S. (1987). Identification and ratings of caricatures: Implications for mental representations of faces. *Cognitive Psychology*, *19*, 473–97.

Rhodes, G., & Tremewan, T. (1994). Understanding face recognition: Caricature effects, inversion, and the homogeneity problem. *Visual Cognition*, *1(2/3)*, 275–311.

Roberts, J.E. (1984). Pigeons experience orientation-contingent chromatic aftereffects. *Perception and Psychophysics*, *36*, 309–14.

Sary, G., Vogels, R., & Orban, G.A. (1993). Cue-invariant shape selectivity of macaque inferior temporal neurons. *Science*, *260*, 995–7.

Scott, T.R., & Powell, D.A. (1963). Measure of a visual motion aftereffect in the rhesus monkey. *Science*, *140*, 57–9.

Shimojo., S, Kamitani, Y., & Nishida, S. (2001). Afterimage of perceptually filled-in surface. *Science*, *293*(5535), 1677–80.

Smith, A., & Over, R. (1975). Tilt aftereffects with subjective contours. *Nature*, *257*, 581–2.

Suzuki, S. (2001). Attention-dependent brief adaptation to contour orientation: a high-level aftereffect for convexity? *Vision Research*, *41*, 3883–902.

Suzuki, S., & Grabowecky, M. (2003). Attention during adaptation weakens negative afterimages. *Journal of Experimental Psychology: Human Perception & Performance*, *29*, 793–807.

Suzuki, S., & Cavanagh, P. (1998). A shape-contrast effect for briefly presented stimuli. *Journal of Experimental Psychology: Human Perception & Performance*, *24*(5), 1315–41.

Taylor, J.G., Schmitz, N., Ziemons, K., Grosse-Ruyken, M.L., Gruber, O., Mueller-Gaertner, H.W. *et al.* (2000). The network of brain areas involved in the motion aftereffect. *Neuroimage*, *11*, 257–70.

Tolias, A.S., Smirnakis, S.M., Augath, M.A., Trinath, T., & Logothetis, N.K. (2001). Motion processing in the macaque: revisited with functional magnetic resonance imaging. *Journal of Neuroscience*, *21*, 8594–601.

Tootell, R.B., Reppas, J.B., Dale, A.M., Look, R.B., Sereno, M.I., Malach, R., Brady, T.J. *et al.* (1995). Visual motion aftereffect in human cortical area MT revealed by functional magnetic resonance imaging. *Nature*, *375*, 139–41.

Tsao, D.Y., Freiwald, W.A., Knutsen, T.A., Mandeville, J.B., & Tootell, R.B. (2003). Faces and objects in macaque cerebral cortex. *Nature Neuroscience*, *6*, 989–95.

Valentine, T. (1991). A unified account of the effects of distinctiveness, inversion, and race in face recognition. *Quarterly Journal of Experimental Psychology. A, Human Experimental Psychology*, *43A*, 161–204.

Valentine, T., & Bruce, V. (1986). The effects of distinctiveness in recognising and classifying faces. *Perception*, *15*(5), 525–35.

van der Smagt, M.J., Verstraten, F.A., Vaessen, E.B., van Londen, T., & van de Grind, W.A. (1999). Motion aftereffect of combined first-order and second-order motion. *Perception*, *28*, 1397–411.

van der Zwan, R., & Wenderoth, P. (1995). Mechanisms of purely subjective contour tilt aftereffects. *Vision Research*, *35*, 2547–57.

Vetter, T., & Troje, N.F. (1997). Separation of texture and shape in images of faces for image coding and synthesis. *Journal of the Optical Society of America A-Optics & Image Science*, *14*, 2152–61.

von der Heydt, R., & Peterhans, E. (1989). Mechanisms of contour perception in monkey visual cortex. I. Lines of pattern discontinuity. *Journal of Neuroscience*, *9*, 1731–48.

Wade, N. (1999). *A Natural History of Vision*. (2nd ed.) Cambridge, Massachusetts: The MIT Press.

Wade, N.J. (1978). Why do patterned afterimages fluctuate in visibility? *Psychological Bulletin, 85,* 338–52.

Watson, T.L., & Clifford, C.W.G. (2003). Pulling faces: An investigation of the face-distortion aftereffect. *Perception, 32,* 1109–16.

Webster, M.A., Kaping, D., Mizokami, Y., & Duhamel, P. (2004). Adaptation to natural facial categories. *Nature, 428,* 557–61.

Webster, M.A., & MacLin, O.H. (1999). Figural aftereffects in the perception of faces. *Psychonomic Bulletin & Review, 6,* 647–53.

Wenderoth, P., & Johnstone, S. (1988). The different mechanisms of the direct and indirect tilt illusions. *Vision Research, 28,* 301–12.

Wenderoth, P., & Smith, S. (1999). Neural substrates of the tilt illusion. *Australian & New Zealand Journal of Ophthalmology, 27,* 271–4.

Wenderoth, P., & van der Zwan, R. (1989). The effects of exposure duration and surrounding frames on direct and indirect tilt aftereffects and illusions. *Perception & Psychophysics, 46,* 338–44.

Wohlgemuth, A. (1911). On the aftereffect of seen movement. *British Journal of Psychology Monograph Supplements, 1,* 1–117.

Wolfe, J.M. (1984). Short test flashes produce large tilt aftereffects. *Vision Research, 24,* 1959–64.

Yin, R.K. (1969). Looking at upside-down faces. *Journal of Experimental Psychology, 81,* 141–5.

Zhao, L., & Chubb, C. (2001). The size-tuning of the face-distortion after-effect. *Vision Research, 41,* 2979–94.

8

Adaptation and Face Perception – How Aftereffects Implicate Norm-Based Coding of Faces

GILLIAN RHODES, RACHEL ROBBINS,
EMMA JAQUET, ELINOR MCKONE, LINDA JEFFERY,
AND COLIN W.G. CLIFFORD

8.1 Introduction

Faces provide vital social information which shapes our interactions. Our response to a person depends on our perception of their identity, sex, age, attractiveness, health, and ethnicity, as well as their emotional and attentional states (Zebrowitz 1997). All of this information is read from the face. Although we do this effortlessly, but not always accurately, our visual system must solve a difficult problem because faces are all very similar as visual patterns.

How does the visual system solve this problem, computationally and neurally? In this chapter we consider whether aftereffects in face perception can help us understand these mechanisms. We suggest that high-level and possibly face-specific aftereffects implicate norm-based, or prototype-referenced, coding of faces and discuss how these aftereffects implicate possible opponent coding of faces and indicate the important dimensions in 'face-space'. We begin by outlining current evidence that suggests specialized processing for faces and a possible innate neural substrate, and then go on to review the role of experience and exposure in developing our prodigious face-processing capabilities. We argue that face aftereffects demonstrate plasticity in adult face perception previously not considered and discuss the role adaptation may play in the fine-tuning of face norms with experience, from momentary shifts (of a few seconds) to longer-term adjustment of norms (see also Webster *et al.*, this volume, for discussion of adaptation over different time scales).

8.1.1 Computational and Neural Coding of Faces

Computationally, faces are coded using subtle configural information about the spatial relations between their component parts, such as the eyes, nose, and mouth. Information about the component parts is also coded, but compared with other objects, face perception relies more on configural information (for recent reviews see Maurer *et al.* 2002; Peterson & Rhodes 2003). Different authors use the term 'configural' in slightly different ways, but here we use it to refer to information about the spatial relations between features.[1] Faces also appear to be represented more holistically than other objects, with less explicit decomposition into component parts (Tanaka & Farah 1993; Tanaka & Sengco 1997). An elegant way to represent faces would be to code how each face deviates from a shared norm or prototype[2] (Diamond & Carey 1986; Rhodes *et al.* 1987; Valentine 1991; Rhodes 1996), although direct empirical support for this hypothesis has proved elusive (see Section 8.2 for further discussion) (Byatt & Rhodes 1998; Rhodes *et al.* 1998).

Neurally, face perception relies on specialized mechanisms that respond more strongly to faces than other stimuli (Haxby *et al.* 2000; Kanwisher 2000; Behrmann & Moscovitch 2001). Furthermore, there may be distinct neural mechanisms for coding invariant aspects of faces, like identity, and for coding changeable aspects, like eye gaze direction and expression (Haxby *et al.* 2000).

These specialized computational and neural mechanisms probably have innate foundations. Newborns prefer to look at faces over other comparable patterns (Johnson *et al.* 1991; Morton & Johnson 1991; but see Turati 2004), they rapidly form prototypes (averages) of seen faces (Walton & Bower 1993) and, within hours of birth, they learn to visually discriminate their mother's face from that of an unfamiliar woman (Bushnell *et al.* 1989). A specialized neural substrate

---

[1] Maurer *et al.* (2002) use 'configural processing' to refer collectively to first-order relational processing (of the basic face structure of two eyes above nose above mouth), second-order relational processing (variations within this basic structure), and holistic coding. We prefer to keep these distinct, using 'configural' to refer to second-order relational processing (see Peterson & Rhodes 2003 for reviews).

[2] We will use the terms 'norm', 'prototype', and 'average' interchangeably.

for face processing may be in place very early, perhaps even at birth. Brain damage at one day of age can produce a lasting prosopagnosia, or inability to recognize faces, in the presence of relatively good object recognition (Farah *et al.* 2000), and by two-months of age (the earliest age tested) faces activate similar brain areas as in adults (Tzourio-Mazoyer *et al.* 2002).

8.1.2 Plasticity and the Role of Experience in Face Perception

Given the importance of reading faces, and the difficult computational problems involved, it may not be surprising that we have evolved specialized neural and computational mechanisms to do so. These mechanisms may rest on innate foundations, but they are certainly shaped by experience. Early visual input is particularly important. Without patterned visual input (particularly to the right hemisphere) in the first six months of life, normal configural face processing never develops (Le Grand *et al.* 2001) and the identification of faces across different viewpoints and expressions is permanently impaired (Geldart *et al.* 2002). Other aspects of face processing seem less dependent on this early experience. For example, there appears to be no impairment in discriminating feature changes in faces (Le Grand *et al.* 2001), in matching facial expressions and direction of gaze, or in lip-reading (Geldart *et al.* 2002). Early visual experience, therefore, seems particularly important for configural coding, which is one of the computational hallmarks of face recognition. Early experience also sharpens the tuning of face processing mechanisms. Six-month olds can discriminate between old and new monkey faces in addition to human faces, whereas nine-month olds can only discriminate old and new human faces (Pascalis *et al.* 2002).

Performance with faces on memory and perceptual tasks improves throughout childhood (Carey *et al.* 1980; Carey 1992; Ellis 1992; Carey & Diamond 1994; Chung & Thompson 1995; Bruce *et al.* 2000; Mondloch *et al.* 2002). Some theorists have attributed this improvement to an increased use of configural or holistic coding, as opposed to analytic, feature-based processing, which continues until 10 or more years of age (Carey & Diamond 1977; Schwarzer 2000; Mondloch *et al.* 2003). However, recent results show that specialized computational face processing mechanisms are present from a young age. Young children show adult levels of both holistic (Pellicano & Rhodes 2003, 4 year-olds) and configural coding (Gilchrist & McKone 2003, 7 year-olds; Pellicano *et al.* 2005, 4 year-olds) and sensitivity to configural information in faces (photographs but not schematic faces) is present as early as eight months of age (Schwarzer & Zauner 2003).

We do not yet know precisely what processing changes are involved in the development of face processing skills. Generic improvements in attention, memory, or executive function may contribute towards its development. So, too may selective improvements in face processing resulting from extensive experience with faces. These could include more detailed representation of face norms (Carey 1996; Pascalis *et al.* 2002), representation of more face dimensions, or more relevant ones for distinguishing individuals (Chung & Thompson 1995), sensitivity to finer differences on those dimensions, and/or better ability to abstract invariant identity-specific information from dynamically changing inputs. More research is needed to determine which of these changes occur during development.

Experience enhances the processing of familiar kinds of faces, such as those from a familiar race, suggesting that we learn how faces vary within populations to which we are exposed. When faces from less familiar races are encountered, people show deficits in recognition memory (Bothwell *et al.* 1989; Meissner & Brigham 2001) and a variety of perceptual judgements (O'Toole *et al.* 1996; Dehon & Brédart 2001; Murray *et al.* 2003). Specialized computational and neural face processing mechanisms also appear to be used less effectively with other-race faces, which are coded less configurally (for a review see Murray *et al.* 2003), less holistically (Tanaka *et al.* 2004), and which produce less activation in face-specific brain areas (Golby *et al.* 2001).

Our adult ability in face processing clearly rests on extensive experience with faces, particularly early in development, and the effects of this experience have been intensively investigated. In contrast, the possibility that experience might continue to affect face processing mechanisms and face perception in adults (beyond simply learning new faces, Bruce & Burton 2002), has received almost no attention. Recently, however, a variety of aftereffects in face perception have been reported, which demonstrate a remarkable degree of plasticity in adult face perception (Webster & MacLin 1999; Leopold *et al.* 2001; MacLin & Webster 2001; Rhodes *et al.* 2003; Watson & Clifford 2003; Webster *et al.* 2004).

In this chapter, we review these face aftereffects and consider their implications for our understanding of face processing. We will argue that these aftereffects indicate that adult face coding mechanisms are continuously and dynamically altered by experience, and that our face norms and preferences are continuously calibrated to fit the faces we see (Section 8.2; see also Webster, *et al.*, this volume). We will also argue that these aftereffects result from adaptation of high-level, and possibly face-specific, mechanisms (Section 8.3). Next we consider a possible functional role for face adaptation, asking whether it enhances discrimination of faces around the adapting distortion (Section 8.4). If it does, then we may have identified a bridge between short-term adaptation effects and longer-range improvements in face processing associated with experience (e.g., with other-race faces). Next we consider whether some dimensions of face-space are more adaptable than others (Section 8.5). In particular we ask whether dimensions that vary more between faces in the natural population are adapted more readily than less variable ones. Finally, we propose a neurally plausible norm-based coding model of face processing which may be useful in understanding the mechanisms that underlie face aftereffects (Section 8.6).

8.2. Face Aftereffects – Norm-based and Opponent Coding

Aftereffects in low-level vision have revealed much about how simple visual attributes, such as orientation, colour, and direction of motion, are coded by the visual system (eg. Frisby 1980; Mather *et al.* 1998; Clifford 2002; other chapters in this volume). We suggest that aftereffects in face perception provide important information about how faces are coded.

Adaptation to systematically distorted faces produces a figural aftereffect in which subsequently viewed faces look distorted in the opposite direction (Webster & MacLin 1999; MacLin & Webster 2001; Rhodes *et al.* 2003; Watson & Clifford 2003), adaptation to a particular identity causes an average face to take on the 'opposite' identity (Leopold *et al.* 2001), and adaptation to a particular gender, race, or expression can cause a previously neutral image to take on the contrasting value (male-female, Caucasian-Japanese, happy-angry) (Webster *et al.* 2004). The appearance of every facial attribute tested so far is affected by which faces have been seen beforehand. But what do these aftereffects suggest about the way in which faces may be represented?

Many theorists have suggested that an elegant and efficient way to mentally represent faces would be to code how each face deviates from a norm or prototype (Hebb 1949; Hochberg 1978; Goldstein & Chance 1980; Diamond & Carey 1986; Valentine & Bruce 1986; Rhodes, *et al.* 1987; Valentine 1991; Rhodes 1996), with each face coded by a unique vector, or point, representing the direction of deviations from the norm on multiple dimensions in 'face-space'. Faces vary in their distance, as well as direction, from the norm, distinctive faces being further from the norm than more 'average' faces, as illustrated in Fig. 8.1(A). Certainly there is evidence that we can abstract norms or prototypes from the faces we see (Reed 1972; Strauss 1979; Solso & McCarthy 1981*a,b*; Bruce *et al.* 1991; Walton & Bower 1992; Inn *et al.* 1993), and the position of faces relative to that norm affects recognition, with distinctive faces recognized better than more typical faces (Going & Read 1974; Light *et al.* 1979;

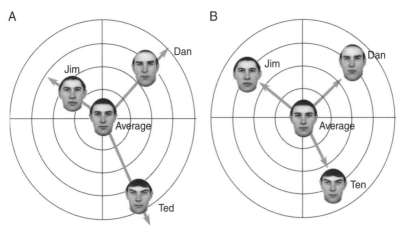

FIG. 8.1 (A) Individual faces represented in a simplified 2-dimensional face-space as unique vectors deviating from the norm or average face at the centre of face-space. Alternatively faces can be thought of as points in the space. More distinctive faces (e.g. Ted) are further from the norm than more average faces (e.g. Jim). (B) Face-space normalized by identity strength, so that all face vectors have unit length, as used by Leopold *et al.* (2001).

Valentine & Bruce 1986; Valentine 1991; Johnston & Ellis 1995). The ease with which we can identify caricatures, which exaggerate how a face deviates from a norm (increasing its distance from the norm along its unique identity vector), also seems to support some form of norm-based coding (Byatt & Rhodes 1998; Rhodes *et al.* 1987, 1998). However, attempts to rule out alternative accounts based on reduced exemplar density around caricatures have proved unsuccessful (Byatt & Rhodes 1998; Rhodes *et al.* 1998). Here we will argue that the face aftereffects described above provide new support for norm-based, or prototype-referenced, coding of faces.

The face identity aftereffect (Leopold *et al.* 2001) provides evidence that faces are coded relative to a norm or prototype. Identification of a face (Dan) is facilitated by adapting, for as little as 5 seconds, to its opposite identity (AntiDan), but not to some other, non-opposite, face (e.g. AntiJim) (see Fig. 8.2.). This effect can be explained if one assumes that exposure to a face (AntiDan) shifts the norm towards that face, perhaps as an initial stage of updating face norms by experience, so that the opposite face (Dan) deviates more from the norm than it did before. The resulting increase in distinctivenes would make Dan easier to recognize, because distinctive faces have an advantage over typical faces in recognition (Going & Read 1974; Light *et al.* 1979; Valentine & Bruce 1986; Valentine 1991*a*; Johnston & Ellis 1995). More direct support for a shift in the norm comes from the finding that after viewing a face (AntiDan), the average (norm) face, which initially has no particular identity, takes on the identity of the opposite face (Dan), consistent with its deviation from the new norm. Finally, adaptation to the average or norm face has little effect on the perception of identity, presumably because this does not induce any shift in the norm (cf Webster & MacLin 1999).

A concern with these identity aftereffect results is that they do not take into account the fact that faces vary in their distances from the norm. In Leopold *et al.* (2001), 'distances' are represented in terms of identity *strength*, with all faces given equal identity strength and shown as equidistant from the norm (see Fig. 8.1(B)). The size of any aftereffect is likely to depend on the perceptual dissimilarity between adapt and test faces, with larger dissimilarities producing larger aftereffects (at least up to some asymptote). Therefore, it is possible that larger aftereffects after adapting to opposite (rather than non-opposite) anti-faces could simply reflect the greater perceptual distance of opposite (compared with non-opposite) adapting faces from the target faces, rather than their location at the opposite end of an axis passing through the norm. For example, in Fig. 8.2, antiDan and Dan are more dissimilar (in regular face-space) than antiJim and Dan, so that adapting to antiDan would produce a larger aftereffect in the perception of Dan than would adapting to antiJim.

We have been able to rule out such an interpretation, however, by showing that the anti-face advantage is maintained when non-opposite adapting faces are matched on perceptual distance, measured by similarity ratings, from the target faces (Rhodes & Jeffery 2005) (see Fig. 8.3, left). The data from one participant is shown in Fig. 8.3, right. It replicates the original identity aftereffect,

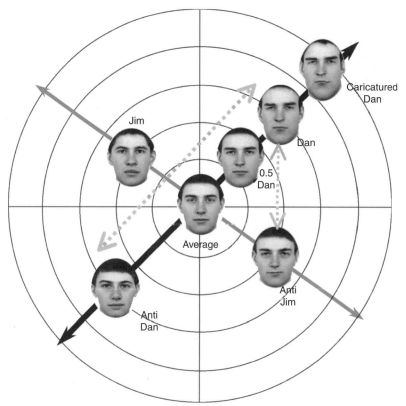

FIG. 8.2 A 2-dimensional representation of face-space showing a morphed continuum representing the Dan Identity Axis (thick black line). The most extreme face is a caricature of Dan, followed by the original face (Dan), a weaker version of the face (0.5 Dan), a norm face in the centre, through to the anti-face (0.8 AntiDan on the opposite side of the norm –NB: The anti-faces were only 0.8 from the norm as limitations in the morph software produce extremely distorted and unnatural images at higher levels), (after Leopold *et al.* 2001). For each face (e.g. Jim) an anti-face (e.g. AntiJim) can be made which has the opposite characteristics to its target face. The anti-face for a given face has the opposite vector in face-space to that face. Note that the distance, shown by grey dotted lines, between Dan and AntiDan is greater than the distance between AntiJim and Dan.

with enhanced recognition of the target face, for anti-face adapting faces, but not for the distance-matched adapting faces.

This result supports Leopold *et al.*'s (2001) interpretation of their identity aftereffects as evidence for some form of 'face-opponent' coding mechanism centred on a prototypical or norm face. 'Opponent coding' is supported by the finding that the aftereffects are largest when the adapt and test faces occupy diametrically opposite locations (relative to the average) in face-space, with little aftereffect for adapt and test faces that are equally far apart but do not occupy

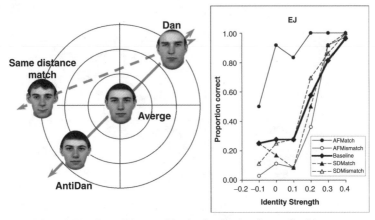

FIG. 8.3 *Left*. The Same-Distance-Match adapting face is equally far
(in face-space) from Dan as is AntiDan, but unlike AntiDan, the Same-Distance-Match
is not diametrically opposite Dan, that is, the axis between Dan and the Same Distance
Match does not go through the norm. *Right*. Representative data from one participant
showing that an identity aftereffect only occurs when the adapting face is diametrically
opposite the target, i.e., when it is the Antiface that matches the target. Proportion correct (the proportion of times the target face is correctly identified) is shown as a function of identity strength, for each type of adapting face. AFMatch = adapt to antiface of
the target (e.g., AntiDan for target Dan), AFMismatch = adapt to antiface of non-target
face (e.g., AntiJim for target Dan), Baseline = no adapting face, SDMatch = adapt
to face that is equally far from the target as its antiface, SDMismatch = adapt to a
non-target face's same-distance matched face.

diametrically opposite locations relative to the average face (Rhodes & Jeffery
2005; see also Leopold & Bondar, this volume).

The best understood opponent-coding system is for colour and, in that
domain, the best evidence for opponent coding is the fact that a colour and its
opponent colour (e.g. red and green or blue and yellow) cannot both be seen
simultaneously (Boynton & Gordon 1965; Abromov & Gordon 1994). One can
see a bluish-green, but not a reddish-green. Therefore, if face identity is also
opponent-coded, then it should be difficult to see opposite identities simultaneously in a face. To test this prediction, we made 50/50 face-blends that combined either opposite identities (i.e. a face and its anti-face) or non-opposite
identities (i.e. a face and its same-distance match) (Fig. 8.4). Participants were
asked to rate the similarity between each blend and its two component faces,
using a seven point scale (1 = not similar at all, 7 = very similar). If opposite
faces cannot be seen simultaneously, then blends made from these faces should
elicit lower (but still above zero, given that all faces resemble each other to
some degree) similarity ratings to their component faces than blends made from
faces and their same-distance matches. This is indeed what we found (Rhodes

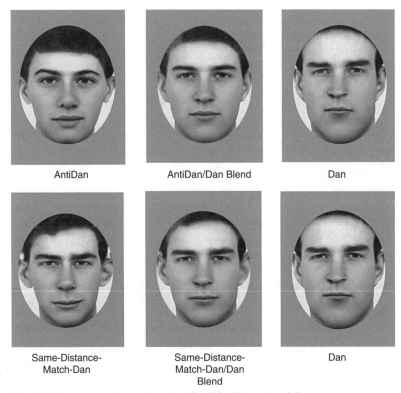

AntiDan   AntiDan/Dan Blend   Dan

Same-Distance-   Same-Distance-   Dan
Match-Dan   Match-Dan/Dan
                        Blend

FIG. 8.4 The top row shows a Face-Anti-face blend (centre) and the two component faces (left and right). The bottom row shows a Same-Distance Blend (centre) and its component faces (left and right).

& Jeffery 2005). Face-Anti-face blends and their components received significantly lower mean ratings (M = 3.5, SE = 0.2) than Face-Same-Distance match blends and their components (M = 4.6, SE = 0.2), F(1, 15) = 55.13, $p < 0.001$. These results are consistent with some form of opponent coding.

In her excellent discussion of the configural distortion and identity aftereffects, Hurlbert (2001) considers alternative explanations to norm-based coding for these face aftereffects. She suggests that faces could be coded as deviations from a small set of exemplars at key locations, with no need for an explicit prototype, in which case the identity aftereffect would result from 'shifts in sensitivity' to these exemplars. This account is logically possible, but it lacks parsimony (admittedly a weak criterion for theory-building) with deviations coded relative to multiple exemplars instead of a single prototype, and in the absence of any specification of what would count as a key location, it lacks precision. Hurlbert also notes that explicit face-anti-face axes need not exist in face-space, and that other dimensions might be used. We agree. The face identity aftereffects show that whatever dimensions are used, they centre on average (prototype) values, and are coded using some form of opponency between values on either side of average (see the final section of this chapter for a more detailed model). But they do not constrain what those dimensions represent. As long as opposite identities receive opposite values on these dimensions, larger aftereffects will be seen for face-anti-face adapt-test pairs, than for other (equally distant) adapt-test pairs.

The face identity aftereffects suggest not only that faces are coded relative to a centrally located norm in a face-space, but also that there is some form of opponent coding on each dimension. Evidence that it is more difficult to see the resemblance between blends of face-anti-face pairs and their component faces than between other blends and their component faces offers further support for this view (Rhodes & Jeffery 2005). A possible form of opponent coding would be for above-average and below-average values on each dimension in face-space to be coded by distinct neural populations which are organized in opponent fashion. We propose an explicit model of this structure in Section 8.6 of the chapter.

Identity is not the only face attribute that appears to be coded in relation to a norm or prototype. Aftereffects also occur in the perception of gender, race, and facial expression (Webster *et al.* 2004). In these studies, Webster and colleagues created morphed face continua that ranged from male to female, from Caucasian to Japanese, and from happy to sad. Viewing one end of the continuum shifted the neutral point, at which faces switch from looking male to female (or Caucasian to Japanese, or happy to sad), towards that end. These results suggest that gender, race, and expression are coded as deviations from, respectively, gender-neutral, race-neutral, and expression-neutral prototypes. Alternatively, a single prototoype derived from all faces (varying on these dimensions) could simultaneously represent neutral values on all these traits.

Also supporting the important role of the 'norm' in face coding are findings that a few-minute exposure to systematically distorted faces (together with re-exposure during testing) can produce a measurable shift of what looks most normal, i.e. the norm, in the direction of that distortion. The appearance of new faces is then judged in relation to the new norm, so that undistorted faces now look distorted in the opposite direction (e.g. Webster & MacLin 1999; Rhodes *et al.* 2003; Watson & Clifford 2003). Apparently the norm has shifted (adapted) in response to a systematic change in the diet of faces, and the distortion perceived in a test face depends on its relation to the new norm (see discussion in MacLin & Webster 2001). The idea that these aftereffects result from adaptation of face norms explains why no aftereffect is seen when undistorted faces are used as adapting stimuli (Webster & MacLin 1999; MacLin & Webster 2001). Undistorted faces simply reinforce the current norm(s), so that there is no change in the norm and therefore no change in the way faces are perceived, i.e. no aftereffect.

Additional support for this view comes from a study that examined the effect of adapting to consistently distorted faces on perceptions of attractiveness (Rhodes *et al.* 2003). Average (norm) faces are attractive (for reviews see Rhodes & Zebrowitz 2002). Therefore, if adaptation to consistently distorted

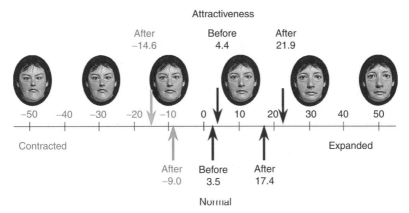

FIG. 8.5 Most attractive (top) and most normal (bottom) distortion levels before and after adapting to contracted and expanded faces.

faces shifts the norm towards that distortion, then there should be a corresponding shift in the faces found most attractive. After adaptation, as predicted, the most attractive distortion level shifted to match the most normal looking distortion level (see Fig. 8.5).

8.2.1 The Duration of Aftereffects and Recalibration of Norms

Face aftereffects suggest that faces are coded in relation to face norms or prototypes, which are constantly calibrated to reflect the properties of the faces we see. However, the duration of the change to the norm may vary as a function of the amount and type of adaptation. Very brief exposures are capable of altering the norm, with a five-second viewing of a single adapting face producing an identity aftereffect in Leopold *et al.* (2001), and even one-second exposures, possibly being sufficient (Leopold *et al.* 2005). Following brief adaptation, recalibration of the norm can be detected at delays of up to 2.4 seconds between adapt and test faces (the longest delay tested by Leopold *et al.* 2001). The relationship between the duration of the adapting stimulus and the decay of the face identity aftereffect resembles classic aftereffects, with longer adapting durations associated with slower decay (Leopold *et al.* 2005).

Little is known about the time course of the figural face aftereffects, first reported by Webster & MacLin (1999), produced by adapting to consistently distorted faces over a period of minutes. Preliminary data from our laboratories (using somewhat different procedures) appear inconsistent. In one case we found that the figural aftereffect induced by adapting to consistently distorted faces (contracted or expanded) for one minute, decays within one minute (Rhodes *et al.* 2005). In another, we found that the aftereffect induced by 2 minutes of adaptation to a different distortion (vertically shifted eyes) (see Section 8.5) can survive a 10–15 min delay, even with intervening exposure to undistorted faces (Robbins *et al.* 2005).

Systematic investigation of the time course of face aftereffects may help to answer the following questions. Do similar mechanisms underlie face aftereffects and classic aftereffects in low-level vision? The investigation of the time course of identity aftereffects by Leopold *et al.* (2005) suggests that they may. Do the same mechanisms underlie different sorts of face aftereffects, such as those following adaptation to identity, configuration, race, gender, etc? How are these face aftereffects related to longer term changes in face norms that result from extended exposure to faces over periods of months or years? It is tempting to suggest some commonality as all may serve to adjust the position of the norm in light of the diet of faces being perceived. Future studies will need to explore the timecourse and robustness of face aftereffects in more detail.

8.2.2 A Single Norm or Multiple Norms Corresponding to Important Face Categories?

Face identity aftereffects suggest that faces are coded in relation to a norm but the exact norm (average) used to make anti-faces in these studies does not appear to be crucial. Leopold *et al.* (2001) used an average face derived from a large set of male and female faces, whereas Rhodes *et al.* (2005*b*) used an average derived from only male faces, with similar results. Given that we can classify faces in a variety of ways – as a face, a male face, a Chinese face, etc – we may well have access to a variety of face norms, which represent the central tendencies of the different face categories that we use. For example, given the salience of race as a visual and social category, it seems likely that people would maintain distinct prototypes for different races (Cosmides *et al.* 2003). Direct support for distinct prototypes for different races comes from findings that caricatures of Caucasian and Chinese faces are recognized best when caricatured against their own-race norms (Byatt & Rhodes 1998). Although it seems likely that we have separate norms for visually distinct and socially meaningful categories, for ease of exposition we will continue to talk about a single face norm.

Given that gender is also a highly salient face category for which we might reasonably expect different norms, it is odd that there is very little difference in the aftereffects for male faces seen after adaptation to anti-faces made using an average of male faces, which would generate *male* anti-faces, and after adaptation to an average of all faces, which would generate *feminized* anti-faces. However, we note that although Leopold *et al.*'s average was created by blending male and female faces, it looks male, which may explain why similar aftereffects are found when a male average is used.

8.3. What is the Neural Locus of Face Aftereffects?

There is no doubt that face aftereffects affect our perception of faces, but do they result from adaptation of specific face-coding mechanisms, as proposed here?

Here we consider whether face aftereffects result from adaptation of low-level coding mechanisms or high-level coding mechanisms, or both, and whether it is possible to make such a distinction.

One possibility is that face aftereffects result from adaptation of low-level mechanisms which code simple visual attributes, such as spatial frequency components, or the shapes of isolated face parts like the eyes and mouth. Any changes to the coding of these simple properties would flow on through the system to affect our perception of faces. We suggest that a *purely* low-level adaptation locus can be ruled out, because these face aftereffects generalize across the changes in retinal position (Leopold *et al.* 2001), size (Zhao & Chubb 2001), and tilt (+/−45 degrees) (Rhodes *et al.* 2003; Watson & Clifford 2003). With these changes, the adapting and test stimuli would activate distinct low-level neural populations, and low-level adaptation would not affect the test faces. Therefore, we conclude that face aftereffects can result from adaptation of relatively high-level neurons whose responses are largely invariant across these kinds of image changes.

But are these face-specific mechanisms? Face-specific mechanisms respond poorly to inverted faces and the visual system treats inverted faces as objects (Yin 1969; Moscovitch *et al.* 1997; Haxby *et al.* 2000). Yet figural and identity aftereffects occur for inverted as well as upright faces, and show some transfer between upright and inverted faces (Webster & MacLin 1999; Leopold *et al.* 2001; Watson & Clifford 2003). These results seem more consistent with adaptation of generic high-level coding mechanisms that respond to objects as well as faces, than with adaptation of face-specific coding mechanisms.

However, we should not rule out the possibility of face-specific adaptation. Functional brain imaging studies show that face-specific brain areas, which respond more strongly to faces than objects, are activated (albeit to a lesser extent) by inverted faces, and that object-specific areas, which respond more strongly to objects than faces, are also activated (to a lesser extent) by upright faces (Haxby *et al.* 2000; Rossion & Gauthier 2002). Therefore, some transfer of aftereffects between upright and inverted faces might occur because face-specific networks respond to inverted, as well as upright faces. However, opposite figural aftereffects can be induced simultaneously in upright and inverted faces, which suggests that there are distinct networks underlying the perception of upright and inverted faces, and that these can be selectively adapted (Rhodes *et al.* 2004).

The discovery of face-selective neurons and regions in temporal cortex, leads naturally to the idea that face-coding is a high-level visual function. However, face perception is actually the result of analysis by an entire visual pathway, and adaptation can occur at any level within that pathway. It may, therefore, be inappropriate to assume that face adaptation has a specific locus. As Leopold *et al.* (2005) suggest, even simple aftereffects cannot be convincingly localized to 'low level' feature analyzing neurons and it may be more apt to think of perceptual aftereffects as reflecting the collective adaptation of a system of neurons at varying levels. What is important is that face aftereffects alter our perception of faces in ways that are illuminating regarding the kind of processing involved.

8.4 Face Adaptation and Face Discrimination

Aftereffects in face perception are compelling visual phenomena. But do they, or the adaptation that produces them, have any functional significance? We conjecture that such adaptation may facilitate discrimination within populations of faces that we experience. Initial transient shifts in face norms following adaptation may, with repetition over time, lead to more enduring changes in the statistics of face-space and in discrimination performance, both during development and when encountering a new population of faces (e.g. other-race faces) as adults. Recalibration of face norms based on our diet of faces may optimize our ability to discriminate among the kinds of faces we see most often, by optimally matching the neural response range to stimulus variation encountered (e.g. Werblin 1973; Wainwright 1999; see also Clifford, this volume; Webster *et al.*, this volume). This would be similar to light adaptation, where our sensitivity to small changes is best around the mean luminance level (Hood 1998). On this view, discrimination should be best for the most commonly experienced stimuli. On a short time scale these would be the adapting faces, or faces with a similar structure, and on a longer time scale they would be stimuli close to the norm, i.e. faces that are typical for a given population.

In low-level vision, adaptation can facilitate discrimination around the adapting stimuli (see Clifford, this volume). Following adaptation, an improved ability to detect small changes near the adapting stimulus has been observed for judgements of grating orientation (Regan & Beverley 1985; Clifford *et al.* 2001), and the direction of motion (Phinney *et al.* 1997). However, improved discrimination ability following adaptation has not been consistently found in low-level vision. Other studies report no improvement in the discrimination of spatial frequency (Regan & Beverley 1983), orientation (Barlow *et al.* 1976), or direction of motion (Hol & Treue 2001).

We were interested in how adaptation affects the discrimination of faces. We asked whether increased exposure to particular kinds of faces in the short-term improves our ability to distinguish among such faces? The idea that increased experience with faces may improve discrimination is not new. Valentine (1991) and others have proposed that it is long-term experience with faces from one's own-race which results in better recognition for these faces, as compared to faces from other, less familiar, races. This type of perceptual learning may be functionally similar to adaptation, in that our perceptions become tuned to the type of faces in the current environment.

We conducted two experiments to investigate how adaptation to consistently distorted faces affects face discrimination (see Fig. 8.6) (Jaquet *et al.* 2005). In the first experiment, participants rated pairs of faces for similarity, before and after adaptation. We asked whether discrimination is facilitated around the

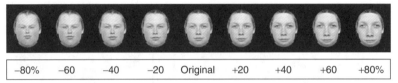

| −80% | −60 | −40 | −20 | Original | +20 | +40 | +60 | +80% |

FIG. 8.6 An example of a continuum of faces used in Experiment 1. Participants adapted to either contracted (−50) or expanded (+50) distortions for one minute. Test images were presented in pairs differing by 20% distortion amounts (e.g. −80 and −60). Each test pair was shown for 2 seconds, alternating with adapting faces shown for 6 seconds, to maintain adaptation. On the far left is the most contracted version (−80%), in the centre is the undistorted face (0%), and on the far right is the most expanded version (80%). Different identities were used for adapting and test faces, which were also presented at different sizes to ensure high-level adaptation.

point of adaptation and whether discrimination is best around the most normal looking distortions. Although these are not face norms, we expected discrimination to be best in this normal range, and to shift as the normal range shifted following adaptation. In the second experiment, we examined whether discrimination thresholds were reduced around the point of adaptation.

The results are shown in Figs. 8.7 (Experiment 1) and 8.8 (Experiment 2). Discriminability was not significantly facilitated at the point of adaptation in either experiment. Nor was it better for more normal than more distorted faces (Experiment 1). In the second experiment, discrimination thresholds decreased after adaptation for both adapted and unadapted pairs, consistent with a general improvement in the ability of the participants to discriminate between face pairs following adaptation. This non-specific increase in sensitivity is likely to reflect the effects of practice at making subtle discriminations amongst faces. However, there was no specific advantage for pairs spanning the point of adaptation.

Taken together, these two experiments offer no evidence that discrimination of particular facial configurations is facilitated by short-term adaptation to similar configurations. These results are surprising given that enhancing sensitivity to variation in the environment would seem to be very useful for face perception. Most faces are composed of two eyes, a nose, and a mouth in approximately the same configuration. Therefore, increased responsiveness to any slight differences in the face environment will facilitate face processing and recognition (Murray *et al.* 2003).

Why might we have failed to find facilitation of discrimination at the point of adaptation? We can rule out failure to adapt, because a preliminary experiment with these exact stimuli and procedures showed significant aftereffects following exposure to both expanded and contracted adapting faces (Jaquet 2002). Rather, it seems possible that adaptation does not in fact facilitate discrimination between commonly experienced faces. Support for this interpretation comes from failure to observe any peak in discrimination performance around the undistorted faces prior to adaptation, although participants would certainly have been adapted to such faces at that time. Webster *et al.*

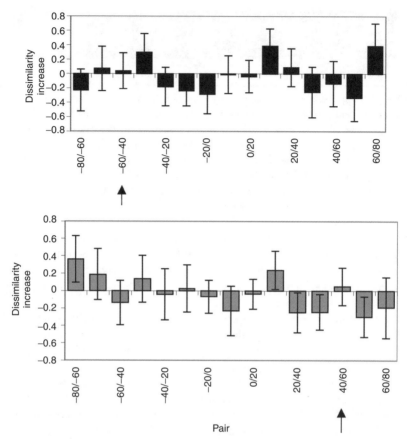

FIG. 8.7 Top: Mean increase in dissimilarity (improved discriminability) after adapting, averaged across participants in the contracted adaptation condition. The arrow indicates the pair (−60/−40 contracted) that spans the point of adaptation. SE bars are shown. Bottom: Mean increase in dissimilarity (improved discriminability) after adapting, averaged across participants in the expanded adaptation condition. The arrow indicates the pair (40/60 expanded) that spans the point of adaptation. SE bars are shown.

(this volume) comment that there is very little clear evidence for enhanced discrimination following adaptation, and suggest that we consider alternative functions for adaptation. In particular, they suggest that the functional role of adaptation may be to direct our attention to the unexpected, rather than to facilitate discrimination of common stimuli.

8.5 Are Some Dimensions in Face-space More Adaptable than Others?

In face-space theories, the many physical properties differentiating faces are specified in terms of a reduced number of underlying dimensions, and each

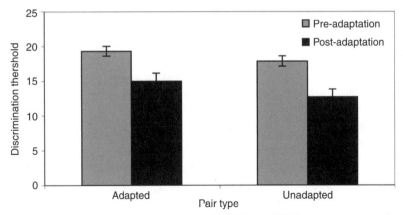

FIG. 8.8 Discrimination thresholds for correctly judging which face was most normal 81.6% of the time before and after adapting, for face pairs around the adapted (e.g. +50) and corresponding unadapted (e.g. −50) point. SE bars are shown.

individual is coded as a point in the resulting space (Valentine & Bruce 1986; Valentine 1991; Busey 1998; Deffenbacher *et al.* 1998). The 'centre' of face-space represents the average face or norm, and a highly atypical individual would lie a long way from this norm on one or more dimensions of face-space. There is currently no agreement on the actual dimensions used to code faces (i.e. the axes of face-space), although the general usefulness of the face-space heuristic is indicated by its ability to explain important empirical results. For example, in face-nonface classification, performance is better for typical faces than distinctive faces (Valentine & Bruce 1986*a*). This is attributed to typical faces being closer to the central norm. In recognition memory, in contrast, performance is better for distinctive faces than typical faces (Valentine & Bruce 1986; Valentine & Endo 1992; Vokey & Read 1992); this is attributed to a distinctive face having a smaller number of nearby neighbours in face-space, thus reducing confusion errors with similar individuals (although see Burton & Vokey 1998).

According to this face-space framework, different aspects of faces are coded as different dimensions. For example, there might exist a dimension which codes the height of someone's eyes within their face[3]. Some of these dimensions have larger variability in the real world than others. As an example, detailed measurement of human faces has shown that, for females, the distance between hair-line and eyebrows has a standard deviation of 6 mm (around a mean of

---

[3] We will use 'dimensions' to mean an aspect of faces that has variability in real-world populations, and for which a norm or centre point can be defined. We are not suggesting that everything we call a dimension is primary, in the sense of having specific populations of cells coding for it (although some may).

52.7 mm), but the distance between lips and chin has a standard deviation of only 3.1 mm (around a mean of 43.4 mm; Farkas *et al.* 1994).

A question of interest then, is whether certain dimensions in face-space might be more affected by adaptation than others. Robbins & McKone (2005) explored this issue using distortions which were somewhat different to the global expansion/contraction of the previous section. Two distortion types were selected, based on dimensions with different amounts of variability in the natural face population. The first was the height of both eyes together in the face; that is, both eyes were moved up or both eyes were moved down (the *symmetric distortion*). The second was the difference in height between the two eyes; that is, one eye was moved up while the other was moved down (the *asymmetric distortion*). Examples are shown in Fig. 8.9.

The symmetric distortion is associated with relatively large variability in the normal face population, given the evidence that the standard deviation of eye-hairline distances is quite large. The variability of the height difference between the eyes has not been reported in published data, but is presumably relatively small given that most people's eyes are fairly symmetrically placed. This is indicated graphically in Fig. 8.10. In face-space terms we assume that these two dimensions would be orthogonal, as they can vary independently.

Robbins and McKone first familiarized subjects with four individuals (Bill, Sam, John, and Fred) in their undistorted form. Distorted versions were then rated for how much each looked like the original, both pre- and post-adaptation. Adapting faces were two of the individuals (Sam and Bill). In the pre-adaptation phase, it was found that the symmetric condition produced broader curves with

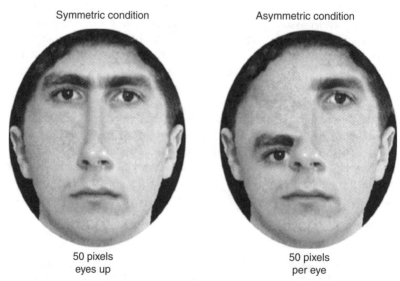

Symmetric condition   Asymmetric condition

50 pixels   50 pixels
eyes up   per eye

FIG. 8.9 An example of the distortions used by Robbins & McKone. Eyes down, and right up/left down, were also tested.

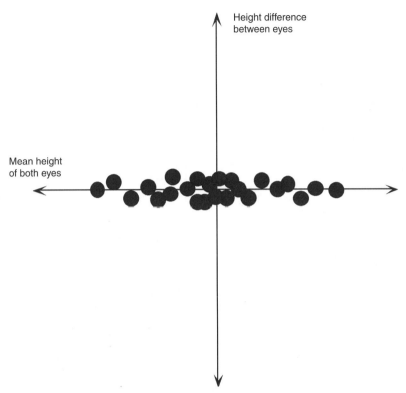

FIG. 8.10 Dimensions in face-space corresponding to symmetric and asymmetric distortions (after McKone & Aitkin 2005). The larger spread for the 'height of both eyes together' dimension indicates larger variability in the natural population of faces, while the smaller spread for 'height difference between eyes' is associated with less variation in the natural population. The centre of each dimension is the norm.

shallower slopes than the asymmetric condition; that is, a wider range of deviations were rated as looking similar to the original person in the symmetric condition. This finding is consistent with the relatively large population variability for the height of both eyes together, and relatively small population variability for asymmetry in height between the two eyes. The question of interest was then whether these differences in sensitivity would correspond to different degrees of adaptability. We measured the amount of adaptation as the shift between the mid-point of the pre-adaptation and post-adaptation curves for each subject. An example for one subject is plotted in Fig. 8.11.

Figure 8.12 shows the amount of shift for each of the four subjects. It can be seen that the shift was greater in the symmetric condition than in the asymmetric condition. That is, there was more adaptation for distortions involving both eyes moved together, than for one eye moved up and the other moved down.

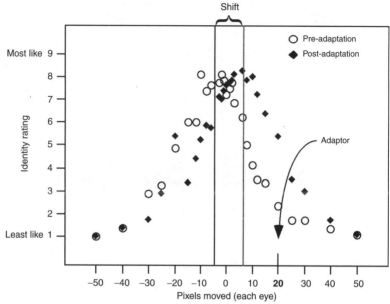

FIG. 8.11 One subject's pre- and post-adaptation curves for the symmetric distortion showing shift towards the adaptor. The adaptor in this case was at +20 pixels. 1 = 'least like the original John/Bill/Fred/Sam', 9 = 'most like the original John/Bill/Fred/Sam'. Adaptors (Bill and Sam, ±20 pixels) were shown for 1 min each, plus a 5 s top-up exposure to an adaptor before each test trial. The adaptor was always smaller than the test faces, and subjects scanned the adaptor faces rather than fixating to encourage high level and not low level adaptation. Direction of adaptor (eyes up versus eyes down for the symmetric condition; left-up-right-down versus right-up-left-down for the asymmetric conditions) had no influence on the pattern of results and data were collapsed over this variable.

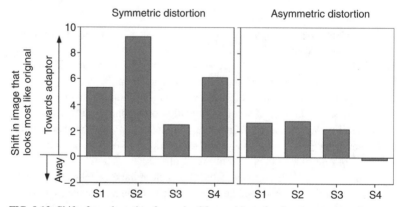

FIG. 8.12 Shift after adaptation for each of four subjects for the symmetric and asymmetric distortions.

Overall, these results provide the first demonstration that some dimensions in face-space are more adaptable than others. The two cases tested so far suggest that dimensions which are associated with more variability in the real world are more adaptable than those associated with less variability (although one would wish to see further dimensions tested to confirm this interpretation). Given that the adaptation seems to produce a simple shift in curve position between the pre- and post-adaptation ratings (rather than any change in shape; see Fig. 8.12), the adaptation is again best thought of as a change in the subject's norm (or average) representation for that dimension. This idea is further supported by an additional finding that adaptation generalized completely from the two faces used as adapting stimuli (Sam and Bill) to the other two faces in the set (John and Fred).

8.6 A Neurally Plausible Model of Face Adaptation and Aftereffects

At a neural level, a change in the position of the subjects' psychological norm might be implemented via a type of population coding previously proposed to explain opponent perceptual aftereffects in early vision (e.g. motion aftereffect; Mather 1980; Clifford, this volume) and in mid-level vision (e.g. shape aftereffects; Regan & Hamstra 1992; Suzuki, this volume). Regan and Hamstra (1992) described a shape aftereffect in which adaptation to a vertically elongated rectangle makes a square appear horizontally elongated. To explain this aftereffect, they hypothesized that at some level in the visual pathway neurons are organized functionally into two pools, one preferentially excited by vertically elongated stimuli, and one preferentially excited by horizontally elongated stimuli.

Our analogy for faces would be that any dimension (e.g. eye height) or combination of dimensions (e.g. expansion/contraction) in face-space could be represented by two pools of broadly tuned cells, with one pool showing peak responsiveness to stimulus values a certain amount below the real world face average, and the other showing peak responsiveness to stimulus values the same amount above the average (see Webster *et al.* this volume, for discussion of the computational and metabolic efficiency of such a system). This architecture is shown for eye height (of both eyes together) in Fig. 8.13.

In this type of model, perception is determined from the population response from all cells. This is commonly modelled as the ratio of Pool 1 output to Pool 2 output, and provides opponency because the 'eyes-above' pool responding more strongly than the 'eyes-below' pool (ratios larger than 1) indicates a perception of eyes higher than the norm, while the 'eyes-below' pool responding more strongly than the 'eyes-above' pool (ratios less than 1) indicates a perception of eyes lower than the norm.

The face perceived as most normal is that which produces equal responses from the two cell sets (a ratio of 1). Prior to adaptation, this stimulus will be a face with average eye height. Adaptation then causes each pool to reduce its firing rate in proportion to its strength of response (Maddess *et al.* 1988). After adaptation to an eyes-up face, therefore, the response of the 'eyes-above'

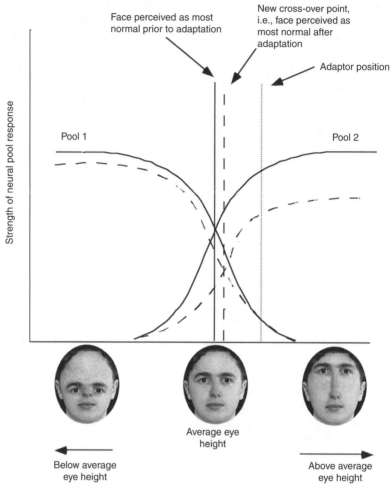

FIG. 8.13 Proposed neural mechanism for coding an opponent dimension such as eye height and an explanation of the adaptation aftereffect. Two pools of cells are used to code deviations above and below the average height. The cross-over point of these then gives the stimulus face perceived as most normal. Solid lines show the response of pools of cells without adaptation. Dashed lines show the response after adaptation, i.e. Pool 2 is reduced by a larger constant than Pool 1. Face images indicate example distortion levels on the eye height axis. Although neural responses are indicated as staying high for large distortions, it is presumably the case that with very extreme distortions (e.g., eyes outside the head) the response of each pool would drop to zero.

pool will be reduced more than the response of the 'eyes-below' pool, shifting the point of equal response levels in the direction of the adaptor (see the dotted lines in Fig. 8.14). This will cause the stimulus that looks most normal to become a face with its eyes shifted up somewhat.

This type of model is also able to explain the finding that adapting to a non-distorted face stimulus does not shift perception (Webster & MacLin 1999; MacLin & Webster 2001). No shift occurs because prolonged exposure to the norm face reduces the firing rate of the 'eyes-above' and 'eyes-below' pools by the same amount. Thus, the stimulus producing equal response levels in the two pools (a ratio of 1) remains the undistorted face.

8.7 Concluding Remarks

Aftereffects have been called the psychologists' microelectrode, because they can be used to probe the neural representation of information (Frisby 1980). Historically, aftereffects have revealed much about the organization of simple, low-level, visual attributes, such as contrast, spatial frequency, line orientation, size, direction of motion, and simple shapes (see earlier chapters, this volume). More recently, a variety of aftereffects has been reported in the perception of complex visual stimuli, most notably faces. At a neural level, we have argued that these aftereffects reflect adaptation of high-level, probably face-specific, coding mechanisms. At a computational level, we suggest that they result from recalibration of face norms or prototypes, which represent the central tendency of the faces that we see. This recalibration occurs rapidly, and continuously, in response to any consistent change in our visual diet of faces. If we are correct, then face aftereffects demonstrate that norms play an important computational role in the perceptual representation of faces, providing new evidence for an old theory (see Rhodes 1996, for a review). Finally, we have presented a preliminary model of norm-based face coding, which accounts for core aspects of the face aftereffects reviewed here.

Acknowledgements

This work was supported by the Australian Research Council. We thank Mark Edwards for helpful discussion of opponent-coding models.

References

Abromov, I., & Gordon, J. (1994). Color appearance: on seeing red – or yellow, or green, or blue. *Annual Review of Psychology*, *45*, 451–85.

Barlow, H.B., MacLeod, D.I., & Van Meeteren, A. (1976). Adaptation to gratings: no compensatory advantages found. *Vision Research*, *16*, 1043–5.

Berhmann, M., & Moscovitch, M. (2001). Face recognition: evidence from intact and impaired performance. In M. Behrmann (ed.), *Handbook of Neuropsychology, Volume 4, Disorders of Visual Behavior* (2nd ed., pp. 181–205). Amsterdam: Elsevier.

Bothwell, R.K., Brigham, J.C., & Malpass, R.S. (1989). Cross-racial identification. *Personality & Social Psychology Bulletin, 15*, 19–25.

Boynton, R.M., & Gordon, J. (1965). Bezold-Brücke hue shift measured by color naming technique. *Journal of the Optical Society of America, 55*, 78–86.

Bruce, V., & Burton, M. (2002). Learning new faces. In M. Fahle, & T. Poggio (ed.), *Perceptual Learning*. Cambridge, MA: MIT Press.

Bruce, V., Campbell, R.N., Doherty-Sneddon, G., Import, A., Langton, S., McAuley, S. et al. (2000). Testing face-processing skills in children. *British Journal of Developmental Psychology, 18*, 319–33.

Bruce, V., Doyle, T., Dench, N., & Burton, M. (1991). Remembering facial configurations. *Cognition, 38*, 109–44.

Burton, A.M., & Vokey, J.R. (1998). The face-space typicality paradox: understanding the face-space metaphor. *The Quarterly Journal of Experimental Psychology, 51A*, 475–83.

Busey, T.A. (1998). Physical and psychological representations of faces: Evidence from morphing. *Psychological Science, 6*, 476–83.

Bushnell, I.W.R., Saï, F., & Mullin, J.T. (1989). Neonatal recognition of the mother's face. *British Journal of Developmental Psychology, 7*, 3–15.

Byatt, G., & Rhodes, G. (1998). Recognition of own-race and other-race caricatures: Implications for models of face recognition. *Vision Research, 38*, 2455–68.

Carey, S. (1992). Becoming a face expert. In V. Bruce, A. Cowey, A.W. Ellis & D.I. Perrett (ed.), *Processing the Facial Image* (pp. 95–102). Oxford: Clarendon Press.

Carey, S. (1996). Perceptual classification and expertise. In R. Gelman & A. Kit-Fong (ed.), *Perceptual and Cognitive Development* (pp. 49–69). San Diego: Academic Press.

Carey, S., & Diamond, R. (1977). From piecemeal to configurational representation of faces. *Science, 195*, 312–4.

Carey, S., & Diamond, R. (1994). Are faces perceived as configurations more by adults than by children? *Visual Cognition, 1*, 253–74.

Carey, S., Diamond, R., & Woods, B. (1980). Development of face recognition – a maturational component? *Developmental Psychology, 16*, 257–69.

Chung, M-S., & Thompson, D.M. (1995). Development of face perception. *British Journal of Psychology, 86*, 55–87.

Clifford, C.W.G. (2002). Adaptation-induced plasticity in perception: motion parallels orientation. *Trends in Cognitive Sciences, 6*, 136–43.

Clifford, C.W.G., Ma Wyatt, A., Arnold, D.H., Smith, S.T., & Wenderoth, P. (2001). Orthogonal adaptation improves orientation discrimination. *Vision Research, 41*, 151–9.

Cosmides, L., Tooby, J., & Kurzban, R. (2003). Perceptions of race. *Trends in Cognitive Sciences, 7*, 173–9.

Deffenbacher, K.A., Vetter, T., Johanson, J., & O'Toole, A. (1998). Facial aging, attractiveness & distinctiveness. *Perception, 27*, 1233–43.

Dehon, H., & Brédart, S. (2001). An "other-race" effect in age estimation from faces. *Perception, 30*, 1107–13.

Diamond, R., & Carey, S. (1986). Why faces are and are not special: An effect of expertise. *Journal of Experimental Psychology: General, 115*, 107–17.

Ellis, H. (1992). The development of face processing skills. In V. Bruce, A. Cowey, A.W. Ellis, & D.I. Perrett (ed.), *Processing the Facial Image* (pp. 105–111). Oxford: Clarendon Press.

Farah, M.J., Rabinowitz, C., Quinn, G.E., & Liu, G.T. (2000). Early commitment of neural substrates for face recognition. *Cognitive Neuropsychology*, *17*, 117–23.

Farkas, L.G., Hreczki, T.A., & Katic, M.J. (1994). Craniofacial norms in North American Caucasians from birth (one year) to young adulthood. In L.G. Farkas (ed.), *Anthropometry of the Head and Face* (2nd ed., pp. 241–335). New York: Raven Press.

Frisby, J.P. (1980). *Seeing: Illusion, Mind and Brain*. Oxford: OUP.

Geldart, S., Mondloch, C.J., Maurer, D., de Schonen, S., & Brent, H.P. (2002). The effect of early visual deprivation on the development of face processing. *Developmental Science*, *5*, 490–501.

Gilchrist, A., & McKone, E. (2003). Early maturity of face processing in children: local and relational distinctiveness effects. *Visual Cognition*, *10*, 769–93.

Going, M., & Read, J.D. (1974). Effects of uniqueness, sex of subject, and sex of photograph on facial recognition. *Perceptual & Motor Skills*, *39*, 109–10.

Golby, A.J., Gabrieli, J.D.E., Chiao, J.Y., & Eberhardt, J.L. (2001). Differential responses in the fusiform region to same-race and other-race faces. *Nature Neuroscience*, *4*, 845–50.

Goldstein, A.G., & Chance, J.E. (1980). Memory for faces and schema theory. *Journal of Psychology*, *105*, 47–59.

Haxby, J.V., Hoffman, E.A., & Gobbini, M.I. (2000). The distributed human neural system for face perception. *Trends in Cognitive Sciences*, *4*, 223–33.

Hebb, D.O. (1949). *The Organisation of Behaviour*. New York: Wiley.

Hochberg, J.E. (1978). *Perception* (2nd ed.). Englewood Cliffs, New Jersy: Prentice-Hall.

Hol, K. & Treue, S. (2001). Different populations of neurons contribute to the detection and discrimination of visual motion. *Vision Research*, *41*, 685–9.

Hood, D.C. (1998). Lower-level visual processing and models of light adaptation. *Annual Review of Psychology*, *49*, 503–35.

Hurlbert, A. (2001). Trading faces. *Nature Neuroscience*, *4*, 3–5.

Inn, D., Walden, K.J., & Solso, R.L. (1993). Facial prototype formation in children. *Bulletin of the Psychonomic Society*, *31*, 197–200.

Jaquet, E. (2002). *Face Adaptation: Investigating the Face Distortion Aftereffect and Discrimination*. Unpublished honours thesis. University of Western Australia.

Jaquet, E., Rhodes, G., & Clifford, C.W.G. (2005). [The face distortion aftereffect and discrimination]. Unpublished raw data.

Johnson, M.H., Dziurawiec, S., Ellis, H., & Morton, J. (1991). Newborns' preferential tracking of face-like stimuli and its subsequent decline. *Cognition*, *40*, 1–19.

Johnston, R.A., & Ellis, H.D. (1995). Age effects in the processing of typical and distinctive faces. *Quarterly Journal of Experimental Psychology*, *48A*, 447–65.

Kanwisher, N. (2000). Domain specificity in face perception. *Nature Neuroscience*, *3*, 759–63.

Le Grand, R., Mondloch, C.J., Maurer, D., & Brent, H.P. (2001). Early visual experience and face processing. *Nature*, *410*, 890.

Leopold, D.A., O'Toole, A.J., Vetter, T., & Blanz, V. (2001). Prototype-referenced shape encoding revealed by high-level aftereffects. *Nature Neuroscience*, *4*, 89–94.

Leopold, D.A., Rhodes, G., Müller, K.-M., & Jeffery, L. (2004). The dynamics of visual adaptation to faces. *Proceedings of the Royal Society of London, Series B*, in press.

Light, L.L., Kayra-Stuart, F., & Hollander, S. (1979). Recognition memory for typical and unusual faces. *Journal of Experimental Psychology: Human Learning & Memory*, *5*, 212–19.

MacLin, O.H. & Webster, M.A. (2001). Influence of adaptation on the perception of distortions in natural images. *Journal of Electronic Imaging, 10,* 100–9.

Maddess, T., McCourt, M.E., Blakeslee, B., & Cunningham, R.B. (1988). Factors governing the adaptation of cells in area-17 of the cat visual cortex. *Biological Cybernetics, 59,* 229–36.

Mather, G. (1980). The movement aftereffect and a distribution-shift model for coding the direction of visual movement. *Perception, 9,* 379–92.

Mather, G., Verstraten, F., & Anstis, S. (1998). *The Motion Aftereffect: A Modern Perspective.* Cambridge, MA: MIT Press.

Maurer, D., Le Grand, R., & Mondloch, C.J. (2002). The many faces of configural processing. *Trends in Cognitive Sciences, 6,* 255–60.

McKone, E., & Aitkin, A. (2005). *Categorical and coordinate relations in faces, or Fechner's law instead? Journal of Experimental Pshychology: Human Perception and Performance,* in press.

Meissner, C.A., & Brigham, J.C. (2001). Thirty years of investigating the own-race bias in memory for faces. *Psychology Public Policy & Law, 7,* 3–35.

Mondloch, C.J., Geldart, S., Maurer, D., & Le Grand, R. (2003). Developmental changes in face processing skills. *Journal of Experimental Child Psychology, 86,* 67–84.

Mondloch, C.J., Le Grand, R., & Maurer, D. (2002). Configural face processing develops more slowly than featural face processing. *Perception, 31,* 553–66.

Morton, J., & Johnson, M.H. (1991). CONSPEC and CONLERN: a two-process theory of infant face recognition. *Psychological Review, 98,* 164–81.

Moscovitch, M., Winocur, G., & Behrmann, M. (1997). What is special about face recognition? Nineteen experiments on a person with visual object agnosia and dyslexia but normal face recognition. *Journal of Cognitive Neuroscience, 9,* 555–604.

Murray, J.E., Rhodes, G., & Schuchinsky, M. (2003). When is a face not a face? The effects of misorientation on mechanisms of face perception. In M.P. Peterson & G. Rhodes (ed.), *Perception of Faces, Objects and Scenes: Analytic and Holistic Processing* (pp. 75–91). Cambridge, MA: Oxford University Press.

O'Toole, A., Peterson, J., & Deffenbacher, K.A. (1996). An "other-race effect" for categorizing faces by sex. *Perception, 25,* 669–76.

Pascalis, O., de Haan, M., Nelson, C.A. (2002). Is face processing species-specific during the first year of life? *Science, 296,* 130–2.

Pellicano, E., & Rhodes, G. (2003). Holistic processing of faces in preschool children and adults. *Psychological Science, 14,* 618–22.

Pellicano, E., Rhodes, G., & Peters, M. (2004). *Are Preschoolers Sensitive to Configural Information in Faces?* Unpublished manuscript.

Peterson, M.P., & Rhodes, G. (ed.) (2003). *Perception of Faces, Objects and Scenes: Analytic and Holistic Processing.* New York: Oxford University Press.

Phinney, R.E., Bowd, C., & Patterson, R. (1997). Direction-selective coding of stereoscopic (cyclopean) motion. *Vision Research, 37,* 865–9.

Reed, S.K. (1972). Pattern recognition and categorization. *Cognitive Psychology, 3,* 382–407.

Regan, D., & Beverley, K.I. (1985). Postadaptation orientation discrimination. *Journal of the Optical Society of America A, 2,* 147–55.

Regan, D., & Beverley, K.I. (1983). Spatial-frequency discrimination and detection: Comparison of postadaptation thresholds. *Journal of the Optical Society of America, 73,* 1684–90.

Regan, D. & Hamstra, S.J. (1992). Shape discrimination and the judgement of perfect symmetry: Dissociation of shape from size. *Vision Research*, *32*, 1845–64.

Rhodes, G. (1996). *Superportraits*: *Caricatures and Recognition*. Hove: The Psychology Press.

Rhodes, G., Brennan, S., & Carey, S. (1987). Identification and ratings of caricatures: Implications for mental representations of faces. *Cognitive Psychology*, *19*, 473–97.

Rhodes, G., Carey, S., Byatt, G., & Proffitt, F. (1998). Coding spatial variations in faces and simple shapes: a test of two models. *Vision Research*, *38*, 2307–21.

Rhodes, G., Clifford, C.W.G., Jeffery, L., & Watson, T. (2005). [Time course of configural face aftereffects]. Unpublished raw data.

Rhodes, G., & Jeffery, L. (2005). [Opponent coding of identity]. Unpublished raw data.

Rhodes, G., Jeffery, L., Watson, T.L., Clifford, C.W.G., & Nakayama, K. (2003). Fitting the mind to the world: Face adaptation and attractiveness aftereffects. *Psychological Science*, *14*, 558–66.

Rhodes, G., Jeffery, L., Watson, T.L., Jaquet, E., Winkler, C., & Clifford, C.W.G. (2005). Orientation-contingent face aftereffects and implications for face coding mechanisms. *Current Biology*, *14*, 2119–23.

Rhodes, G., & Zebrowitz, L.A. (ed.) (2002). *Facial Attractiveness*: *Evolutionary, Cognitive and Social Perspectives*. Westport, CT: Ablex.

Robbins, R., Anderson, R., & McKone, E. (2005). [Duration of aftereffects following adaptation to face dimensions]. Unpublished raw data.

Robbins, R., McKone, E., & Edwards, M. (2005). Are some dimensions in face-space more adaptable than others? In preparation.

Rossion B., & Gauthier, I. (2002). How does the brain process upright and inverted faces. *Behavioral and Cognitive Neuroscience Reviews*, *1*, 63–75.

Schwarzer, G. (2000). Development of face processing: The effect of face inversion. *Child Development*, *71*, 391–401.

Schwarzer, G., & Zauner, N. (2003). Face processing in 8-month-old infants: evidence for configural and analytic processing. *Vision Research*, *43*, 2783–93.

Solso, R.L., & McCarthy, J.E. (1981a). Prototype formation of faces: A case of pseudomemory. *British Journal of Psychology*, *72*, 499–503.

Solso, R.L., & McCarthy, J.E. (1981b). Prototype formation: Central tendency models vs. attribute frequency model. *Bulletin of the Psychonomic Society*, *17*, 10–11.

Strauss, M.S., (1979). Abstraction of prototype information by adults and 10-month-old infants. *Journal of Experimental Psychology*: *Human Learning & Memory*, *5*, 618–32.

Tanaka, J.W., & Farah, M.J. (1993). Parts and wholes in face recognition. *The Quarterly Journal of Experimental Psychology*, *46A*, 225–45.

Tanaka, J.W., Bukach, C.M., & Kiefer, M. (2004). A holistic account of the own-race effect in face recognition: evidence from a cross-cultural study. *Cognition*, *93*, B1–B9.

Tanaka, J.W., & Sengco, J.A. (1997). Features and their configuration in face recognition. *Memory and Cognition*, *25*, 583–92.

Turati, C. (2004). Why faces are not special to newborns: An alternative account of the face preference. *Current Directions in Psychological Science*, *13*, 5–8.

Tzourio-Mazoyer, N., de Schonen, S., Crivello, F., Reutter, B., Aujard, Y., & Mazoyer, B. (2002). Neural correlates of woman face processing by 2-month-old infants. *NeuroImage*, *15*, 454–61.

Valentine, T. (1991). A unified account of the effects of distinctiveness, inversion and race on face recognition. *Quarterly Journal of Experimental Psychology*, *43A*, 161–204.

Valentine, T., & Bruce, V. (1986). The effects of distinctiveness in recognising and classifying faces. *Perception, 15*, 525–35.

Valentine, T. & Endo, M. (1992). Towards an exemplar model of face processing: The effects of race and distinctiveness. *Quarterly Journal of Experimental Psychology, 44A,* 671–703.

Vokey, J.R. & Read, J.D. (1992). Familiarity, memorability, and the effect of typicality on the recognition of faces. *Memory and Cognition, 20,* 291–301.

Wainwright, M.J. (1999). Visual adaptation as optimal information transmission. *Vision Research, 39,* 3960–74.

Walton, G.E., & Bower, T.G.R. (1993). Newborns form "prototypes" in less than 1 minute. *Psychological Science, 4,* 203–5.

Watson, T.L., & Clifford, C.W.G. (2003). Pulling faces: an investigation of the face distortion aftereffect. *Perception, 32,* 1109–16.

Webster, M.A., Kaping, D., Mizokami, Y., & Dumahel, P. (2004). Adaptation to natural face categories. *Nature, 428,* 558–61.

Webster, M.A., & MacLin, O.H. (1999). Figural aftereffects in the perception of faces. *Psychonomic Bulletin & Review, 6*(4), 647–53.

Werblin, F.S. (1973). The control of sensitivity in the retina. *Scientific American, 228,* 70–9.

Yin, R. (1969). Looking at upside-down faces. *Journal of Experimental Psychology, 81,* 141–5.

Zebrowitz, L.A. (1997). *Reading Faces.* Boulder, CO: Westview Press.

Zhao, L., & Chubb, C. (2001). The size-tuning of the face-distortion after-effect. *Vision Research, 41,* 2979–94.

9

Adaptation and the Phenomenology of Perception

Michael A. Webster, John S. Werner,
and David J. Field

9.1 Introduction

To what extent do we have shared or unique perceptual experiences? We examine how the answer to this question is constrained by the processes of visual adaptation. Adaptation constantly recalibrates visual coding so that our vision is normalized according to the stimuli that we are currently exposed to. These normalizations occur over very wide ranging time scales, from milliseconds to evolutionary spans. The resulting adjustments dramatically alter the appearance of the world before us, and in particular, alter visual salience by highlighting how the current image deviates from the properties predicted by the current states of adaptation. To the extent that observers are exposed to and thus adapted by a different environment, their vision will be normalized in different ways and their subjective visual experience may differ. These differences will be illustrated by considering how adaptation influences properties which vary across different environments. To the extent that observers are exposed and adapted to common properties in the environment, their vision will be adjusted toward common states, and in this respect they will have a common visual experience. This will be illustrated by considering the effects of adaptation on image properties that are common across environments.

In either case, it is the similarities or differences in the stimuli – and not the intrinsic similarities or differences in the observers – which largely determine the relative states of adaptation. Thus, at least, some aspects of our private internal experience are controlled by external factors that are accessible to objective measurement.

In 2001, a controversial new portrayal of Queen Elizabeth II was unveiled by the painter Lucian Freud. Freud, the grandson of Sigmund, has been hailed as the greatest living portrait artist in England, and had clearly labored carefully over a work that included 70 sittings by the Queen. However, the painting was not well-received. Reviews in the press ranged from muted disappointment ("while she is no longer the heartbreakingly beautiful young woman she was, she is still easy on the eye") to open hostility ("Freud should be locked in the tower"). Many editorials pointed to distortions in the representation ("the chin has what can only be described as a six o'clock shadow, and the neck would not disgrace a rugby prop forward"). But perhaps, the most telling comment was that "she should have known what to expect," for the painting bears Freud's distinctive style and – to the untrained eye – the face depicted seems notably similar to his own self-portrait. Apparently, many in the public saw the painting in a way that the artist did not. In this chapter, we argue that they *literally saw* the painting differently. This is not to suggest that Freud thought that the work actually looked like a faithful copy of the Queen, an error of logic known as the El Greco fallacy (Anstis 1996). Rather, we explore the possibility that Freud might have seen the painting differently, simply because he had spent so much time looking at it.

What might the world look like if we could see it through the eyes of another? Such questions are central to the debate over the nature of perceptual experience and sensory qualia, or what it "feels" like to see. Because we have access only to our own private experience, we cannot directly observe whether it is similar in others. A classic example of this limitation is Locke's inverted spectrum (Locke 1689, 1975). Even if two observers completely agree on how they label the hues of the spectrum, we cannot be certain that their experiences agree, for the subjective sensation of redness in one might correspond to the sensation of greenness in the other. Arguments about phenomenology must instead rely on inferences from indirect observations. For example, arguments against a phenomenally inverted spectrum have pointed out that this possibility would be inconsistent with asymmetries in the properties of color perception (Hardin 1997; Palmer 1999).

In this review, we consider how the nature of subjective experience is constrained by the processes of sensory adaptation. Adaptation adjusts visual sensitivity according to the set of stimuli an observer is exposed to. As the many chapters in this book illustrate, such adjustments are a built-in feature of visual coding and probably regulate most if not all aspects of visual perception. Indeed, adaptation may represent a fundamental "law" of cognition and behavior, a point most forcefully argued by Helson (1964). Here we focus on how specific presumed properties of visual adaptation might be expected to influence visual phenomenology. Studies of adaptation aftereffects have shown that changes in the state of adaptation have dramatic consequences for how the world appears. The states of adaptation may therefore play a fundamental role in determining whether the world looks the same or different to others.

9.2 Adaptation and Response Normalization

The use of information theory has provided major insights into our understanding of sensory coding. By understanding the statistics of the environment and relating those statistics to response properties of sensory neurons, we have learned that these sensory neurons are providing a highly efficient representation of the environment (Atick 1992; Field 1994; Simoncelli & Olshausen 2001). It seems reasonable to assume that the processes of perceptual adaptation contribute to this efficiency in coding (Wainwright 1999). To understand how the phenomenology of adaptation might bear on such coding, we first consider the influence of adaptation on individual neurons and then on the distribution of responses across neurons.

Neurons have a limited dynamic range, and because they are noisy, can reliably signal only a relatively small number of response levels (Barlow & Levick 1976). To maximize the information a neuron can carry, these levels should be matched to the distribution of levels in the stimulus. This principle closely predicts evolutionary adaptations such as the sigmoidal shape of a neuron's response function (Laughlin 1987). Most points in a scene have a brightness and color that are close to the modal level, and thus the optimal response function should be steep near the mode, to allow fine discrimination among frequently occurring stimulus values, while shallow at the tails, where signals are rare. This effectively expands the representation of data near the modal level and compresses those data near the outliers (Fig. 9.1).

The same considerations also predict the need for short-term adaptations, since the variation within any scene will be less than the variation between scenes. Therefore, a system that can "float" the sensitivity range can maximize the information carrying capacity of a neuron. An obvious example is the enormous variation in the average light level during the course of the day. The intensity variations within a scene (in the range of 300 to 1) are much less than the intensity variations across scenes (on the order of 10^{14} to 1). Therefore, a system that can recalibrate to the individual scene can reduce the required dynamic range by several orders of magnitude. Without this adaptation, any given neuron with its limited dynamic range, would be silent or saturated most of the time (Walraven et al. 1990).

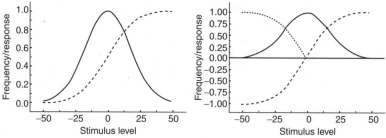

FIG. 9.1 Fitting the response to the stimulus. (Left panel) For a Gaussian distribution of stimulus levels, the optimal response curve will be steepest near the mean, where stimuli are frequent, while asymptoting at the tails, where signals are rare. (Right panel) For an opponent mechanism the response curve signals deviations (positive or negative) from the mean; this opponency can also be realized in all-positive response curves by splitting the response into separate on and off mechanisms.

By adjusting to the average stimulus, the visual system could represent information in the form of deviations from the average. This gives special importance to the mean because it defines the reference point to which other responses are now relative. One way to realize this reference in the neural response is to use an opponent code, in which the responses can be of opposite sign. For example, the intensity response of a mechanism can be recoded so that there is zero response to the mean intensity, and darker or brighter stimuli are represented by negative or positive values, respectively (Fig. 9.1). Opponent processing is a hallmark of color vision: color-opponent mechanisms receive inputs of opposite sign from different cone types and thus their outputs represent a comparison of the relative activity across the cones (De Valois 2003). It may be that opponent processing is more generally a central property of perception because of the general need to make comparisons (Hurvich & Jameson 1974). A consequence of opponency is that the neuron is silent to the average. Thus, a "red versus green" mechanism does not respond to "white," or importantly, to the average color that it is exposed to. This average is thus represented only implicitly, by the absence of a signal. Note that within a single neuron, responses of opposite sign are relative to the neuron's background activity. However, these opposing responses may instead be instantiated within separate "on" and "off" mechanisms. This split code can improve efficiency by increasing the signal-to-noise ratio over a pair of neurons that instead both spanned the full dynamic range, (MacLeod & von der Twer 2003) while opponency itself increases the metabolic efficiency by greatly reducing the average firing rate of cells.

To realize its full capacity, a neuron's operating curve should be matched not only to the average stimulus, but also to the range of stimulus levels or available contrasts. A clear example of this optimization is in color coding. Color vision depends on comparing the responses across different classes of cone. Yet, because the spectral sensitivities of the cones overlap, this difference signal is necessarily smaller than the range of available luminance signals (which instead depend on adding the cone signals). If the post-receptoral neurons encoding luminance and color had similar dynamic ranges, then they would again be silent or saturated most of the times. Instead, chromatic sensitivity is much higher than luminance sensitivity, consistent with matching responses to the available gamut (Chaparro et al. 1993). However, in this case again, the environment can vary in the range of stimulus contrasts, and thus short-term adaptations would again be necessary if the neurons are to be appropriately tuned to the scenes before us. This form of adjustment, known as contrast adaptation, is well-established psychophysically as well as in individual neurons (Webster 2003). Thus, for example, sensitivity to contrast is reduced in the presence of high contrast stimuli (though the precise form of the response changes or their functional consequences are less clear than for light adaptation). Our first point then, is that it is plausible to expect adaptation to play a pervasive role in normalizing neural responses and that these adjustments should operate in similar ways across observers. Whether or not two observers have similar subjective experiences should therefore be in part predictable from whether or not they are under similar states of adaptation.

At least in the early stages of the visual system, it is common to assume that information is encoded by channels that are selective for different values along a stimulus dimension. For example, color is initially encoded by three channels – the cones – that differ in their selectivity to wavelength. How should the responses across these channels be distributed? Assuming that neurons involved in different computations have a roughly similar dynamic range, we can predict that if we shift to a new set of axes (e.g. an opponent system), then we can expect the magnitudes along the different axes to be roughly similar (Fig. 9.2). This predicts that the channel gain should be inversely proportional to the strength of the stimulus component for which each channel is selective. One example of this principle in color vision is the gain of signals derived from S cones. The S cones make up only a small fraction of the total number of cone receptors and the wavelengths to which they respond are more strongly filtered by the lens and macular screening pigments, yet their signals are greatly amplified in the visual cortex so that the response to different hues is more effectively "spherized" (De Valois et al. 2000).

A second example of matching channel gain to the stimulus distribution is provided by the spatial statistics of images, which have less contrast at fine scales (high spatial frequencies) than coarse scales (low frequencies). Cortical mechanisms tuned to different spatial scales may vary in sensitivity in such a way that compensates for the stimulus bias so that the response across scale is the same on average (Field & Brady 1997). Both of these examples could reflect the evolutionary adaptations of the visual system in response to more or less stable attributes of the visual environment. Yet in

Alignment   Repulsion   Multi-channel

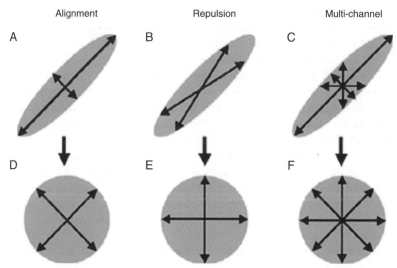

FIG. 9.2 Three ways in which a set of channels might selectively adapt to sphere the responses. (A) and (D) alignment of the response axes along the principal stimulus axes and gain control; (B) and (E) repulsion of the axes relative to the principal axis; (C) and (F) independent gain changes within multiple channels tuned to different stimulus directions.

both cases, we consider below how these stimulus properties can routinely change because of changes in the environment or the observer, and thus short-term adaptive adjustments would again be important for maintaining the balance across the channels. In fact, the processes that adjust each neuron to the average stimulus level it is exposed to, will serve to balance the responses across neurons. Thus, our second point is that adaptation will normalize visual responses to adjust to the specific biases in the observer's environment.

A final prediction is that the responses of different neurons should be as independent as possible. If two neurons are redundantly carrying the same information, then together they will require greater information capacity than if the data were represented independently. For example, the signals from different cone classes are highly correlated. Postreceptoral neurons remove much of this redundancy by recoding the cone signals into their sums or differences (Buchsbaum & Gottschalk 1983). In a similar way, the center-surround organization of retinal receptive fields can be viewed as a strategy for removing the correlations between the receptor responses to nearby regions of space, which tend to have similar brightness and color (Srinivasan et al. 1982). However, although the channels may be largely uncorrelated when considering the population of all images, any given image or environment may have relatively strong correlations. Furthermore, there are likely to be correlations between different stimulus dimensions (e.g. between brightness and color) that will vary between environments. Thus, a channel structure that will allow the system to dynamically tune its responses to different environments will provide a means of making maximal use out of the limited dynamic range of the system.

To remove the correlations between a set of channels, it is obviously not enough to equalize their responses – instead, the actual tuning of the channels must change, and there is evidence that adaptation can influence not just the gain, but also the stimulus selectivity of individual neurons (Carandini *et al.* 1997; Movshon & Lennie 1979; Dragoi *et al.* 2002). How might adaptation adjust the neural representation to achieve independence? It turns out that there are many possible strategies, and these are illustrated in Fig. 9.2 for a pair of mechanisms encoding an elliptical stimulus distribution. One way would be to rotate the preferred axes of the mechanisms to align them with the principal axes of the stimulus variance (Fig. 9.2(A)). This process, called Principal Components Analysis (PCA), has been used to predict the realignment of the cone axes along separate luminance and color-opponent channels (Buchsbaum & Gottschalk 1983), and a rotation followed by scaling (Fig. 9.2(D)) would effectively sphere the responses. However, note that after sphering, the vectors will remain independent for any orthogonal rotation. Thus, decorrelation alone places weak constraints on the choice of axes. An alternative principle is to select the channels in order to capture the separate components contributing to the distribution. This method, known as Sparse Coding or Independent Components Analysis, is more effective for non-elliptical stimulus distributions (e.g. composed of multiple ellipses from multiple sources), and has been found to closely predict the receptive field properties of cells in striate cortex (Olshausen & Field 1996). Both of these processes may be important in longer-term evolutionary adaptations of visual coding, and it is an intriguing question whether similar types of adjustments – and specifically, adjustments that align the channel axes along the stimulus axes – can occur through short-term adaptation. The signature of these might be changes in the "labels" carried by the channels. However, short-term visual aftereffects have instead been interpreted in terms of response changes within channels whose labels are fixed.

Barlow and Földiák (Barlow & Földiák 1989; Barlow 1990) suggested that perceptual adaptation might reflect mutual inhibition that builds up between channels whenever they respond together, thus biasing their preferred axes by setting up a mutual repulsion between them (Fig. 9.2(B and E)). Note that this results in a different pair of channels than the pair predicted by PCA, because the response vectors are biased relative to the stimulus axes rather than aligned with them. Their model provides a physiologically plausible mechanism for decorrelation and could in particular account for the phenomenon of "contingent adaptation." For example, in the McCollough Effect

(McCollough 1965), color aftereffects are elicited that are contingent on the orientation of the adapting grating, and the sensitivity changes may reflect adaptive adjustments that are designed to remove the correlation between color and orientation.

However, a problem arises when the set of data axes and the number of channels (i.e. vectors) is overcomplete, or in other words, when a larger number of output vectors is used to span a smaller number of input dimensions (e.g. Fig. 9.2(C)). For example, for the plane in Fig. 9.2, it is not possible to have an overcomplete set of vectors in addition to keeping them uncorrelated. Field (in preparation) argues that with certain forms of non-linearity the family of vectors can be both uncorrelated and overcomplete. The details are beyond the scope of this chapter. However, the issue of overcomplete coding and its relationship to optimal mapping is an important issue. The number of neurons in the visual cortex is at least an order of magnitude larger than the number of inputs into it. For instance, signals from the three cone classes appear to be carried within more than three types of color channels in the cortex (Lennie 1999), and thus simple linear operations cannot remove the correlations between them. Moreover, in practice, the aftereffects predicted by linear decorrelation are similar to the changes predicted by an independent adaptation within multiple channels (Fig. 9.2(C and F)). That is, both predict a selective loss in sensitivity to the principal axis of the stimulus even though the basis for this loss is entirely different (Webster & Mollon 1994). Thus it has proven difficult to distinguish between different models of the adaptation. Nevertheless, in each of these cases the selective aftereffects can be thought of as sphering the representation of the environment, and thus the principle of sphering remains a powerful predictor of the consequences of adaptation for visual experience.

9.3 Adaptation to a Colored Environment

The implications of these adaptive adjustments for the problem of other minds can be illustrated by considering the simple case of adapting to the average color of a scene. Suppose that two otherwise identical observers are placed in a pair of identical rooms, except that in one room the average color is white while in the other it is red (Fig. 9.3). Adaptation will adjust the gains of the cones so that their average responses are equated in each room, a process that in the case of color vision is known as von Kries scaling (von Kries 1970). As a result, over time both observers should report that their room is more nearly achromatic, and if the adaptation were complete then the color difference would be completely factored out. However, if they were suddenly able to look through each others' eyes then their perceptions would not agree, for what the observer in the reddish room perceived as white, would appear red to the other. Thus, two observers who are intrinsically the same will perceive the same stimulus differently if they are adapted to different environments.

"White room"   "Red room"

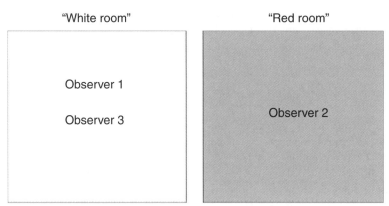

FIG. 9.3 Adaptation to different colored environments. Observers 1 and 2 are assumed
to be physiologically identical but will experience color differently because they are
adapted to "white" and "red" worlds. Observers 1 and 3 are assumed to
have different spectral sensitivities but will have similar color experiences because
they are adapted to the same world.

Now suppose a third observer is placed in the white room, and that the
spectral sensitivity of this observer differs from that of the first. For example,
this individual might have a higher density of lens pigment, reducing the
amount of shortwave light reaching the observer's retina. However, von Kries
scaling should again adjust their perception so that the room appears achromatic. The first and the third observer would therefore agree about the color
of the room, and in this sense would have a common perceptual experience.
Thus, even if two observers are physiologically different, their phenomenal
experience may be similar in important ways if they are adapted to the same
environment.

These two cases illustrate a fundamental asymmetry in the adaptation.
Specifically, the visual system is adjusting to the properties of the environment,
or as stated by Hecht, "the stimulus adapts the organism to itself" (Hecht 1923,
p. 577). This means that in order to predict whether the observers have common
or different perceptual experiences it may often be more important to characterize the environment than the observer.

It turns out that we do not have to imagine these examples in the minds of
others, for we can each readily experience them in our own visual systems. The
afterimages we experience when we look at a dark or colored form, and then
shift our gaze to a uniform field are the lingering aftereffects of an adjustment
that serves to normalize sensitivity to the brightness and color of the adapting
stimulus. As the stimulus changes, our color perception is shifted accordingly.
Alternatively, as we look at a uniform field we do so through a retina which is
highly inhomogeneous, yet our subjective impression often gives little hint of

this pronounced physiological variation. It may be that this is in part because the physiologically different areas of the retina have nevertheless been normalized through adaptation to roughly the same external stimulus.

9.4 Varieties of Perceptual Constancy

It is instructive to reconsider color experience within the two rooms of Fig. 9.3 from the perspective of perceptual constancy. Constancy refers to the stable perception of object properties despite changes in the viewing conditions. Most discussions of constancy focus on how the visual system can discount or compensate for variations in the stimulus. Yet the notion of constancy can also be applied to the problem of discounting variations within the observer, and by extension, can be generalized to variations between observers. These different aspects of constancy are illustrated in Table 9.1 and are discussed in turn.

9.4.1 Compensating for Variations in the Stimulus

Many forms of stimulus constancy, such as veridical judgments of size despite changing distance or of shape despite changing viewpoint, may not involve adaptation in a direct or obvious way. However, color vision is a case in which adaptation plays a widely recognized role. Under most natural viewing conditions the perception of color is more closely correlated with an object's reflectance properties than with the distribution of wavelengths the object is currently reflecting. The latter is a product of both the reflectance function and the incident illuminant, and the problem for color constancy is how to factor out the contribution to color from the illuminant (Lennie & D'Zmura 1988; Zaidi chapter, this volume). The human visual system is only approximately color-constant and employs many different strategies to achieve this, but a simple mechanism that works to promote color constancy is von Kries scaling of the cone signals (Brainard & Wandell 1992). In Fig. 9.3, suppose we change the white room into a red room simply by changing the illuminant. We have already seen that an observer in this room will renormalize to the new mean

Table 9.1 Forms of perceptual constancy. Constancy can compensate for changes in the stimulus (e.g. a change in the color of the illuminant) or the observer (e.g. a change in spectral sensitivity with aging), and thus could also compensate for environmental or physiological differences between observers

	Environmental variation	Observer variation
Within-observer	E.g. illuminant change	E.g. aging lens
Between-observers	E.g. two observers under two different illuminants	E.g. two observers that differ in lens density

chromaticity, so that the average color appears achromatic. As a result of this adjustment, the spectral bias introduced by the new illuminant is partially discounted. For example, for the surfaces with a flat reflectance function, the spectrum of the reflected light will mirror the illuminant, and thus without adaptation, would appear as the color of the illuminant. Yet, to the extent that adaptation renormalizes the cone signals to "flatten" the response to this spectrum, the surface itself will appear spectrally flat ("gray") and thus, will be the same under either illuminant.

In what sense does observer 1 maintain constant color experience if the lighting is changed to red, when we had argued previously that (as observer 2) their color perception does change when the room itself is red? The difference is because we have assumed that their subjective experience refers to the object reflectances. In either case, von Kries adaptation will adjust to the average chromaticity. Yet when the lighting changes, this adaptation removes the illuminant color and thus preserves the same response to the same reflectance, while in the previous case it is the objects themselves that have changed, and thus the perception of object reflectance changes. [Note that to illustrate these points we have considered only a simple adjustment to the mean chromaticity. In actual practice, the visual system can exploit differences in how color signals vary with changes in reflectance versus lighting in order to disambiguate between them, and thus can exhibit better constancy for both reflectances and illuminants than that predicted by von Kries adaptation alone (Golz & MacLeod 2002)].

In general, adaptation should lead toward constancy when it factors out extraneous sources of variation in the stimulus. Again, in the case of color or lightness constancy, these arise because of variations in the spectral content or intensity of the illuminant. The visual system may also exhibit contrast constancy, and perhaps blur constancy, in scenes with reduced visibility as when we view them through fog (Brown & MacLeod 1997). All of these cases represent situations in which the extraneous variable is the light medium. Are there analogous cases in other domains of perception, in which adaptation can compensate for irrelevant sources of stimulus variance? For example, in face or speech perception, the stimulus is shaped by both individual factors (e.g. identity, fitness, or expression) and more global factors (e.g. familial or ethnic characteristics). If adaptation allows the visual system to parse out and compensate for these more global population characteristics, then it is meaningful to suppose that it provides a form of "face constancy" for individual characteristics. For example, discounting the average characteristics of a population (by normalizing for these characteristics) may allow the observer to maintain stable perceptual criteria (e.g. "average" features) for judging properties of individual faces such as attractiveness (Rhodes *et al.* 2003).

9.4.2 Compensating for Variations in the Observer

What will happen if observer 1 changes over time to become observer 3, because properties of their visual system change? Here again, we see that adaptation should adjust to compensate for these physiological differences. From the perspective of constancy, this means that the observers should continue to maintain a stable perception of the world even though they have themselves changed. This is accomplished by factoring out extraneous sources of variation which are now due to the observer. This recalibration may represent one of the most important and general forms of perceptual constancy. The genetic specification of visual pathways is unlikely to provide more than a broad outline for coding, leaving much to be shaped by experience. The problem of calibrating the channel structure is obviated by the processes of adaptation, since these adjust visual sensitivity in order to match it to the environment. Thus, the adaptation represents a form of "error-correction" in the observer (Andrews 1964). In the same way, these processes should correct for the errors that could arise in the course of normal development and aging, during which there are profound changes throughout the visual system (Werner 1998). As we describe below, studies of color perception across the lifespan provide powerful evidence for perceptual constancy despite the dramatic changes in visual pathways with aging.

9.4.3. Interobserver Constancy

If we accept that adaptation can maintain a stable perceptual experience despite changes within an observer, then it is perhaps not too far a leap to suppose that the same processes can contribute to constancy between observers. This "interobserver constancy" means that the world should look similar to different observers in important ways. The states of adaptation may not speak to the nature of qualia. For example, they do not require that what white looks like to one will be similar to another. However, they do strongly influence what stimulus appears white, or more generally, what stimuli appear perceptually neutral to an observer, and thus whether these perceptual landmarks are equivalent in others. These shared perceptions are possible when observers are adapted to similar worlds, or when the adaptation factors out the differences between their worlds (e.g. differences in illumination); but should break down when observers are instead normalized for different properties of their (different) environments.

9.5 Variation and Constancy in the Visual Environment

9.5.1 Color and the Natural Environment

In the previous sections, we explored the consequences of adaptation by asking how we might be adapted if we lived in different colored rooms. But to what extent do our color worlds actually vary? A number of studies have examined the color statistics of natural images (Burton & Moorhead 1987; Webster & Mollon 1997; Párraga et al. 1998; Ruderman et al. 1998). Short-term color differences routinely arise from differences in illumination, but more long-term differences also result from differences in the settings themselves. One principal source of variation is between arid and lush scenes, which can contribute to differences both across environments and within the same environment over time. For example, Fig. 9.4 shows measurements from a set of scenes from a single valley in rural India during the monsoon (wet) and winter (dry) seasons (Mizokami *et al.* 2003). The changes in vegetation shifted the mean color from green to yellow, and shifted the principal axes of the distributions from near the S axis of cone-opponent space to a bluish-yellowish axis intermediate to the S and LM axes. Note that these mean color shifts were large compared to the differences in the illuminants during the two seasons. Thus, different environments can in fact vary widely in their color properties.

Are these differences large enough to induce different states of adaptation? Webster and Mollon (1997) exposed observers to a sequence of colors drawn from different measured scenes, and then used a matching task to measure changes in the appearance of a set of test colors. Adaptation altered the perceived color by adjusting to both the average color in the scene and to the contrast axis defining the scene. For example, after viewing the colors from an arid yellowish scene that varied primarily along a blue-yellow axis, the mean color

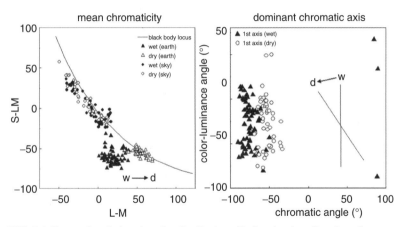

FIG. 9.4 Seasonal variations in color distributions. Each point describes the color properties of one image taken within the same vicinity during wet or dry seasons in Nashik district, India. The color values are represented according to a scaled version of the MacLeod-Boynton/Derrington-Krauskopf-Lennie color space, which forms a sphere with "gray" at the origin. Color coordinates correspond to the distance from the origin along the three cardinal axes of postreceptoral color coding (representing variations in luminance or in color along axes that vary in activity in L versus M cones or the S cones versus the sum of L and M cones). (Left) Average color in the scenes. Seasonal changes in vegetation cause the average color to shift along the L-M axis from green to yellow; these shifts in reflectance are large relative to the seasonal differences in illumination (shown by the small symbols for sky); (Right) Principal axis of the image colors. The principal directions of the color distributions also rotate over time, varying primarily along a bluish-greenish axis (the vertical S versus LM axis in the color space) during the wet monsoon, while along a bluish-yellowish axis (~ -60 deg) during the dry winter.

for this distribution appeared whiter, and there was a selective loss in the perceived saturation of blues and yellows compared to other hues (Fig. 9.5). This is consistent with an adjustment to the mean color through chromatic adaptation and with an adjustment to the relative variance in different color directions through contrast adaptation. These selective shifts in color appearance were also found with a hue-scaling task for colors presented on spatially varying backgrounds (Webster *et al.* 2002b). Thus, the color differences across scenes are in principle sufficient to hold observers under different adaptation states. However, it ultimately remains to be demonstrated whether individuals who actually live in different settings would show differences in color perception that can be linked to different states of adaptation (Webster *et al.* 2002c). The strongest test of this possibility might be to measure the white point for populations immersed in characteristically different environments.

9.5.2 Adaptation to Faces

A second example where stimuli might vary across environments and thus shape perception in different ways is in the perception of faces. Adaptation to

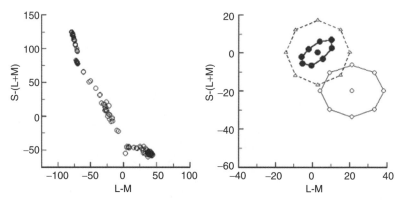

FIG. 9.5 Adaptation to natural color distributions. (Left) color distribution measured from an arid scene in the Sierra Nevada mountains, plotted within the scaled MacLeod-Boynton diagram. Symbols plot the chromaticities of points sampled from different locations within the same scene. The set of colors in the scene is largely confined to a bluish-yellowish (sky and earth) axis varying around the yellowish mean, lying at an orientation of roughly −55 deg within the color plane. (Right) shifts in color appearance after adapting to a rapid sequence of colors drawn from this distribution. Test colors (unfilled circles) were a set of stimuli centered on the adapting mean, and all appeared yellowish under neutral adaptation (to the reference white). After adaptation (filled circles), the average color instead appeared white (consistent with normalizing for the adapting mean), and stimuli along the blue-yellow axis appeared less saturated (consistent with normalizing for the adapting contrasts). Open triangles are the color changes that would be predicted if adaptation adjusted only to the average color, and not the color contrast, through independent gain changes within each cone class (von Kries scaling).

faces is reviewed in detail in other chapters of this volume. Here we focus only on the evidence that these adaptation effects are large for the natural variations that characterize human faces and that they can strongly affect the kinds of perceptual judgments that we normally make when we look at faces. These include such categorical judgments as the identity, gender, expression, or ethnicity of an individual. To explore these, Webster *et al.* (2004) took images of actual faces from different categories (e.g. a male and female face), and then morphed between them to form a finely graded series of intermediate images. Subjects varied these images to estimate the boundary between the two perceived categories (e.g. the point at which the image stopped looking "male" and started looking "female"). These ratings were strongly and rapidly biased by prior adaptation to one of the original faces. Thus after viewing the male image, intermediate morph levels were more likely to be perceived as a female, and consequently the category boundary shifted toward the adapting image (Fig. 9.6). These perceptual shifts are consistent with a renormalization of face perception so that the face we are currently exposed to appears more neutral.

Similar aftereffects were found for faces that differed in ethnicity or expression. Moreover, the aftereffects also transferred across different faces. Thus exposure to a sequence of female faces biases the gender boundary between male and female images that were not part of the adapting set. Such results suggest that adaptation can – and probably routinely does – strongly shape our face perception. Again, faces are interesting in this regard precisely because they vary across individuals. Yet these variations are not random. We are each exposed to a different diet of faces because we live in environments peopled by different distributions of individuals, ages, genders, and ethnic groups. To the extent that our perception is normalized for the specific characteristics of these distributions, our perception of faces should differ.

9.5.3 Color Vision and Aging

The preceding two examples illustrate the possibility that individuals see the world differently because they are adapted to different worlds. Can we identify reasonable instances where physiologically different individuals may perceive in similar ways because they are adapted to the same world? One instance can again be drawn from color vision, and specifically, from measures of color appearance across the life span.

Sixty years after Wright (1928–29) discovered that age-related brunescence (i.e. yellowing) of the lens of the eye causes rather substantial changes in color matching, he posed the question: "Why do the colors of familiar objects look exactly the same to me now as they did when I was a boy?" (Wright 1988, p. 138). In addition to the lenticular pigment changes that Wright knew about, there are numerous other age-related changes in the eye, the photoreceptors and the visual pathways. Of most interest, however, is the lens itself, for its effect on the visual stimulus is well-understood; it selectively attenuates short wavelengths, and as a consequence, the relative excitation of the three different classes of cone photoreceptors. The effect

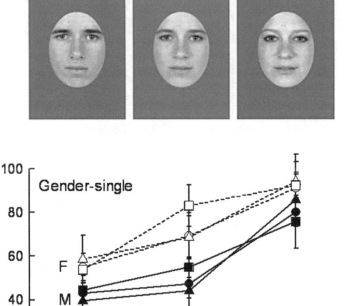

FIG. 9.6 Adaptation to natural variations in faces. Subjects were shown a graded
set of 100 images formed by morphing between a male and female face, and chose the
point along the continuum that divided the images into "male" or "female". The three
images at the top show an example of one of the male and female face pairs and the
intermediate morphed image between them. Curves plot the settings for a female
(F, open symbols) or male (M, closed symbols) subject, each tested with three different
morph pairs (square, circle, triangle). Note that each subject chose a boundary closer to
their own gender. After adapting to a male (female) face, the blended images appear
more female (male), shifting the perceived neutral point toward the adapting gender.

is quite substantial, as shown in Fig. 9.7 where the change in excitation of S-, M-,
and L-cones is plotted as a function of changes associated with age (due to increasing
lens density) and phases of daylight illumination (or correlated color temperature).
While the changes in cone excitation are similar for aging and changes in the color
of the ambient illumination, they take place on different time scales, and the visual
system adapts to them on different time scales, as discussed in the next section.

Wright's (1988) suggestion that colors appear the same over a wide range of
ages, despite changes in the retinal stimulus and the visual system, was based
on introspection, but has been supported by a variety of color appearance studies.

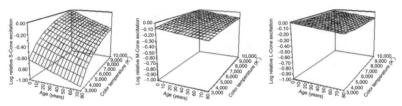

FIG. 9.7 Relative excitation of the S-, M-, and L-cones is plotted as a function of two variables, age (or the changes in the optical density of the lens correlated with age) and phases of daylight illumination (correlated color temperature). From J.S. Werner, N.N. Olsborne, and J. Chade (ed.) (1996). Visual problems of the retina during ageing: Compensation mechanisms and colour constancy across the life span. *Progress in Retinal and Eye Research*, **15(2)**, p. 627. Reproduced with permission of Elsevier.

Consider, for example, the locus in color space of the stimulus that appears achromatic. This stimulus represents the balance point of all color mechanisms and so, ought to be sensitive to changes in that balance in any direction in color space whether those imbalances originate in receptoral or postreceptoral pathways. In Fig. 9.8, the arrow shows predictions which result from an experiment

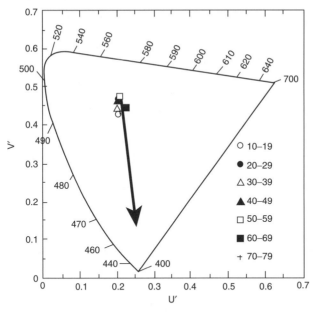

FIG. 9.8 The origin of the arrow represents the location of a theoretical achromatic point for a 10-year-old observer plotted in the CIE 1976 U',V' chromaticity diagram (a standard color space in which equal distances are roughly equal perceptual steps). The arrowhead shows the expected shift in this point (an additive mixture of short- and long-wave monochromatic light) resulting from changes in the ocular media from age 10 to 80. The overlapping data points represent average achromatic loci of different age groups. (Data from Werner and Schefrin 1993. Reproduced with permission of the Optical Society of America.)

in which subjects were asked to adjust a light mixture until it appeared achromatic. The origin of the arrow denotes the location of a theoretical achromatic point for a 10-year-old observer, the ratio of short-wave and long-wave lights adjusted to appear devoid of all hue. Because aging of the lens progressively reduces the amount of short-wave light that reaches the retina, more of it will be needed as the person becomes older. The head of the arrow shows how the stimulus would have to be changed to maintain the same retinal stimulus for the same observer at age 80. In other words, the achromatic point at age 80 would be quite blue at age 10. This is not what happens. As shown by the data points representing the average of about seven observers in each age group, the stimulus that appears achromatic is relatively constant. Stability of the achromatic point would not be possible in a static visual system, but is obtained by the visual system renormalizing itself for changes in the retinal stimulus and any age-related physiological changes.

Lens density increases across the life span, but the rate depends on many factors. Especially important in modulating lens aging is the exposure to ultraviolet-B (UV-B) radiation. Higher exposure to UV-B radiation due to more sunlight exposure or living at latitudes closer to the equator is associated with more rapid lens aging (Young 1991). This implies that the relative reduction in S-cone stimulation associated with normal aging is accelerated in people residing at lower latitudes. The color lexicon is also different in many cultures closer to the equator in that some lack separate terms for "green" and "blue." The combined term is sometimes called "grue." Lindsey and Brown (2002) have hypothesized that this is due to their increased exposure to UV-B radiation leading to premature lens brunescence and a loss in the ability to see "blue" due to a reduction in short-wave light reaching the retina. They demonstrated that when the short-wave energy in stimuli was reduced in a manner that simulated an older lens, individuals were significantly less likely to use the color term "blue." This result suggests that adaptation to age-related changes in the lens is not complete even within the normal range before cataract formation. However, we now know that long-term adaptation to brunescence of the lens may be different from short-term adaptation in simulated aging. To test this hypothesis, Hardy *et al.* (2005) examined color-naming patterns in native English speakers with a wide range of ocular media densities (a logarithmic scale); ten were younger (18–35 y.o.) and ten were older (65–85 y.o.), but all had normal color vision. Lens density was measured for each individual prior to tests in which 40 stimuli (simulated Munsell chips) were presented on a computer screen as $2°$ disks on a gray (illuminant C) background. The same set of stimuli was also presented but with a modification such that the older subjects viewed stimuli that simulated chips filtered through the ocular media of an average younger observer, while younger subjects viewed stimuli that simulated chips filtered through the ocular media of an average older observer. As expected from Lindsey and Brown (2002), younger subjects used "blue" significantly less often in the simulated aging condition. However, for the first set of stimuli, older subjects used "blue" just as often as younger subjects did. In fact, color naming in the younger and older groups was virtually identical for the first set of stimuli. As shown in Fig. 9.9,

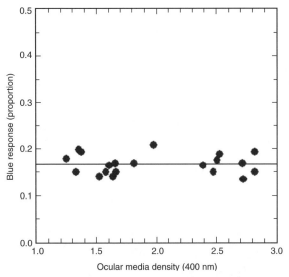

FIG. 9.9 The proportion of blue responses to 40 simulated Munsell chips presented on a computer screen is plotted as a function of ocular media density. The density range shown here spans the lowest values typically found in an adult population to values typically diagnosed as early-stage cataract. From J.L. Hardy, C.M. Frederick, P. Kaye, & J.S. Werner. Colour naming, lens aging, and grue: What the optics of the aging eye can teach us about colour language. *Psychological Science* (in press). Reproduced with permission of Blackwell Publishing Ltd.

there was no correlation between the proportion of "blue" responses and density of the ocular media. Thus, while lens brunescence is likely to be accelerated in individuals with higher UV-B exposure, this does not explain the existence of "grue" in high UV-B areas. Indeed, the visual system adapts to these changes in the retinal stimulus, at least over a large range, to maintain constancy of color appearance across the life span.

9.5.4 Adaptation and Blur

A second example where adaptation to a common environment may factor out large intrinsic differences between observers is in the perception of image blur. Blur is an important dimension of image quality, and like face recognition, is a stimulus that we make intuitive and natural judgments about all of the time. There is no question that blur is also a property to which the visual system is constantly adjusting. However, most studies examining these adjustments have focused on the accommodative changes in the eye's optics. Yet the neural visual system also adjusts to image blur (Fig. 9.10). Webster *et al.* (2002a) measured blur adaptation using methods similar to the ones described earlier to examine face adaptation. Images were blurred or sharpened by "distorting" the ratio of low to high frequency content in the images (or specifically, by varying the slope

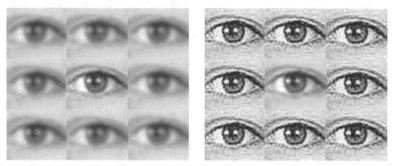

FIG. 9.10 An illustration of visual adjustments to image blur (after Webster *et al.* 2002*a*). The two eyes at the center of each array are identical and physically focused, yet the right eye appears blurrier because it is embedded in a sharpened surround.

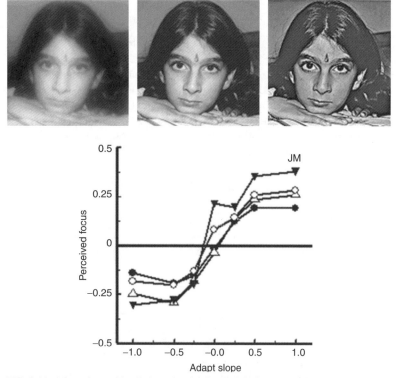

FIG. 9.11 Adaptation to blur. Points plot the slope of the image amplitude spectrum that appeared best-focused after adapting to images with different spectral slopes. Steeper slopes (negative values) reduce the amplitude of higher frequencies more than lower frequencies and thus blur the images. Shallower slopes (positive values) boost the higher frequencies more than lower frequencies and thus sharpen the image. The four curves are for four different images. Prior adaptation to blurry images causes the original image to appear too sharp, and thus shifts the point of subjective focus toward the blurry adapting stimulus. Sharpened adapting images induce the opposite aftereffect.

of the image amplitude spectra). Subjects adapted by viewing these biased images for a few minutes, and then adjusted the frequency spectrum of target images until they appeared properly focused. After viewing a blurry or sharpened image, a physically focused image appeared too sharp or too blurry, respectively (Fig. 9.11). Thus, the point of subjective focus shifted toward the adapting image. This also appears to happen in natural settings as clinicians seldom correct large refractive errors at once. Instead, patients with severe defocus or astigmatism prefer to have their optical aberrations corrected incrementally over time. Once again, these effects are consistent with a renormalization of perception, so that the currently viewed stimulus becomes the new prototype for proper image focus.

Like color, we can appreciate these effects in our own experience by considering the large changes in sensitivity across the visual field. Spatial resolution falls precipitously in the periphery, yet we do not experience the peripheral world as blurred (Galvin et al. 1997). Adaptation could again perceptually discount the optical and physiological variations because the responses at each retinal region will be normalized for the same external stimulus.

With regard to the themes we have been emphasizing, there are two important aspects in the compensations for optical differences between observers. The first is that we have better clues in the case of color or blur about the "priors" that the visual system is adjusting to (at least relative to the priors involved in processes like face recognition). As noted above, a number of studies have shown that the spatial statistics of natural images have a characteristic property (e.g. Burton & Moorhead 1987; Field 1987; Tolhurst et al. 1992; van der Schaaf & van Hateren 1996). Specifically, the amplitude spectrum of images falls inversely with spatial frequency (or as $1/f$), or in other words has a strong low-frequency bias. This scaling property of images is a common (though not universal) property of the physical world, and spatial sensitivity of the visual system is matched to it in many ways. A convincing perceptual demonstration of this can be seen when we look at filtered noise patterns.

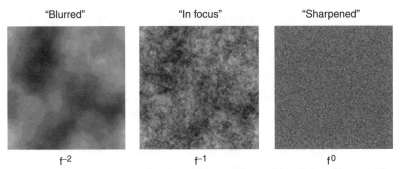

| "Blurred" | "In focus" | "Sharpened" |
| f^{-2} | f^{-1} | f^{0} |

FIG. 9.12 The match between visual sensitivity and the spatial statistics of images. The white noise image at the right has a flat amplitude spectrum but perceptually appears to contain information only at fine scales. The middle image has a $1/f$ spectrum characteristic of natural images and instead appears to have equal energy at all scales.

As Field and Brady (1997) noted, $1/f$ noise has salient structure at all spatial scales, while white noise, for which the amplitude is physically equal at all scales, instead appears dominated by the high-frequency components (Fig. 9.12).

The second important aspect is that for the eye's optics we have a good understanding of how individuals differ, and where we can be confident that these individual differences are very large. Specifically, we know that blur in the retinal image can vary widely because of differences in refractive errors, and that spectral sensitivity can vary widely because of the differences in the density of the lens pigment. Yet, individuals are often unaware of the changes in their optics, and when they become aware these are experienced as a failure of acuity or color discrimination rather than as a subjective experience that the world has changed. Arguably, this is because adaptation adjusts neural responses to maintain the balance of cortical responses to color and space, thus compensating for the imbalances introduced in the retinal image.

9.6 Time Scales and Types of Adaptation

Our review has focused on relatively dynamic perceptual adaptations, but it is important to emphasize that these are only one part of a wide array of different mechanisms that serve to adapt different aspects of visual coding. Table 9.2 lists some commonly recognized forms of visual plasticity ordered roughly in terms of the time scales over which they operate. (Note that this is only a subset from a still broader notion of plasticity that might include such phenomena as attention and priming.) While these involve very different mechanisms they may share a common functional role in shaping visual responses to fit properties of the world. Obviously, the properties that each adjusts to must vary depending on the time over which the information is integrated, and characterizing the relevant scene statistics over these integration times could provide important clues about the operating states that the visual system is trying to achieve. Yet the question of time scales is an aspect of adaptation that still remains very poorly defined. Some of the response changes associated with adaptation are extremely rapid, changing sensitivity with each brief fixation (Muller *et al.* 1999), and often only a few seconds of viewing are sufficient to induce powerful visual aftereffects. However, there is also evidence for much slower perceptual adjustments.

Table 9.2 Mechanisms for perceptual plasticity and the time scales over which they may operate

Adjustment	Time scale
Evolution	Multiple life spans
Development	Months to years
Long term light and pattern adaptation	Minutes to months
Short term light and pattern adaptation	Milliseconds to minutes
Gain control	Milliseconds
Perceptual learning	?

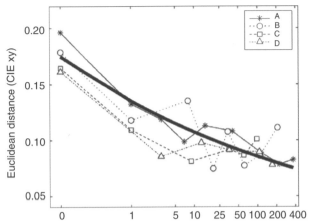

FIG. 9.13 Changes in the white point following cataract surgery. Points plot the change in the achromatic settings (as distance in the standard CIE chromaticity diagram) for 4 observers as a function of post-operative days. Bold curve is the best fitting exponential function. From P.B. Delhunt, M.A. Webster, L. Ma, & J.S. Webster. Long-term renormalization of chromatic mechanisms following cataract surgery, *Visual Neuroscience* (in press). Reprinted with permission of Cambridge University Press.

Delahunt *et al.* (2004) examined the changes in color appearance following lens replacement in cataract patients. As pointed out above, the cataractous lens strongly filters short wavelength light, and thus immediately after the operation many patients report that the world appears bluish. Delahunt *et al.* tracked the changes in this perception by measuring the achromatic point at different times after surgery. Notably, white points in these subjects took weeks to return to values close to their pre-surgery settings (Fig. 9.13), even though changes in chromatic sensitivity were almost immediate. Long-term changes in color appearance have also been reported following exposure to biased light environments (Neitz *et al.* 2002). Neitz *et al.* exposed subjects to colored or filtered illuminants for several hours at a time, and found that this led to biases in perceived hue that could last for several days after observers returned to unbiased lighting. There are also reports of very long-term effects on spatial vision in patients with chronic cataracts. Fine *et al.* (2002) examined blur perception in an individual who had cataracts most of his life. After their removal, edges to him appeared to be too sharp, and this "aftereffect" showed little sign of diminishing even after months, suggesting that it might reflect a calibration fixed during development.

Webster *et al.* (2004) tested for analogous long-term adjustments in the perception of faces. They formed a series of images by morphing between a Japanese and a Caucasian face, and then asked subjects to select the boundary between the two ethnicities (i.e. the point at which the blended morph stopped looking Japanese and started looking Caucasian). These neutral points turned out to be very different for Asian and Caucasian observers, with each choosing a boundary closer to their own ethnic category (Fig. 9.14). Webster *et al.* used this difference to compare whether the settings might shift when individuals entered a new environment. For this, they compared the neutral points for Asian students

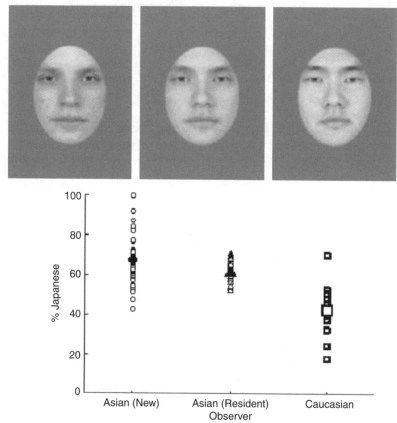

FIG. 9.14 Changes in face perception. Each point shows the ethnicity boundary chosen by an individual subject in morphs between a Caucasian and Japanese face, as illustrated at the top by a Caucasian-Japanese face pair and an intermediate morphed image between them. Caucasian students in the US (points at right) chose a boundary closer to the Caucasian face, as if this face were more neutral to them. Newly arrived Asian students showed the opposite bias (points at left). Asian students who were resident in the US for a year or more show weak but significant shifts toward the Caucasian students' boundaries (middle points).

who had either just arrived in the US or who had been resident for a year or more. The latter group had a mean ethnicity boundary that was weakly but significantly shifted toward the mean settings for the Caucasian students. Moreover, these shifts in the direction of the Caucasian settings were positively correlated with their self-reports of the length of time in the US and with the proportion of time they interacted with Caucasian individuals while in the US. Each of these results is consistent with a gradual renormalization to their new face environment.

In order to probe these long-term adjustments, it is important to measure the neutral points in the absence of the relevant adapting stimulus. That is, to track the patient's achromatic locus the testing is best done while the subject is dark adapted. What if the cataract patient instead first stares at a colored field, or if a Japanese observer stares at a Caucasian face? In these cases there is a very rapid adjustment to the current stimulus. For example, as shown before, viewing one face from a pair quickly and strongly biases the perceptual boundary in the morph between them, and a chromatically biased field quickly appears less saturated. Thus, when these stimuli are presented they rapidly capture the visual system and reset their sensitivity, but their effects also dissipate rapidly when the adapting stimulus is removed. There are other adaptation effects which have a much longer persistence. For example, the McCollough Effect can last for days, and this has suggested that the aftereffects do not passively decay, but instead are actively extinguished by exposure to a different stimulus (Stromeyer 1978). However, the problem remains that for at least some adaptive adjustments there appear to be at least two distinct rates of sensitivity change, and possibly many. One represents an "extrinsic" state of adaptation that is controlled by the stimuli currently in front of us. However, underlying this is a more slowly drifting "intrinsic" state that integrates over a much longer time frame and thus over a much larger ensemble of stimuli. Very little is currently known about the dynamics and function of these long-term adjustments.

It is interesting to speculate that the extrinsic and intrinsic states might reflect adjustments to different aspects of visual coding. For example, most models of visual aftereffects depend on the notion of labeled lines – that the activity in a channel is associated with specific perceptual qualities. The aftereffects arise because adaptation selectively alters the distribution of responses across the channels (Webster 2003). However, it is possible that longer-term adjustments might involve changes in the *interpretation* of these responses, or in other words, in the labels the channels carry, and thus might reflect forms of "learning" that are very distinct from short-term adaptation. For example, one way to adapt to color would be to rescale the cone sensitivities so that the stimulus satisfies the "fixed" rule for white changes (e.g. so that the stimulus that equates responses across the three cone types changes). Another way is to change the rule, for instance by changing how the cone signals might be weighted within post-receptoral channels (Neitz *et al.* 2002).

9.7 Limits to Adaptation

Can we adapt to anything, so that aftereffects tell us only about the general malleability of perception, or does the presence of a specific aftereffect reveal something specific about the underlying skeletal structure of the visual system? Negative results have a tendency to go unreported, but as the number of new aftereffects continues to grow it may become increasingly interesting to identify situations in which the visual system fails to adapt. Such cases are important both for understanding which aspects of the environment are shaping our perception, and for understanding the extent to which adaptation can be used as a tool for characterizing visual mechanisms.

One apparent limit is suggested by the finite selectivity of adaptation after-effects. Exposure to a particular stimulus reduces sensitivity not only to that stimulus but also to similar ones, and thus this restricts the ways in which perception could be altered by adaptation. For example, in chromatic adaptation, the sensitivity changes are largely limited to independent response changes within a small number of chromatic mechanisms ("pi mechanisms"), which have spectral sensitivities that are similar (though not identical) to that of the photoreceptors (Stiles 1959). Similarly, after viewing a vertical grating, thresholds are elevated for a range of orientations around vertical, and these tuning curves have a bandwidth that is at least in rough correspondence with the average orientation selectivity of V1 cells (Blakemore & Campbell 1969). The limited selectivity of adaptation effects suggest that it should be possible to define "adaptation metamers," or physically different stimuli that induce identical aftereffects, even though the two stimuli might be visually distinct. Such metamers should be specific for particular properties of the environment and to the particular visual mechanisms that adjust to those properties. As such, they provide a tool for isolating different stages of adaptation. For example, equivalent states of light adaptation can be induced by a steady field or a flickering field of the same mean luminance, since the property that light adaptation is adjusting to is effectively only the time-averaged mean (Webster & Wilson 2000). However, these two stimuli look very different, and lead to very different adaptation effects in mechanisms that respond to luminance contrast, or to how light levels are varying around the mean. Thus the response changes of contrast adaptation are isolated by holding the state of light adaptation constant. Indeed, in studies of spatial pattern-adaptation, it is a routine procedure to move the stimulus over the retina in order to eliminate afterimages owing to local differences in light adaptation, and this is done in the hope of teasing out response changes that are specific to contrast adaptation. It is possible that similar techniques could be used to form pattern or contrast metamers to isolate still higher stages of adaptation. For example, it is possible in principle to specify different sets of colors that are perceptually distinct but result in equivalent changes of color contrast adaptation (e.g. identical aftereffects to those shown in Fig. 9.5). However, because these are perceptually different, there may be other ways in which the visual system adapts differently to the two distributions (e.g. changing how noticeable or salient different colors are after adapting to either distribution), and thus such pairs might isolate adaptive adjustments that are more closely tied to the phenomenal appearance of the stimuli.

A further possible constraint concerns the nature of contingent adaptation. As we noted before, the McCollough Effect (ME) is usually interpreted as a color afterimage that is contingent on orientation. A number of studies have explored whether analogous aftereffects can be induced by pairing color with more arbitrary spatial patterns. Strong ME's have been reported for a variety of geometrical patterns (e.g. concentric rings versus radial spokes) (Humphrey *et al.* 1985). Conversely, spatial aftereffects can be made contingent on color. An intriguing case was reported by Durgin (1996), in which texture density aftereffects were selective for the color of a surrounding frame. Such results suggest that the visual system can adapt to a potentially wide range of associations, and there are arguments that contingent aftereffects may actually represent a form of learning rather than sensory adaptation (Siegel & Allan 1992). However, it remains controversial whether a ME can be formed with any pattern. For example, reports of ME's for different printed words have been difficult to replicate (Humphrey *et al.* 1994). Yamashita *et al.* (in press) tested for ME's when red and green were paired with a contracted or expanded face. No aftereffects were visible, even though the spatial differences between the two adapting patterns were very obvious. Thus the ME's that can be formed may say something non-arbitrary about visual coding.

A final important but largely unexplored limit to adaptation may be individual differences in the degree or form of the adaptation. We have assumed for the present arguments that adaptation is uniform across different individuals, but to the extent that two observers differ in their adaptability, they should be held in phenomenally different worlds even within the same environment. A particularly intriguing case to consider is adaptation in the aging visual system. As noted above, adaptation may play a crucial role in maintaining perceptual constancy despite the large optical and neural changes that accompany normal aging. Surprisingly, very little is known about how the processes of adaptation – and in particular how cortical processes of pattern-selective adaptation – might themselves age. Deficits in adaptation could have significant and unfavorable consequences for perception, for as we have seen, discrimination is best around the stimulus levels we are adapted to. Failures to adjust this level to the appropriate environment might hinder perceptual distinctions (e.g. leaving the individual with a perpetual "other-race effect"), and could be visually discomforting by inflating stimulus salience (e.g. if the world always appeared noticeably blurred). Studies of adaptation in the aging visual system might also shed light on the underlying mechanisms of the response changes. For example, to the extent that adaptation reflects passive fatigue, then factors that compromise visual function might result in more pronounced adaptation. Alternatively, if the sensitivity changes depend on an active mechanism for calibrating neural sensitivity, then factors that weaken efficiency should reduce adaptation.

9.8 Adaptation and the Contents of Visual Awareness

The preceding sections explore the possibility that the states of adaptation vary in more or less predictable ways, and that these variations constrain whether two different observers have similar or different subjective experiences. In this section, we consider how adaptation might influence the actual content of their experience. Visual aftereffects are among the most striking phenomena in perception, and can quickly alter the appearance of the world in dramatic and startling ways – the sensation of a contracting world after watching an expanding spiral arouses the curiosity of even the most apathetic observer. Yet it has thus far proven surprisingly difficult to demonstrate that these perceptual shifts are accompanied by equally dramatic shifts in visual performance. Most performance measures have focused on the ability to discriminate changes in the stimulus following adaptation (e.g. detecting a difference in contrast or orientation). Better discrimination is predicted if adaptation shifts the response curves of visual mechanisms so that they are steepest and thus most sensitive around the adapting level. This clearly occurs in the case of light adaptation, where it is easy to show that we can discriminate the contrasts in a scene better after we adjust to the average brightness (Whittle 1992); and in individual neurons, which have limited dynamic range for intensity and contrast (Ohzawa *et al.* 1985). But whether similar improvements in pattern discrimination occur following adaptation to patterns remains controversial, and even where these have been reported, they seem weak compared to the sheer magnitude of the perceptual shifts (e.g. Regan & Beverley 1985; Greenlee & Heitger 1988; see also the chapter by Rhodes *et al.*, this volume). This suggests that some of the principal consequences and functions of adaptation may lie in how they influence phenomenology. The startle and awe that visual aftereffects engender may turn out to be the best measure of their utility.

9.8.1 Perceptual Norms

Adaptation produces a number of interrelated effects on phenomenology. One set of effects concerns how we experience the adapting stimulus itself, while a second set concerns our perception of new stimuli, to which we are not adapted. As we have stressed throughout, one of the chief consequences of adaptation is to normalize visual coding relative to the stimuli that we have been exposed to. Through this adjustment, the adapting stimuli define the neutral points of visual coding. But there is also a strong sense in which they become the neutral points of visual experience. The white point has a special status in color perception because it provides the chromatically neutral reference point or norm against which other stimuli can be contrasted. It represents the average or expected color percept. Yet again what appears gray is to a large extent the average of the set of colors that we have encountered.

Calibrating the perception of different observers relative to a common external reference may prove to be an essential precursor to the ability to communicate about our perceptions with others, and could underlie some important aspects of norms and aesthetics within a population that might instead be attributed to a common culture. That is, these collective norms may reflect shared perceptions rather than shared criteria. Judgments of facial attractiveness are an example of this. A number of studies have found that faces that are physically average tend to be rated as more attractive than more distinctive faces (Langlois & Roggman 1990). However, we are all exposed to a different distribution of faces, and thus the average that is important to any individual may be the average of the particular distribution they have seen. Rhodes *et al.* (2003) recently showed that exposure to a set of distorted faces biased the rated attractiveness of a different set of test faces. These shifts are consistent with renormalizing face coding with respect to the adapting faces, so that these faces appeared less distorted and thus, more attractive. This could also conceivably explain the sometimes-striking tendency of spouses and partners to look alike. They may be visually attracted to individuals that match the facial configurations to which they are adapted, for example because of exposure to a particular community or their relatives or themselves. Perceptual adjustments could also provide a simple sensory explanation of how judgments of attractiveness might change when an individual is exposed to a new visual environment, as the following description of the anthropologist Malinowski's experiences suggests:

"Malinowski (1929) makes the intriguing observation that after he had lived in the Trobriand Islands for some time his judgments of Trobriand beauty began to agree with the Trobrianders' judgments." (Symons 1979, p. 196).

Within the present framework, it was not so much Malinowski's perception of beauty that changed. Rather, what changed was the physical stimulus that induced that perception, through the changed state of adaptation to his new environment.

It is important to note that perceptual norms may be important not only for judging the average stimulus, but also for categorizing stimuli. For example, in the perception of a facial quality like gender, images corresponding to the mean may be rare. Yet adaptation to the population mean may nevertheless be important for defining the category boundary. It is possible that in contexts where the distribution of males and females is highly skewed (e.g. in some institutionalized settings), judgments of gender would become perceptually skewed because of adaptation-induced shifts in the category boundaries.

9.8.2 Perceptual Gamuts

A second consequence of renormalization may be to expand perceptual space in order to match it to the range of levels in the stimulus. This is similar to the notion of sphering in visual coding, so that equal perceptual weight is given to the variance along different stimulus dimensions. Distorting the range of perceptual responses may not affect the ability to discriminate between different stimulus levels, for simply boosting the gain of a mechanism will not improve sensitivity if it increases both signal and noise. Thus, the impact of these adjustments on perception may not be readily captured in measures of visual sensitivity. An interesting example is provided by the perceptual experience of anomalous trichromats. The difference in spectral sensitivity between their L and M cone pigments is much smaller than in color normals, and thus their color discrimination is much poorer. Yet they may not "experience" the world as desaturated because this signal is amplified in postreceptoral channels (MacLeod 2003). In the same way, we noted previously that in normal observers the signals from S cones are amplified, and this perceptually spheres color space even though it does not undo sensitivity limits imposed by the paucity of S cones.

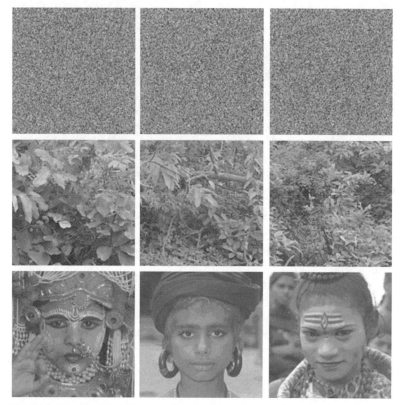

FIG. 9.15 Perceptual distortions of stimulus space. Top row: three examples of white noise. Though these images are statistically very different they appear very similar and are difficult to discriminate. Middle row: three examples of foliage. Natural images share a great deal of common statistical structure, but their differences are much more readily perceived. Bottom row: three examples of faces (devotees at the Nashik Kumbh Mela). Faces are highly similar physically, but differences between them are more salient than most other image classes.

Figure 9.15 is a further possible illustration of these perceptual distortions. The top row shows three examples of white noise, in which the value of each pixel is chosen at random. These images are physically quite different. That is, their RMS difference (i.e., their Euclidean distance) is quite large. However, perceptually they appear quite close. In contrast, the three middle images of outdoor scenes are conspicuously different, yet their statistics are highly constrained. In fact, the set of all natural images fills only a tiny fraction of the state space of all possible images, yet the visual system distorts this space by expanding the response to natural images (and by perceptually compressing the responses to images that fall outside the natural gamut) (Field 1994). In the same way, we can find distortions across different classes of natural images. For example, the bottom row shows three examples of faces. The set of possible faces again occupies only a miniscule volume within the space of natural images, yet the differences between faces are often much more conspicuous and much easier to remember than for other classes of objects. These perceptual differences may reflect both evolutionary and short-term adaptations that amplify visual responses to the characteristic properties of the visual environment.

The principle of perceptual expansion can be applied at a still finer level by comparing visual responses within the category of face images. An example is the "other race" effect, or the tendency to easily distinguish among the kinds of faces we are used to seeing while finding it difficult to distinguish among individuals from other groups (Furl *et al.* 2002). If adaptation matches face coding to the specific gamut of faces we encounter, then this will serve to highlight the differences between faces around the average. This predicts that for physically equivalent stimulus differences, judgments of phenomenal similarity would increase for images that are far removed from the average face, a behavior consistent with the other-race effect.

What are the advantages of biasing phenomenal differences if they do not lead to comparable improvements in visual discrimination? The answer may be that they do help discriminations, but not of the type that are usually measured. The classic work of Miller (Miller 1956) illustrated that perceptual judgments are limited to a finite number of categories. Adjusting the response gamut might aid perception by making the full range of categories available.

9.8.3 Perceptual Salience

A second way in which adaptation could aid perception is by highlighting how a stimulus differs from the stimuli we are adapted to. Barlow (1990) proposed that adaptation reflects a form of learning about the associations underlying the structure of the visual world. This is important for coding efficiency because adjusting to these associations allows us to encode the world within mechanisms whose signals vary independently. But another effect of this is to draw attention to new associations, or "suspicious coincidences" in the world. That is, according to Barlow, adaptation is a process that brings new properties of the environment to our notice. Note that these novel properties are the very stimuli we experience in visual aftereffects. In a red world a flat spectrum stands out as green, and in a world of expanded faces a neutral face will appear conspicuously contracted. Note also that when we experience an adaptation effect, it is the aftereffect that strikes us much more than any perceptual changes in the adapting stimulus itself. For example, when we stare at a waterfall we are largely unaware of the changes in motion sensitivity, but these changes are overwhelming when we switch our gaze to the novel properties of the surrounding static scene. Yet we are always adapted, and thus we are always experiencing an adaptation effect. Thus, much of the content that reaches our conscious awareness may be a visual aftereffect.

Another way to conceptualize these perceptual consequences is from the perspective of predictive coding (Srinivasan *et al.* 1982; Mumford 1994).

The current state of adaptation is in a sense a prediction about the current state of the world. This prediction may be represented only implicitly in our conscious awareness, for it forms a template that filters out the expected stimulus structure and thus passes only the errors. These errors represent the novel properties of the image, and these become accessible only by first discounting the properties that are old. One implication of this is that as we adapt to a new environment we should become better at detecting novel features within it. Consistent with this, Webster *et al.* (1998) found in a visual search task that observers were faster at finding a colored target if they were first adapted to the colored backgrounds on which they had to search. Similarly, this would predict that in "change blindness" tasks, which measure the failures to detect alterations in scenes, (Rensink *et al.* 1997) the changes observers do or do not notice should depend in part on whether or not they are adapted to properties of the scenes.

The role of adaptation in modulating visual salience suggests that there is a close relation between adaptation and attention, and there are many examples of interactions between them (Boynton 2004). Other chapters in this book discuss the role of attention in modulating the magnitude of perceptual adaptation. Here we note that, conversely, the state of adaptation may strongly modulate what aspects of the world we attend to.

With these thoughts in mind, we can now return to Freud's portraits. The very act of exploring the face as he created it may have strongly adapted him to it, so that he perceived it – visually – in a way that perhaps no one else can. While at first glance others are struck by salient distortions and stylistic similarities, in his eye the same stimulus properties might be dulled by a process that calibrates normal only according to the history of stimulation. This is in fact a common anecdotal impression. Faces that appear striking to us when we first see them typically lose their distinctiveness over time, and this can be parsimoniously accounted for by actual shifts in perception. Our analysis of Freud's paintings is not intended as an aesthetic judgment about the work, for we instead suggest that differences in aesthetics may have roots in perceptual differences. Nor do we mean to preclude the possibility that the artist chose to emphasize or perhaps exaggerate certain traits that are perceptually obvious to him. We used the work merely as an example to say that, if we could look at the painting through his eyes, it would not look the same.

9.9 Measuring Conscious Experience

The central problem in the phenomenology of perception is that it is a private experience, and thus we have access only to our own. In this chapter, we have argued that this private experience is shaped in important ways by processes of adaptation, and have assumed that these physiological processes are similar in important ways within different individuals (in that the common effect of adaptation is to normalize neural activity). We have also argued that we are always adapted to specific properties of our environment, and that it is these properties that ultimately control the states of adaptation. Thus, some aspects of our inner private experience depend on outer public variables. To measure what world an observer would experience as physically focused (i.e. not blurred), we may not need to measure the observer. We can instead measure the spatial statistics of their environment. To ask whether you and I have different experiences, we can measure whether our environments differ. There is a rapidly growing interest in characterizing natural scene statistics because they hold the promise of revealing much about visual coding. Ultimately, these measurements may also reveal much about visual experience.

9.10 Epilogue

At the time of this writing, news was focused on another royal portrait, this time of Prince Phillip. Commissioned by the Royal Society for the Encouragement of the Arts, Manufactures and Commerce, of which Phillip is President, the portrait was painted by the artist Stuart Pearson Wright, and showed a bare-chested Phillip with cress growing out of his finger (a strand for each child) and a bluebottle fly resting on his shoulder (to signify mortality). Phillip refused further sittings after seeing the work in progress. The painting was rejected by the RSA, and Wright instead provided a second image showing the Prince only from the neck up, but the controversy recently resurfaced when the original was put on the market. We note it here because it again bears on the theme of whether different individuals see the world in similar ways. Asked by Wright if he had caught his likeness, the Prince replied "I bloody well hope not!"

Acknowledgments

Supported by the National Eye Institute (EY10834), the National Institute on Aging (AG04058), and a Jules and Doris Stein RPB Professorship to JSW. Parts of this chapter are based on Webster (2002).

References

Andrews, D.P. (1964). Error-correcting perceptual mechanisms. *Quarterly Journal of Experimental Psychology, 16*, 104–15.

Anstis, S.M. (1996). Was El Greco astigmatic? *Investigative Ophthalmology and Visual Science, 37*, S697.

Atick, J.J. (1992). Could information theory provide an ecological theory of sensory processing? *Network, 3*, 213–51.

Barlow, H.B. (1990). A theory about the functional role and synaptic mechanism of visual aftereffects. In C. Blakemore (ed.), *Vision: Coding and Efficiency* (pp. 363–75). Cambridge, UK: Cambridge University Press.

Barlow, H.B., & Földiák, P. (1989). Adaptation and decorrelation in the cortex. In R. Durbin, C. Miall, & G.J. Mitchison (ed.), *The Computing Neuron* (pp. 54–72). Wokingham: Addison-Wesley.

Barlow, H.B., & Levick, W.R. (1976). Threshold setting by the surround of cat retinal ganglion cells. *Journal of Physiology, London B, 212,* 1–34.

Blakemore, C., & Campbell, F.W. (1969). On the existence of neurones in the human visual system selectively sensitive to the orientation and size of retinal images. *Journal of Physiology, 203,* 237–60.

Boynton, G.M. (2004). Adaptation and attentional selection. *Nature Neuroscience, 7,* 8–10.

Brainard, D.H., & Wandell, B.A. (1992). Asymmetric color matching: how color appearance depends on the illuminant. *Journal of the Optical Society of America A, 9,* 1433–48.

Brown, R.O., & MacLeod, D.I.A. (1997). Color appearance depends on the variance of surround colors. *Current Biology, 7,* 844–9.

Buchsbaum, G., & Gottschalk, A. (1983). Trichromacy, opponent colours and optimum colour information transmission in the retina. *Proceedings of the Royal Society London B, 220,* 89–113.

Burton, G.J., & Moorhead, I.R. (1987). Color and spatial structure in natural scenes. *Applied Optics, 26,* 157–70.

Carandini, M., Barlow, H.B., O'Keefe, L.P., Poirson, A.B., & Movshon, J.A. (1997). Adaptation to contingencies in macaque primary visual cortex. *Philosophical Transactions of the Royal Society of London B: Biological Sciences, 52,* 1149–54.

Chaparro, A., Stromeyer, C.F.I., Huang, E.P., Kronauer, R.E., & Eskew, R.T.J. (1993). Colour is what the eye sees best. *Nature, 361,* 348–50.

De Valois, R.L. (2003). Neural coding of color. In L.M. Chalupa, & J.S. Werner (ed.), *The Visual Neurosciences.* (Vol. 2., pp. 1003–16). Cambridge, MA: MIT Press.

De Valois, R.L., Cottaris, N.P., Elfar, S.D., Mahon, L.D., & Wilson, J.A. (2000). Some transformations of color information from lateral geniculate nucleus to striate cortex. *Proceedings of the National Academy of Sciences, 97,* 4997–5002.

Delahunt, P.B., Webster, M.A., Ma, L., & Werner, J.S. (2004). Long-term renormalization of chromatic mechanisms following cataract surgery. *Visual Neuroscience, 21,* 301–7.

Dragoi, V., Sharma, J., Miller, E.K., & Sur, M. (2002). Dynamics of neuronal sensitivity in visual cortex and local feature discrimination. *Nature Neuroscience, 5,* 883–91.

Durgin, F.H. (1996). Visual aftereffect of texture density contingent on color of frame. *Perception and Psychophysics, 58,* 207–23.

Field, D.J., & Brady, N. (1997). Visual sensitivity, blur, and the sources of variability in the amplitude spectra of natural images. *Vision Research, 37,* 3367–83.

Field, D.J. (1987). Relations between the statistics of natural images and the response properties of cortical cells. *Journal of the Optical Society of America A, 4,* 2379–94.

Field, D.J. (1994). What is the goal of sensory coding? *Neural Computation, 6,* 559–601.

Fine, I., Smallman, H.S., Doyle, P., & MacLeod, D.I.A. (2002). Visual function before and after removal of bilateral congenital cataracts in adulthood. *Vision Research, 42,* 191–210.

Furl, N., Phillips, P.J., & O'Toole, A.J. (2002). Face recognition algorithms and the other-race effect: computational mechanisms for a developmental contact hypothesis. *Cognitive Science, 26,* 797–815.

Galvin, S.J., O'Shea, R.P., Squire, A.M., & Govan, D.G. (1997). Sharpness overconstancy in peripheral vision. *Vision Research, 37,* 2035–9.

Golz, J., & MacLeod, D.I.A. (2002). Influence of scene statistics on colour constancy. *Nature, 415,* 637–40.

Greenlee, M.W., & Heitger, F. (1988). The functional role of contrast adaptation. *Vision Research, 28,* 791–7.

Hardin, C.L. (1997). Reinverting the spectrum. In A. Byrne & D. Hibert (ed.), *Readings on Color, Volume 1: The Philosophy of Color* (pp. 289–301). Cambridge, MA: MIT Press.

Hardy, J.L., Frederick, C.M., Kay, P., & Werner, J.S. (2005). Color naming, lens aging, and grue: What the optics of the aging eye can teach us about color language. *Psychological Science, 16,* 321–7.

Hecht, S. (1923). Sensory adaptation and the stationary state. *Journal of General Physiology, 5,* 555–79.

Helson, H. (1964). *Adaptation-Level Theory.* New York: Harper and Row.

Humphrey, G.K., Dodwell, P.C., & Emerson, V.F. (1985). The roles of pattern orthogonality and color contrast in the generation of pattern-contingent color aftereffects. *Perception and Psychophysics, 38,* 343–53.

Humphrey, G.K., Skowbo, D., Symons, L.A., Herbert, A.M., & Grant, C.L. (1994). Text-contingent color aftereffects: a reexamination. *Perception and Psychophysics, 56,* 405–13.

Hurvich, L.M., & Jameson, D. (1974). Opponent processes as a model of neural organization. *American Psychologist, 29,* 88–102.

Langlois, J.H., & Roggman, L.A. (1990). Attractive faces are only average. *Psychological Science, 1,* 115–21.

Laughlin, S.B. (1987). Form and function in retinal processing. *Trends in Neuroscience, 10,* 478–83.

Lennie, P. (1999). Color coding in the cortex. In K. Gegenfurtner & L.T. Sharpe (ed.), *Color Vision: From Genes to Perception* (pp. 235–47). Cambridge, UK: Cambridge University Press.

Lennie, P., & D'Zmura, M. (1988). Mechanisms of color vision. *CRC Critical Reviews of Neurobiology, 3,* 333–400.

Lindsey, D.T., & Brown, A.M. (2002). Color naming and the phototoxic effects of sunlight on the eye. *Psychological Science, 13,* 506–12.

Locke, J. (1689, 1975). *An Essay Concerning Human Understanding.* Oxford: Clarendon Press.

MacLeod, D.I.A. (2003). Colour discrimination, colour constancy, and natural scene statistics. In J.D. Mollon, J. Polorny, & K. Knoblanch (ed.), *Normal and Defective Colour Vision.* Oxford: Oxford University Press.

MacLeod, D.I.A., & von der Twer, T. (2003). The pleistochrome: optimal opponent codes for natural colors. In R. Mausfeld & D. Heyer (ed.), *Colour Perception: Mind and the Physical World* (pp. 155–84). Oxford: Oxford University Press.

McCollough, C. (1965). Color adaptation of edge-detectors in the human visual system. *Science, 149,* 1115–16.

Miller, G.A. (1956). The magic number seven, plus or minus two: some limits on our capacity for processing information. *Psychological Review, 63,* 81–97.

Mizokami, Y., Webster, M.A., & Webster, S.M. (2003). Seasonal variations in the color statistics of natural images. *Journal of Vision, 3,* 444.

Movshon, J.A., & Lennie, P. (1979). Pattern-selective adaptation in visual cortical neurones. *Nature, 278,* 850–2.

Muller, J.R., Metha, A.B., Krauskopf, J., & Lennie, P. (1999). Rapid adaptation in visual cortex to the structure of images. *Science, 285*, 1405–8.

Mumford, D. (1994). Neuronal architectures for pattern theoretic problems. In C. Koch & J.L. Davis (ed.), *Large Scale Neuronal Theories of the Brain* (pp. 125–52). Cambridge, MA: MIT Press.

Neitz, J., Carroll, J., Yamauchi, Y., Neitz, M., & Williams, D.R. (2002). Color perception is mediated by a plastic neural mechanism that is adjustable in adults. *Neuron, 35*, 783–92.

Ohzawa, I., Sclar, G., & Freeman, R.D. (1985). Contrast gain control in the cat's visual system. *Journal of Neurophysiology, 54*, 651–67.

Olshausen, B.A., & Field, D.J. (1996). Emergence of simple-cell receptive field properties by learning a sparse code for natural images. *Nature, 381*, 607–9.

Palmer, S.E. (1999). Color, consciousness, and the isomorphism constraint. *Behavioral and Brain Sciences, 22*, 923–89.

Párraga, C.A., Brelstaff, G., Troscianko, T., & Moorehead, I.R. (1998). Color and luminance information in natural scenes. *Journal of the Optical Society of America A, 15*, 563–9.

Regan, D., & Beverley, K. (1985). Postadaptation orientation discrimination. *Journal of the Optical Society of America A, 2*, 147–55.

Rensink, R.A., O'Regan, J.K., & Clark, J.J. (1997). To see or not to see: the need for attention to perceive changes in scenes. *Psychological Science, 8*, 368–73.

Rhodes, G., Jeffery, L., Watson, T.L., Clifford, C.W.G., & Nakayama, K. (2003). Fitting the mind to the world: face adaptation and attractiveness aftereffects. *Psychological Science, 14*, 558–66.

Ruderman, D.L., Cronin, T.W., & Chiao, C-C. (1998). Statistics of cone responses to natural images: implications for visual coding. *Journal of the Optical Society of America A, 15*, 2036–45.

Siegel, S., & Allan, L.G. (1992). Pairings in learning and perception: Pavlovian conditioning and contingent aftereffects. In D. Medin (ed.), *The Psychology of Learning and Motivation* (Vol. 28, pp. 127–60). New York: Academic Press.

Simoncelli, E.P., & Olshausen, B.A. (2001). Natural image statistics and neural representation. *Annual Review of Neuroscience, 24*, 1193–216.

Srinivasan, M.V., Laughlin, S.B., & Dubs, A. (1982). Predictive coding: a fresh view of inhibition in the retina. *Proceedings of the Royal Society of London B, 216*, 427–59.

Stiles, W.S. (1959). Color vision: the approach through increment-threshold sensitivity. *Proceedings of the National Academy of Sciences, 45*, 100–14.

Stromeyer, C.F.I. (1978). Form-color aftereffects in human vision. In R. Held, H.W. Leibowitz, & H.L. Teuber (ed.), *Handbook of Sensory Physiology*, (Vol. VIII, pp. 97–142). New York: Springer-Verlag.

Symons, D. (1979). *The Evolution of Human Sexuality*. New York : Oxford University Press.

Tolhurst, D.J., Tadmor, Y., & Chao, T. (1992). Amplitude spectra of natural images. *Ophthalmology Physiological Optics, 12*, 229–32.

van der Schaaf, A., & van Hateren, J.H. (1996). Modelling the power spectra of natural images: statistics and information. *Vision Research, 36*, 2759–70.

von Kries, J. (1970). Chromatic adaptation, in Festschrift der Albrecht-Ludwigs-Universitat (Fribourg, 1902). Trans. D. L. MacAdam (ed.), *Sources of Color Science* (pp. 109–19). Cambridge: MIT Press.

Wainwright, M.J. (1999). Visual adaptation as optimal information transmission. *Vision Research, 39*, 3960–74.

Walraven, J., Enroth-Cugell, C., Hood, D.C., MacLeod, D.I.A., & Schnapf, J.L. (1990). The control of visual sensitivity: receptoral and postreceptoral processes. In L. Spillmann & J.S. Werner (ed.), *Visual Perception The Neurophysiological Foundations* (pp. 53–101). San Diego, CA: Academic Press.

Webster, M.A. (2002). Adaptation, high-level vision, and the phenomenology of perception. In B.E. Rogowitz, & T. Pappas (ed.), *Human Vision and Electronic Imaging VII* SPIE Proceedings, *4662*. (pp. 1–11).

Webster, M.A. (2003). Pattern-selective adaptation in color and form perception. In L.M. Chalupa, & J.S. Werner (ed.), *The Visual Neurosciences*, (Vol. 2, pp. 936–47). Cambridge, MA: MIT Press.

Webster, M.A., Georgeson, M.A., & Webster, S.M. (2002a). Neural adjustments to image blur. *Nature Neuroscience, 5*, 839–40.

Webster, M.A., Kaping, D., Mizokami, Y., & Duhamel, P. (2004). Adaptation to natural facial categories. *Nature, 428, 558–61*.

Webster, M.A., Malkoc, G., Bilson, A.C., & Webster, S.M. (2002b). Color contrast and contextual influences on color appearance. *Journal of Vision, 2*, 505–19.

Webster, M.A., & Mollon, J.D. (1994). The influence of contrast adaptation on color appearance. *Vision Research, 34*, 1993–2020.

Webster, M.A., & Mollon, J.D. (1997). Adaptation and the color statistics of natural images. *Vision Research, 37*, 3283–98.

Webster, M.A., Raker, V.E., & Malkoc, G. (1998). Visual search and natural color distributions. In B.E. Rogowitz, & T. Pappas (ed.), *Human Vision and Electronic Imaging III* SPIE Proceedings, *3299* (pp. 498–509).

Webster, M.A., Webster, S.M., Bharadwaj, S., Verma, R., Jaikumar, J., Madan, G., *et al.* (2002c). Variations in normal color vision III. Unique hues in Indian and United States observers. *Journal of the Optical Society of America A, 19*, 1951–62.

Webster, M.A., & Wilson, J.A. (2000). Interactions between chromatic adaptation and contrast adaptation in color appearance. *Vision Research, 40*, 3801–16.

Werner, J.S. (1998). Aging through the eyes of Monet. In W.G.K. Backhaus, R. Kliegl, & J.S. Werner (ed.), *Color Vision: Perspectives from Different Disciplines* (pp. 3–41). Berlin: de Gruyter.

Werner, J.S., & Schefrin, B.E. (1993). Loci of achromatic points throughout the life span. *Journal of the Optical Society of America A, 10*, 1509–16.

Whittle, P. (1992). Brightness, discriminability, and the 'Crispening Effect'. *Vision Research, 32*, 1493–1507.

Wright, W.D. (1928–29). A re-determination of the trichromatic coefficients of the spectral colors. *Transactions of the Optical Society, London, 30*, 141–64.

Wright, W.D. (1988). Talking about color. *Color Research and Application, 13*, 138–9.

Yamashita, J.A., Hardy, J.L., De Valois, K.K., & Webster, M.A. Stimulus selectivity of figural aftereffects for faces. *Journal of Experimental Psychology: Human Perception and Performance*, in press.

Young, R.W. (1991). *Age-related Cataract*. New York: Oxford University Press.

Section III

Attention and awareness

10

Adaptation as a Tool for Probing the Neural Correlates of Visual Awareness: Progress and Precautions

RANDOLPH BLAKE AND SHENG HE

10.1 Adaptation and the Study of the Neural
Correlates of Consciousness

Adaptation within sensory systems broadens the dynamic range of those systems, making it possible for organisms to function efficiently over a wide variety of environmental conditions. To maximize efficiency sensory adaptation is characteristically 'selective' for different stimulus attributes, as it should be in order to promote adaptive changes in neural representations of environmental stimuli. Because of this stimulus selectivity, sensory adaptation has been characterized as the "psychophysicist's microelectrode" (Frisby 1980), the idea being that aftereffects of adaptation isolate neural mechanisms selectively responsive to given stimulus features. Thus, for example, staring for a minute or so at contours moving upward subsequently causes stationary contours to appear to drift downward for a few seconds, the well-known motion aftereffect (MAE). The MAE, like other kinds of adaptation aftereffects, presumably reflects a temporary reduction in the sensitivity of neural mechanisms responsive to the adaptation stimulus (Mather 1980). By studying stimulus conditions that generate aftereffects and the conditions that modulate the magnitude of those aftereffects, one can discover properties of those neural mechanisms responsible for coding aspects of objects and events.

A number of chapters in this volume outline the rationale underlying the study of adaptation and visual aftereffects, amply document the various forms that these aftereffects can take, discuss the adaptive/computational benefits subserved by adaptation, and offer reasoned accounts of the neural bases of various forms of adaptation. The present chapter has little additional to offer in consideration of these issues. Instead, the aim of this chapter is to consider several simple but potentially revealing questions about adaptation aftereffects, and interrelated questions that attempt to get at the neural bases of perceptual awareness:

- What happens when a visual adapting stimulus falls outside of conscious awareness for a substantial portion of the adaptation period, thereby dissociating phenomenal perception from physical stimulation?

- What transpires within the visual nervous system when a given stimulus takes on different appearances owing to visual adaptation?

Before surveying evidence bearing on these questions, we should justify why, in the first place, these questions are worth asking and, then, consider how one can go about trying to answer them.

10.2 Why Study Adaptation Outside of Awareness?

So, let's start with the "why" question – what's the purpose of studying the role of awareness in visual adaptation? The answer grows out of neuroscience's zealous effort to learn as much as possible about the neural concomitants of conscious awareness, dubbed the "NCC" by Crick and Koch (1995). What goes on inside our brains when we consciously perceive an object or an event in our environment? Pursuing an answer to this question has captured the minds and imaginations of some of the leading figures in neuroscience (Sperry 1970; Changeux 1985; Edelman 1992; Gazzaniga 1992; Crick 1994; Logothetis 1998; Ramachandran & Blakeslee 1998; Damasio 1999), and among these individuals it is generally agreed upon that efforts to study the problem require paradigmatic phenomena for manipulating consciousness and assessing the consequences of that manipulation.

Among the strategies available for pursuing the NCC are those utilizing visual adaptation. After all, the visual consequences of adaptation are reasonably well-established and lawfully related to the duration of adaptation. And in at least some instances, plausible neural sites of adaptation have been identified. This knowledge, in turn, makes it feasible to infer something about the neural concomitants of awareness, by studying the extent to which certain types of visual adaptation can proceed outside of awareness – this represents a major theme of much of the work described in this chapter.

In a related vein, there is a category of fascinating visual phenomena – collectively known as bistable perception – wherein visual awareness fluctuates over time even though the evoking stimulus remains invariant (Leopold & Logothetis 1999). Well-known examples include the Necker cube, the vase/face ambiguous figure and binocular rivalry. It is commonly believed that fluctuations in perception when viewing bistable or rival figures result from neural adaptation, such that the neural activity instantiating the currently dominant perceptual inter-pretation weakens over time and eventually gives way to an alternative pattern of activity favoring another perceptual interpretation (Kohler 1940; Orbach *et al.* 1963; Kawamoto & Anderson 1985; Mueller 1990; Nawrot & Blake 1991; Wilson 1999). While other factors may also be involved in bistable perception (Leopold *et al.* 2002), it is reasonable to assume that neural adaptation plays a critical role in this class of phenomena. For this reason, the study of adaptation may well bear on our understanding of visual awareness as revealed in bistable perception, par-ticularly since it is possible to measure cortical activity accompanying fluctuations in bistable perception in humans (e.g. Tong *et al.* 1998; Andrews *et al.* 2002) and in alert, behaving animals (Andersen & Bradley 1998; Dodd *et al.* 2001).

10.3 How Can We Study Adaptation Outside of Awareness?

This brings us to the second question: what strategies are available for studying the relation between conscious awareness and visual adaptation? Here, students of visual perception have at their disposal several reliable, relatively easy means by which to erase an ordinarily visible stimulus from conscious awareness. Probably the most widely used of these techniques is visual masking, wherein one briefly presented visual stimulus, the "target," is rendered invisible by the brief pres-entation of another stimulus, the "masker" (Breitmeyer 1984). Visual masking has been widely used in cognitive studies of object and word recognition, some-times yielding evidence for the enduring efficacy of a visual target masked to invisibility (e.g. Marcel 1983). Similar in format to visual masking is the atten-tional blink (Raymond *et al.* 1992) wherein the appearance of one briefly pre-sented "target" makes it more difficult to detect a second "target" presented in close temporal proximity. And related to the attentional blink is inattentional blindness (Mack 2003) wherein a highly visible stimulus goes completely unnoticed when attention is diverted to another object or location within the visual field. All three of these phenomena – masking, attentional blink, and inat-tentional blindness – can be quite effective at dissociating physical stimulation from visual awareness. All three, however, usually entail brief presentations of multiple visual events occurring closely in time, stimulus conditions unfavorable to the study of visual adaptation, which requires more prolonged durations of stimulus presentation. To satisfy these conditions, we must turn to other techniques for dissociating stimulation and perception, techniques that are described in the next several sections. By way of preview, we are going to consider two general strategies for dissociating physical stimulation and perceptual experience (strategies summarized schematically in Fig. 10.1). In one case, the *same* pattern of visual stimulation (dissimilar forms viewed dichoptically by the two eyes)

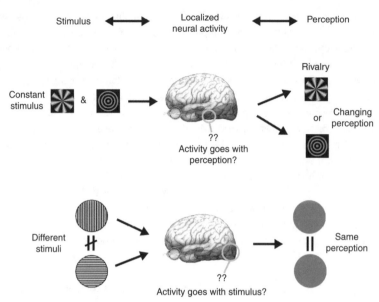

FIG. 10.1 Schematic depictions of two approaches that dissociate physical stimulation and perception. Top panel shows the scenario of binocular rivalry in which unchanging stimulation leads to alternating perception. Neurons whose activity follows changes in perception are potential candidates for NCC. Bottom panel shows a case where two different stimuli (horizontal and vertical gratings) are not perceptually resolved and thus are perceived to be identical. Logically, neurons that respond differently to these two stimuli are not directly supporting the viewer's visual experience.

produces *different* visual perceptions (binocular rivalry, in this example); in the other case, *different* visual stimuli produce the *same*, unchanging perceptual state.

10.4 Adaptation and Binocular Rivalry

To create relatively prolonged dissociation of physical stimulation and phenomenal awareness, binocular rivalry does an especially effective job (Blake 1997). During rivalry, the two eyes view dissimilar monocular stimuli that resist fusion and, instead, undergo alternating periods of perceptual dominance and suppression. During suppression periods a normally visible, potentially salient stimulus is erased from conscious awareness for several seconds at a time (Fig. 10.2(A)). Thus, we may use rivalry to uncouple physical stimulation and phenomenal awareness. The strategy applied in the case of visual adaptation is seemingly simple. To quote from Blake and Fox (1974), where this strategy was first introduced:

"Imagine that an aftereffect-inducing stimulus impinges on an eye for a certain duration, but at the same time is phenomenally suppressed for a substantial portion

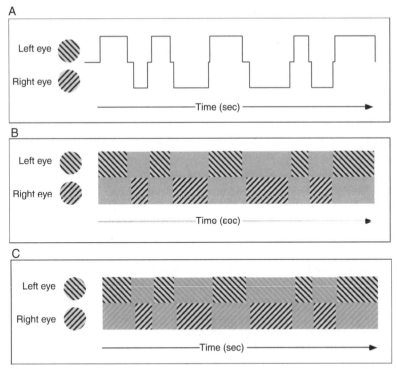

FIG. 10.2 Alternative conceptualizations of the "effective" strength of two rival patterns as they undergo dominance and suppression. (A) Schematic showing a typical sequence of alternations in dominance between orthogonally oriented gratings viewed dichoptically. An observer presses one of two keys to indicate which pattern is currently dominant exclusively and presses neither key when dominance is mixed. The trace illustrates (i) the initial brief period of mixed dominance at the onset of rivalry, (ii) the irregularity in duration among successive dominance periods, and (iii) the very brief periods at transition points during which mixed dominance may be experienced. For the purposes of this chapter, the important point to note is the dissociation between physical stimulation (which is constant for each pattern) and phenomenal visibility (which is intermittent for each pattern). It is simple to adjust the contrast and spatial configuration of rival targets to ensure that each is visible only about 50% of the total viewing period. (B) To mimic the appearance and disappearance of a pair of rival targets, one can physically turn them on and off in a reciprocal fashion whose time-course matches that indicated by tracking results from rivalry episodes such as the one shown in (A). This "mimic" condition is valid as a rivalry analog only to the extent that rivalry suppression intermittently abolishes neural activity associated with a given rival target. (C) Alternatively, rivalry suppression may be characterized as involving an attenuation in effective contrast, in which mimicking rivalry is achieved by intermittently reducing the contrast of each pattern. Most studies of rivalry's effect on visual adaptation have been based on the assumption embodied in (B), but recent evidence (Sobel *et al.* 2004) implies that the assumption embodied in (C) is a more appropriate characterization for at least some aftereffects.

of that time because of binocular rivalry. If the inducing stimulus remains effective while suppressed, the magnitude of the aftereffect will correspond to the duration of physical stimulation. But if the stimulus is rendered ineffective by suppression the aftereffect will be weakened, and its magnitude will correspond to the duration of phenomenal viewing." (p. 488)

Thus Blake and Fox envisioned one of two possible outcomes from experiments deploying this strategy: one outcome – a weakened aftereffect – would imply that suppression transpires prior to the site of adaptation, and the other outcome – a full strength aftereffect – would imply that adaptation transpires prior to suppression. In their study using two, related spatial frequency adaptation aftereffects, Blake and Fox found no evidence for an attenuating influence of suppression on adaptation, leading them to conclude that spatial frequency information arrives full strength at the locus of adaptation even during suppression.

Over the last several decades, almost a dozen other studies have deployed the same strategy to assess suppression's effect on a host of other visual aftereffects. Results from those studies reveal that some forms of visual adaptation survive suppression unscathed while others are diminished in strength by suppression – a summary of those studies appears in Table 10.1. The emerging pattern of results seems to point to a tidy conclusion: visual aftereffects arising within "early" stages of processing, most likely V1, are immune to rivalry suppression whereas more complex aftereffects arising from neural adaptation within "higher" extrastriate stages of processing are vulnerable to the effects of suppression (Blake 1995; Logothetis 1998). It would seem, therefore, that the

Table 10.1 Published studies measuring effect of binocular rivalry suppression on the magnitude of various visual adaptation aftereffects

Publication	Aftereffect studied	Effect of suppression
Blake & Fox (1974)	Grating threshold elevation/spatial frequency shift	None
Lemkuhle & Fox (1975)	Translational motion	None
Blake & Lehmkuhle (1976)	Grating threshold elevation	None
Wade & Wenderoth (1978)	Tilt orientation (direct component)	None
Blake & Overton (1979)	Interocular grating threshold elevation	None
O'Shea & Crassini (1981)	Interocular translational motion	None
Blake & Bravo (1985)	Spatial phase/triangle illusion	Weakens
Wiesenfelder & Blake (1990)	Spiral motion	Weakens
Lehky & Blake (1991)	Grating threshold elevation	Weakens
Wiesenfelder & Blake (1992)	Storage of translational motion adaptation	Weakens
Van der Zwan et al. (1993)	Plaid motion	Weakens
Van der Zwan & Wenderoth (1994)	Tilt orientation (subjective contours)	Weakens

physiological concomitants of binocular rivalry suppression transpire at an intermediate neural site sandwiched between "early" and "late" stages of visual processing. This was the view championed for a number of years by one of us (Blake 1989, 1995, 1997), but there is now reason to believe that this view is probably wrong. In the following paragraphs, we consider reasons why this interpretation may be oversimplified and should be replaced by a model in which suppression results from a cascade of neural events distributed over multiple stages of processing. Our argument is based on several converging lines of evidence concerning rivalry as well as on a reinterpretation of the logic underlying the strategy developed by Blake & Fox (1974).

Considering first some psychophysical results, several aspects of rivalry are difficult to reconcile with a single site of suppression located at an "intermediate" stage of processing. First, there are results implying that information about "eye of origin" is retained within the rivalry process. Specifically, when suppressed and dominant rival targets are swapped between the eyes, the dominant pattern immediately disappears and the previously suppressed pattern suddenly appears in visual awareness (Blake *et al.* 1980). Evidently, then, it is a region of one eye that is dominant at any moment in rivalry, not a particular stimulus. This, in turn, implies that the brain "knows" which eye contains which stimulus during rivalry ("eye of origin" information), even though perceptually observers have no sense of seeing with one eye or the other. Now it is generally thought that neurons in extrastriate visual areas are exclusively binocular and, therefore, insensitive to the "eye of origin" information. So the swapping results would seem to point to the involvement of striate cortex in binocular rivalry, contrary to the conclusion based on visual adaptation.

A second characteristic of rivalry pointing to an "early" stage is the nonselective loss of visual sensitivity that accompanies rivalry suppression. So long as abrupt transients are avoided, normally conspicuous changes in a suppressed stimulus go completely unnoticed until its spontaneous return to dominance. These can include changes in spatial frequency, orientation, or direction of motion (reviewed by Blake 2001); indeed, even biologically salient events such as changes in facial expression fail to be seen when they occur during suppression (Kim *et al.* 2002; Pasley *et al.* 2004). The all-encompassing nature of suppression, like the swapping results described above, suggest that suppression is operating on a given region of an eye and not on a limited set of stimulus features defining the initially suppressed target.

Turning next to neurophysiological evidence, several studies have recorded neural activity from single cells in alert, behaving monkeys trained to track perceptual fluctuations in rivalry (Logothetis & Schall 1989; Leopold & Logothetis 1996; Sheinberg & Logothetis 1997). Results from these studies imply that the neural concomitants of suppression are progressively amplified along the visual pathways, with no single visual area representing *the* site of suppression. Thus, the majority of V1 neurons continue to respond to their preferred stimulus even when the monkey's response indicates that this stimulus is suppressed from visual awareness. Within extrastriate areas, however, an increasingly larger percentage of neurons exhibit activity fluctuations that mirror the monkey's phenomenal report, with essentially *all* neurons sampled in inferotemporal cortex correlating with rivalry alternations. The same kind of graded increase in the neural strength of suppression is seen in several human brain imaging studies, with the reduction in blood oxygen level dependent signals being progressively larger within successively higher visual areas (Tong *et al.* 1998; Polonsky *et al.* 2000; Lee & Blake 2002; but see Tong & Engel 2001). Considered together, the results from single-unit measurements and brain imaging studies seem to imply that suppression, although phenomenologically an all-or-none event, arises from inhibitory events that are graded across the visual hierarchy. In view of these other results, it is worth reconsidering the assumptions underlying measurements of suppression's effect on visual adaptation.

To reiterate briefly the logic underlying the deployment of binocular rivalry and adaptation, it is assumed that intermittent visibility during adaptation should reduce the magnitude of an adaptation aftereffect if the suppression producing intermittency transpires prior to the site of adaptation. Of course, for this logic to be valid it is necessary that the magnitude of the aftereffect under study vary with the total duration of adaptation – thus, for example, 30 total seconds of adaptation distributed intermittently over a 60-second period must yield a weaker aftereffect than 60 seconds of continuous adaptation (see Fig. 10.3). Moreover, it is important to verify this precondition empirically, because the curve describing adaptation strength as the function of adaptation duration exhibits a strong compressive nonlinearity (Rose & Lowe 1982). For most of the aftereffects studied to date, test conditions have been arranged to satisfy this condition. Of course, for well-designed studies that do find a measurable reduction in aftereffect strength following adaptation with suppression (e.g. Wiesenfelder & Blake 1990), the conclusion is uncomplicated: suppression weakens neural signals arriving at the site of adaptation. The complication arises for those studies reporting *no* effect of suppression on the build-up of adaptation (e.g. Lehmkuhle & Fox 1975). Here it is incumbent upon the investigators to document that intermittent adaptation does weaken the resulting aftereffect, thereby confirming that suppression could, in principle, have reduced aftereffect strength. All studies reporting negative results (i.e. no reduction in aftereffect magnitude by suppression) have satisfied this constraint.

But in addition to these considerations about the lawful relation between adaptation duration and aftereffect strength, there is an additional assumption lurking in the background, an assumption that depends crucially on our conceptualization of suppression. The Blake and Fox strategy as outlined above tacitly assumes that if suppression occurs prior to adaptation then the reduction in adaptation strength should be proportional to the fraction of time a stimulus is suppressed. In other words, the strategy implicitly assumes that, at the site of suppression, the neural events underlying suppression are equivalent to the neural signals associated with physical absence of that stimulus (Fig. 10.2(B)). That is precisely why investigators have used intermittent presentation to "mimic" the putative effect of suppression.

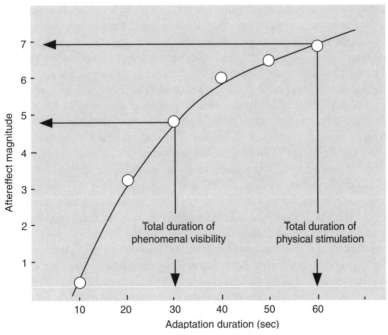

FIG. 10.3 Schematic graph showing general form of the function relating adaptation duration and visual aftereffect strength. The particulars of the compressive non-linearity depend on the particular aftereffect under study, but for several visual aftereffects the magnitude of the adaptation aftereffect asymptotes after a minute or so of adaptation. The lines and arrows denote two possible outcomes following a 60-second period of adaptation during which the adapting stimulus is presented to one eye and a competing, rival target is presented to the other eye. With appropriate adjustment of stimulus contrast and size, the aftereffect-inducing pattern can be suppressed from visual awareness for at least half of the total viewing period. If suppression completely blocks input to the neural site of adaptation, the strength of the resulting aftereffect should be reduced to a level corresponding to the total duration of phenomenal visibility, not the duration of physical stimulation. If, on the other hand, neural signals arrive unattenuated at the adaptation site even during suppression, the resulting aftereffect should be equivalent in strength to that obtained without rivalry.

But the assumption that an adaptation stimulus is rendered completely ineffective during suppression may be wrong. Perhaps, at least at early stages of visual processing, suppression involves a *weakening* of neural signals but not their *complete abolishment* (Fig. 10.2(C)). This is certainly an implication one can draw from the neurophysiological results described above. If "weakening" rather than "abolishment" were true, then it is misleading to gauge suppression's expected consequence based on intermittent physical removal of an adaptation stimulus. Perhaps to mimic suppression's effect, one should turn "down" the adaptation stimulus intermittently, but not turn it off. This concern is exacerbated by the realization that the magnitude of most aftereffects is sensitive not only to the duration of adaptation but also to the "strength" of the adaptation stimulus, where "strength" is typically defined in terms the intensity or the contrast of that stimulus. Re-examining those studies that failed to find an effect of suppression on aftereffect build-up (see Table 10.1), one sees that relatively high contrast adaptation stimuli were employed in all cases. And it is well-established that the magnitude of several of these visual aftereffects grows with contrast but only within limits, saturating at contrast values a log-unit or two above threshold. Let's consider the implication of this compressive nonlinearity for assessments of suppression's effect on aftereffect strength.

The open symbols connected by the solid line in Fig. 10.4 show the contrast/response function for the translational MAE, with the duration of adaptation always being 60 seconds (unpublished results from the Vanderbilt Vision Research laboratory). The exponent summarizing the growth in aftereffect strength will, of course, vary with stimulus conditions, but for our purposes the specific value of this exponent is not crucial. Now, suppose we present this adaptation stimulus to one eye while, at the same time, exposing the other eye to a salient rival target that suppresses the adaptation stimulus for a substantial fraction of the 60-second adaptation period. Moreover, the assumption is that suppression involves a weakening – not an abolishment – of neural signals arriving at the site of adaptation. What would happen if one were to employ a relatively high contrast adapting pattern? The effective contrast of the adapting stimulus would remain substantial throughout the adaptation period, even though the stimulus itself was only intermittently visible. Consequently, intermittent weakening of that pattern's effective contrast would have essentially no effect on the subsequent aftereffect. And the absence of an effect of suppression could lead one erroneously to conclude that the neural events underlying suppression transpire at a site *after* the locus of adaptation.

These considerations led Sobel *et al.* (2004) to reassess the effect of suppression on the growth of the MAE. Earlier work (Lehmkuhle & Fox 1975; O'Shea & Crassini 1981) had found that a moving stimulus rendered intermittently invisible by rivalry nonetheless generated a full-blown MAE. This finding was interpreted to imply that suppression occurs after the site of motion adaptation. In the context of the present discussion, it is noteworthy that both studies employed relatively high contrast, moving adaptation stimuli. Sobel and colleagues replicated this result using a high contrast, drifting grating, finding that intermittent suppression had minimal influence on the strength of the MAE. However, they went on to show that suppression *does* retard growth of the MAE when the contrast of the adaptation grating is purposefully set to an intermediate or a low value. (Sobel *et al.* measured the entire contrast/response function for the MAE and used that function to guide their selection of adapting contrasts.) Furthermore, they showed that this reduction in MAE strength could be mimicked by intermittently reducing the contrast of the moving grating by approximately 0.3 log-units. From this, Sobel *et al.* concluded that suppression *does* weaken, but does not abolish, neural signals at the site of

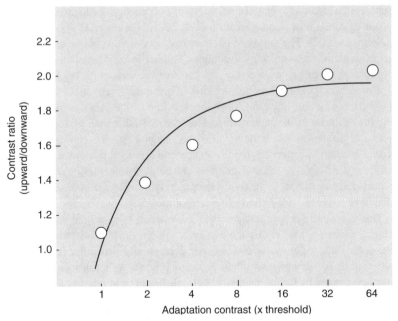

FIG. 10.4 Motion aftereffect strength (measured using a nulling technique, described by Tadin *et al.* 2003) increases with the contrast of the adapting stimulus, within limits. Each data point is the average of four staircase estimates of the contrast ratio (upward drifting/downward drifting) at which a counterphase flickering test grating appeared to drift neither upward nor downward. For each staircase estimate, the observer initially adapted for 60 seconds to a grating moving upward and then received brief test trials interspersed with 5 second periods of readaptation to upward motion. On each test trial a counterphase grating (sum of an upward and a downward drifting grating) was presented and the observer indicated in which direction it appeared to drift. Over trials the contrast of the upward component was varied to find the contrast ratio where responses were evenly distributed between upward and downward. The order of adapting contrasts was randomized across trials, and the contrast of the downward drifting component of the test grating was always 16X the contrast detection threshold for that stimulus; adaptation contrast is expressed in units relative to its own contrast threshold. As observed by other laboratories (e.g. Nishida *et al.* 1997), MAE strength saturates once adaptation contrast reaches a moderate to high level.

motion adaptation. A similar pattern of results was reported by Lehky and Blake (1991) in the case of the grating threshold elevation aftereffect.

In view of these considerations, we believe it is necessary to re-evaluate the conclusions drawn from studies reporting that suppression has *no* effect on visual adaptation. In at least some instances, this outcome may well be contrast-dependent. And if this proves to be true, we would then be in a position to reconcile the adaptation findings with results from other psychophysical and neurophysiological studies, results implying that the neural events underlying suppression are first expressed at an early stage of processing and grow ever more potent at subsequent stages (Freeman *et al.* 2005; Nguyen *et al.* 2001; Blake & Logothetis 2002). The notion of distributed suppression would be entirely consistent with the finding that more complex, "higher-level" adaptation aftereffects are susceptible to suppression (e.g. Van der Zwan & Wenderoth 1994).

Before wrapping up this consideration of binocular rivalry and adaptation, it is worth noting that one can reverse the direction of the causal arrow underlying the rationale of the strategy discussed above. Rather than asking how suppression influences the build-up of visual adaptation, one can ask whether visual adaptation influences the instigation and temporal dynamics of binocular rivalry. Answers to this question, too, can help pinpoint the sites of action of rivalry and adaptation. In the following paragraphs, we describe several studies that have examined adaptation and rivalry in this way.

One potentially revealing tactic is to ask whether two, normally compatible stimuli viewed separately by the two eyes will trigger binocular rivalry when those left- and right-eye stimuli *appear* perceptually dissimilar by virtue of adaptation. To see how this might be accomplished, let's consider an experiment performed by Ramachandran (1991). He began by alternately adapting his left eye and his right eye to opposite directions of motion for a period of time sufficient to generate opposing monocular MAEs (Fig. 10.5). When viewing a static test pattern with either eye alone, Ramachandran experienced a vivid MAE whose direction was opposite that of the adapting motion used for that eye; the two eyes on their own, in other words, experienced MAEs in

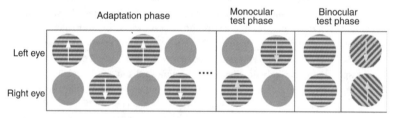

FIG. 10.5 Schematic of stimulus conditions employed by Ramachandran (1991) to learn whether binocular rivalry is experienced when the two eyes experience motion aftereffects in opposite directions. He sequentially adapted his left eye and his right eye to opposite directions of motion (upward and downward, respectively) for several minutes, and then observed the resulting motion aftereffects. Viewing a stationary test pattern, he experienced downward motion when viewing the pattern with his left eye and upward motion when viewing the pattern with his right eye. When he viewed the test pattern with both eyes simultaneously, it "usually looked stationary" (implying that the two aftereffects cancelled). But when he viewed orthogonally oriented, stationary gratings that underwent pattern rivalry, the two gratings also appeared to "drift" in one of two directions, depending on which grating was dominant; the perceived direction of illusory drift was appropriate for the eye whose oriented grating was currently dominant.

opposite directions. Would these two opposing MAEs engage in rivalry when a test pattern was viewed with both eyes open? According to Ramachandran, the answer was "no" – the test pattern viewed with both eyes did not fluctuate in perceived direction of motion but, instead, appeared perfectly stationary with no hint of either monocular MAE. Blake *et al.* (1998) replicated this observation using a static test pattern, but they went on to show that opposite-direction MAEs could generate rivalry when the MAE was evoked using dynamic test stimuli.

Possible implications of these findings are discussed elsewhere (He *et al.* 2005). For our purposes, we simply wish to point out that this strategy – generating opposing adaptation aftereffects in the two eyes – is clever in principle but difficult to implement in practice, because most aftereffects show substantial interocular transfer. Thus left-eye and right-eye adaptation aftereffects tend to cancel one another, undermining the conditions required to observe opposing monocular aftereffects. One exception to this rule is the McCollough effect (McCollough 1965), which exhibits little, if any, interocular transfer (Murch 1972). Capitalizing on this property of the McCollough effect, Kim and Blake (2004) found that the illusory color associated with a given contour orientation strongly influences the incidence of exclusive dominance by one figure or another during binocular rivalry.

Another strategy for examining adaptation's influence on rivalry is illustrated by an experiment performed by Blake and Overton (1979). Before having observers track alternations in rivalry dominance, they adapted one eye to a high-contrast version of the pattern to be viewed by that eye during rivalry. In the subsequent rivalry tracking task, this period of monocular adaptation temporarily reduced the percentage of time that the "adapted" rival pattern was dominant. Moreover, this reduction in predominance came about by a lengthening of the average duration of suppression of that pattern, implying that adaptation had temporarily reduced the effective contrast of the rival pattern. This same strategy has been used by Blake *et al.* (2003) to test the hypothesis that adaptation of the dominant stimulus is responsible, in part, for switches in dominance during rivalry.

So we conclude that binocular rivalry coupled with visual adaptation can provide revealing glimpses into the NCC. In the following section, we turn to another, complementary strategy for dissociating physical adaptation from perceptual awareness, one that exploits the visual system's limited spatial frequency sensitivity.

10.5 Adaptation to Patterns Beyond the Resolution Limit

The ability to perceive spatial patterns is limited to a range of spatial and temporal frequencies (Robson 1966). This means, therefore, that spatial patterns too finely modulated in space or too rapidly modulated in time are lost to our conscious vision. Taking spatial vision as an example, we can see spatial frequency patterns as fine as 50–60 cycles/deg under conditions of bright illumination;

patterns with spatial frequency beyond this limit are indistinguishable from an uncontoured, uniform field. Imagine, then, that stimulus *A* is a horizontal grating at 65 cycles/deg and stimulus *B* is a vertical grating at 65 cycles/deg. An observer will be unable to differentiate these two gratings, for both will appear to be uncontoured. This is true even when a laser interferometer is used to generate the gratings directly on the observer's retina, thus bypassing the spatial frequency cutoff imposed by the eye's optics (Campbell & Green 1965; Williams 1985). So when gratings are formed on the retina using a laser, we can safely conclude that the neural representation of the physical difference between gratings *A* and *B* is lost somewhere within the visual processing stream. Are there neural stages where these differences are nonetheless registered, meaning that visual neurons at some level(s) of processing actually "know" the difference between these two stimuli (horizontal versus vertical)? Without putting an electrode into an observer's brain, how can we tell whether neural responses evoked by these two "invisible" patterns are different at some stage(s) of neural processing?

True to the spirit of adaptation being the psychophysicist's microelectrode, visual aftereffects provide a gauge for measuring whether patterns rendered invisible by virtue of resolution limits are nonetheless registered at adaptation sites within the neural processing stream. To illustrate how this measurement gauge works, let's consider one of the better understood visual aftereffects: orientation-specific adaptation (Gibson & Radner 1937; Blakemore & Campbell 1969). Because orientation selectivity is a unique property of cortical (not retinal or thalamic) neurons, it is generally believed that orientation-specific adaptation transpires within the visual cortex, most probably in area V1 (Movshon & Lennie 1979). Given this likelihood, a successful demonstration of orientation-selective adaptation from two invisible orientations would lead to the inference that orientation information, although unavailable to conscious awareness, is nonetheless represented within V1, the site of orientation adaptation. What, then, actually happens when this kind of experiment is performed?

He and MacLeod (2001) obtained evidence for just such an orientation-specific aftereffect following adaptation to a grating rendered invisible owing to limited spatial resolution. They first adapted observers to a horizontal or a vertical grating slightly above the resolution limit (and, therefore, invisible) and then measured the contrast threshold for a "test" grating slightly lower than the resolution limit. The test grating was more difficult to see (i.e. its contrast threshold was elevated) when the test orientation matched the "invisible" adapting grating; test grating visibility was unaffected when the test and adaptation orientations were different (Fig. 10.6). Moreover, the "invisible" adaptation grating also temporarily affected the perceived orientation of a visible test pattern (i.e. the well-known tilt-aftereffect), even though observers were completely unable to resolve the adaptation grating during adaptation.

Based on these two findings, we can conclude that an invisible adaptation grating still activates orientation selective neurons, presumably in visual area V1. This activation, however, is insufficient to support visual awareness of that pattern, as evidenced by the observer's inability to recognize the pattern's orientation. But why is grating orientation impossible to see if the pattern activates V1 neurons?

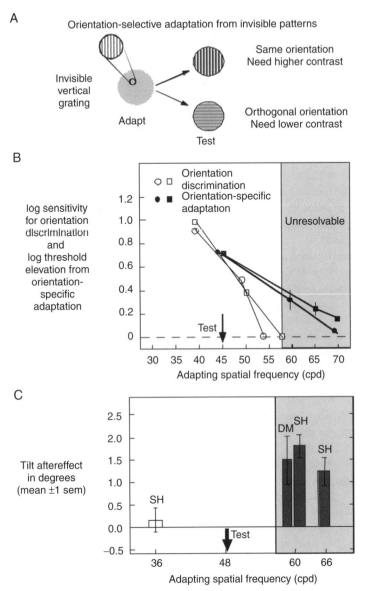

FIG. 10.6 Orientation-selective adaptation produced by gratings too fine to be visible.
(A) Schematic depiction of the orientation adaptation paradigm and the expected results.
(B) Gratings beyond 60 cycles/deg were no longer resolvable perceptually, as evidenced by
the fact that orientation discrimination was only possible for gratings under 60 cycles/deg
(open symbols). Yet adapting to invisible gratings (60–70 cycles/deg) resulted in orientation-
selective threshold elevation for resolvable test gratings (filled symbols). Squares and
circles are for two different observers. (C) The classic tilt aftereffect could also be induced
by adapting to full contrast invisible gratings (60 and 66 cycles/deg). Control stimuli in the
resolvable frequency range (36 cycles/deg) with matched effective contrast did not lead to
significant tilt aftereffect, suggesting that it is not a simple sub-threshold effect.

One could surmise that very high spatial frequency information fails to activate higher visual areas because neurons in those areas have coarser spatial resolution attributable to their larger sized receptive fields (Lennie 1998). However, it is not necessarily true that larger receptive fields of neurons in higher visual areas automatically obliterate fine patterns. After all, humans *can* see spatial frequencies much higher than what would be predicted by the receptive field sizes of neurons in extrastriate cortical areas. Perhaps within these higher visual areas, fine spatial patterns are represented in a more abstract, location invariant fashion. In any case, the implication of these adaptation experiments seems clear: activity in V1 neurons is not sufficient to support conscious visual awareness. A similar conclusion was reached by Gur and Snodderly (1997) based on V1 neural responses to fast temporal modulations recorded from V1 in non-human primates (Gur & Snodderly 1997). In that study, color opponent neurons in monkey V1 continued to respond to chromatic flicker at rates beyond the value where flicker could be resolved perceptually. It is worth noting that these findings are consistent with the view advanced by Crick and Koch (1995), stating that activation within V1 provides an insufficient basis for the NCC.

Now, one might object that studying adaptation at and beyond the limits of vision represents a highly artificial situation that has no bearing on normal visual perception. However, adaptation to invisible patterns has also been observed under conditions employing ordinarily visible patterns rendered invisible by spatial crowding (He *et al.* 1996, 1997). To obtain a strong crowding effect, the adapting stimulus was presented in the near visual periphery, but the pattern's spatial frequency and contrast were adjusted to ensure that it was clearly visible when viewed on its own. When the normally visible adapting stimulus was flanked by similar gratings of randomly selected orientations, observers could no longer discern the orientation of the adapting grating. Nonetheless, this indistinct grating still induced an orientation-selective elevation in contrast threshold comparable in strength to that produced when this adapting grating was presented on its own and was, therefore, clearly visible (Fig. 10.7). Rajimehr and colleagues (2003, 2004) have reported a similar pattern of results for "crowded" orientations created by subjective contours. The enduring adaptation potency of a grating rendered invisible by crowding implies that adaptation can transpire outside of awareness.

To draw more refined conclusions from these results, however, we need to know more about the neural bases of crowding. Lateral inhibition probably contributes to some extent to crowding but cannot fully explain crowding in the periphery (Levi *et al.* 2002 a,b). The fact that crowding occurs when target and flankers are presented dichoptically implicates a cortical locus for the crowding effect (Toet & Levi 1992). One possibility is that crowding arises from limited attentional resolution (He *et al.* 1997). Whatever the neural bases of crowding, it is clear that orientation-selective adaptation survives crowding's deleterious effect on pattern visibility. In this regard, it is noteworthy that motion adaptation, unlike orientation adaptation, *is* susceptible to crowding (He & Cavanagh 1996, but see Rajimehr *et al.* 2004 for apparent motion).

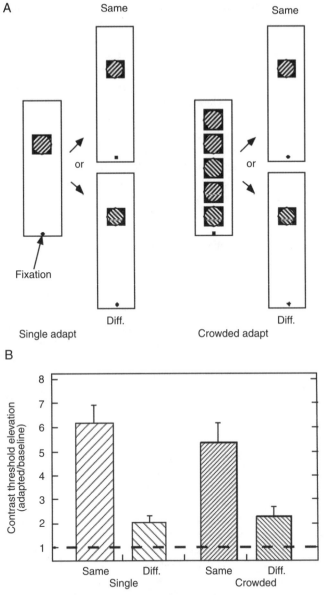

FIG. 10.7 Orientation-selective adaptation from invisible grating due to crowding.
(A) Adaptation stimulus could be either a single grating (left) or a grating flanked by
similar distracters (right, crowded condition). In the crowded condition, the orientation
of the critical adapting grating was not available to conscious vision. (B) Following
adaptation to either a single grating or to the "invisible" crowded grating, the magnitude
of orientation-selective threshold elevation for a test grating was comparable for the
two conditions. These results suggest that orientation-selective adaptation transpired at
full strength without the observer's knowing which orientation was being viewed.

Evidence that orientation information can be processed in the absence of conscious awareness comes from other sources, too. For example, Rajimehr *et al.* (2004) were able to show that change in the orientation of gratings rendered invisible by motion-induced blindness (MIB) (Bonneh *et al.* 2001) could truncate MIB. In addition, certain forms of brain damage reveal dissociations between conscious awareness of orientation and visually guided, orientation-sensitive motor behavior: Goodale and Milner (1992) studied a patient with occipital lobe damage who exhibited impaired perceptual recognition of object orientation while, at the same time, exhibiting normal manual grasping behavior dependent on object shape. Even the McCollough effect, an orientation-contingent color aftereffect, could be elicited in a patient unable to perceive contour orientation because of extensive damage in extrastriate cortical areas (Humphrey *et al.* 1995).

10.6 Different Perceptual Experiences from the Same Stimulus because of Adaptation

So far we have discussed the effects on adaptation when an adapting stimulus is rendered invisible either intermittently (because of binocular rivalry) or continuously (owing to spatiotemporal limitations of the visual system or to crowding). Now we turn our attention to adaptation's ability to cause a temporary change in the appearance of a stimulus. This means, in other words, that the same stimulus can take on one of several appearances, depending on the adaptational state of the observer. Using adaptation to alter the appearance of a stimulus provides another powerful means for identifying the neural correlates of different perceptual states independent of changes in the physical stimulus. To illustrate this strategy in action, consider once again the MAE.

As noted earlier, a stationary pattern appears to move when presented immediately following a prolonged period of adaptation to a given direction of motion (Wohlgemuth, 1911; Anstis *et al.* 1998). Thus, the same visual stimulus – a stationary pattern – can take on one of two appearances – stationary versus moving – depending on the state of adaptation of the visual system. Can we identify regions of the brain where these two perceptual states are mirrored by distinct neural states? To answer this question, several research groups have used functional brain imaging to identify neural correlates of the MAE by comparing cortical activation to the same static stimulus with and without motion adaptation (Tootell *et al.* 1995; He *et al.* 1998; Culham *et al.* 1999). These studies have consistently found that motion sensitive cortical areas, in particular area MT, are more active when an observer is experiencing the MAE than when not, even though in both cases the physical stimulus remains the same (Fig. 10.8). Moreover, Culham *et al.* and He *et al.* also observed a small elevation in MT activity during the storage period between the adapting phase and the testing phase when no motion was experienced (no stimulus was presented), leading them to conclude that activity in MT maybe a necessary, but insufficient,

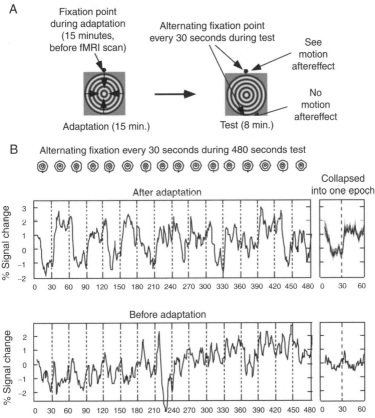

FIG. 10.8 Same stimulus creates two perceptual experiences due to motion adaptation. (A) In this example, the observer fixated just above the contracting concentric circles during adaptation, then shift fixation between the point just above and a point just below the static test pattern. A vivid MAE was clearly seen when fixation was the same in test and adapt conditions, but no MAE was seen when fixation was shifted away. (B) visual area MT showed clear modulation to the perceived change in appearance following adaptation even though the stimulus itself was stationary.

condition for perceiving motion. This tentative conclusion was more firmly supported by a recent transcranial magnetic stimulation (TMS) study in which the sensation of motion generated by TMS applied to a region of the scalp overlaying visual area MT could be wiped out by a subsequent TMS pulse targeting visual area V1 (Pascual-Leone & Walsh 2001)[1]. This outcome

---

[1] In the last decade, we have seen that TMS can selectively disrupt or even induce neural activity at particular stages in the processing stream. Already this new technique has provided some surprising results that question the wisdom of a bottom-up hierarchy of visual information processing (Pascual-Leone & Walsh 2001; Juan *et al.* 2004), and one can imagine a synergistic combination of TMS and visual adaptation leading to hybrid localization strategies.

suggests that MT activity alone is insufficient for motion perception. Returning for a moment to the brain imaging results, it should be acknowledged that attention may contribute to (but we do not believe can account for) increased brain activation measured following motion adaptation (Huk *et al.* 2001), but even when attention is explicitly controlled one finds evidence for motion adaptation in MT as well as in early visual cortex (Huk *et al.* 2001).

10.7 Implications, Caveats, and Final Thoughts

We have reviewed several different types of experiments in which the consequences of visual adaptation to a stimulus have been measured while manipulating the state of the visual awareness of that stimulus. And we have seen how results from those experiments can illuminate details of the architecture of the neural circuitry underlying adaptation as well as shed light on the neural correlates of conscious visual awareness (NCC). But, as we have argued, conclusions from these kinds of experiments are based on assumptions whose validity may be questionable. In this final section, we consider some of those assumptions in more detail.

First, when using adaptation as a tool for identifying the NCC, the strategy of ruling out a given site of adaptation as necessary for consciousness could, in principle, result in all sites being excluded. For each form of adaptation, one might find conditions wherein activity within this site, as evidenced by an adaptation aftereffect, does not lead to conscious visual experience. To put it in other words, visual awareness may always require the participation of multiple visual areas with both feedforward and feedback connections (Lamme & Roelfsema 2000; Lamme 2001; Pascual-Leone & Walsh 2001; Ro *et al.* 2003; Juan *et al.* 2004). On such a model, no given area by itself is sufficient to support visual awareness. We should not rule out a given cortical area as a participant in the NCC, just because an adaptation aftereffect presumably arising in that area is generated under conditions where the inducing stimulus cannot be seen.

Another complication associated with this approach is that neurons within an area are generally heterogeneous in terms of their response properties. Thus, one cannot make claims about the involvement of an entire area (e.g. V1 or MT) in NCC. As a rule, results from psychophysical and functional neuroimaging experiments cannot distinguish among different neuronal populations within a given visual area. By the same token, psychophysical and neuroimaging results cannot differentiate between effects occurring at the synaptic input level to a cortical area and effects occurring consequent to the spiking activity among neurons in that area. This limitation means, again, that claims about the role of a visual area in NCC could be attributable to the input to that area or to the output from that area. Consider, for example, the orientation-selective adaptation experiments reviewed earlier in this chapter. Results from those experiments can be construed to mean that V1 activity is independent of visual awareness. But, on the other hand, brain imaging studies tracking V1 activity during binocular rivalry suggest that V1 activity is closely correlated with perception (Polonsky *et al.* 2000; Tong & Engel 2001; Lee & Blake 2002; Ress & Heeger 2003). How do we reconcile these seemingly discrepant results? Perhaps the different experiments, because of their methodologies, are tapping into different sub-populations of V1 neurons, into different cortical layers or even into different intrinsic signal sources (Logothetis 2002).

Some of the experiments discussed in this chapter also rely on the assumption that awareness is blocked at a given stage of processing which, in turn, leads to the notion of adaptation occurring before versus after that stage of processing. But, as discussed earlier, this putative site of blockage may not be identified with a single neuroanatomical site but, instead, may arise from distributed sites along the visual hierarchy (Blake Logothetis 2002). Moreover, it is entirely possible that not all aspects of visual processing are susceptible to "blockade" in the first place (He *et al.* 2005).

Finally, when a visual stimulus is erased from conscious awareness owing to rivalry, crowding or limited visual resolution, observers are unable to attend to that stimulus because it is not visible. Yet we know that attention plays a pervasive role in cortical visual processing. For example, the aftereffects of motion adaptation are significantly influenced by attention (Chaudhuri 1990; Rees *et al.* 1997; Alais & Blake 1999). Given attention's normal potency, it becomes tricky to draw firm conclusions about weakened visual aftereffects when visual awareness is manipulated during adaptation. Are such reductions in aftereffect strength attributable to the absence of awareness of the adapting stimulus *per se* or to the inevitable absence of attention paid to that stimulus? Of course, in the final analysis, attention and visual awareness may be two sides of the same coin, in which case the argument becomes semantic in nature.

To close on a positive note, the utility of adaptation as a tool for studying visual awareness lies in its generality as well as its specificity. Almost all neural systems and components are adaptable, making adaptation a very versatile tool. At the same time, adaptation is typically rather specific, thus endowing this tool with its "electrode-like" character. The experiments reviewed in this chapter focused primarily on rather simple visual stimuli (e.g. oriented contours) generally thought to be preferred stimuli for "early" visual areas. However, there is no reason that the same general strategy cannot be applied to adaptation of more complex stimuli directed toward "higher" visual processes such as face recognition (a topic reviewed in other chapters in this volume). Moreover, some aftereffects exhibit a so-called storage effect, defined by the delayed onset of an aftereffect when presentation of a test pattern is postponed for some time following adaptation. One can envision exploiting this storage phenomenon to reveal something about the neural mechanisms underlying recovery from adaptation (see, for example, Wiesenfelder & Blake 1992). Thus, imagine presenting the test pattern immediately following adaptation but erasing it from conscious perception for a period of time, thereby imposing a "phenomenological" delay before actually seeing the test pattern. Would storage still transpire, or is physical stimulation alone outside of awareness sufficient to preclude storage?

In conclusion, visual adaptation provides a psychophysical "tool" for determining whether certain processes have transpired even when the normal flow of visual information is interrupted by neural events underlying binocular rivalry, crowding, or other phenomena wherein visual awareness is dissociated from physical stimulation. Like any good tool, adaptation should be employed with prudence, intelligence, and forethought, especially when using this "tool" to construct an account of the NCC. And like all structures built with available tools, today's emerging theory of NCC may appear solid, but we should not be surprised when it eventually collapses. And when that happens, recall an old maxim: "It is a poor workman who blames failure on his tools."

10.8 Summary

This chapter has described and critiqued several strategies that have been employed to learn what types of visual adaptation transpire in the absence of visual awareness. These strategies exploit phenomena such as binocular rivalry and crowding to dissociate phenomenal perception from physical stimulation. After reviewing studies that have employed this strategy and summarizing conclusions that can be drawn from those studies, we raise some questions about assumptions underlying the strategy, questions that may limit the scope of conclusions that can be drawn concerning the neural correlates of consciousness as revealed by adaptation.

Acknowledgments

Supported by EY13358, EY015261, and an award from James S McDonnell Foundation. We thank Tony Raissian for his careful reading of this manuscript.

References

Alais, D., & Blake, R. (1999). Neural strength of visual attention gauged by motion adaptation. *Nature Neuroscience*, 2, 1015–18.

Andersen, R., & Bradley, D. (1998). Perception of three-dimensional structure from motion. *Trends in Cognitive Sciences*, 2, 222–8.

Andrews, T.J., Schluppeck, D., Homfray, D., Matthews, P., & Blakemore, C. (2002). Activity in the fusiform gyrus predicts conscious perception of Rubin's vase-face illusion. *Neuroimage*, 17, 890–901.

Anstis, S., Verstraten, F., and Mather, G. (1998). The motion after-effect. *Trends in Cognitive Sciences*, 2, 111–17.

Blake, R. (1989). A neural theory of binocular rivalry. *Psychological Review*, 96, 145–67.

Blake, R. (1995). Psychoanatomical strategies for studying human vision. In T. Papathomas, C. Chubb, E. Kowler, & A. Gorea (ed.), *Early Vision and Beyond*. Cambridge, MA: MIT Press.

Blake, R. (1997). What can be perceived in the absence of visual awareness? *Current Directions in Psychological Science*, 6, 157–62.

Blake, R. (2001). A primer on binocular rivalry, including current controversies. *Brain and Mind*, 2, 5–38.

Blake, R., & Bravo, M. (1985). Binocular rivalry suppression interferes with phase adaptation. *Perception & Psychophysics, 38,* 277–80.

Blake, R., & Fox, R. (1974). Adaptation to "invisible" gratings and the site of binocular rivalry suppression. *Nature, 249,* 488–90.

Blake, R., & Lehmkuhle, S. (1976). On the site of strabismic suppression. *Investigative Ophthalmology, 15,* 660–3.

Blake, R., & Logothetis, N.K. (2002). Visual competition. *Nature Reviews Neuroscience, 3,* 13–21.

Blake, R., & Overton, R. (1979). The site of binocular rivalry suppression. *Perception, 8,* 143–52.

Blake, R., Sobel, K., & Gilroy, L.A. (2003). Visual motion retards alternations between conflicting perceptual interpretations. *Neuron, 39,* 869–78.

Blake, R., Westendorf, D., & Overton, R. (1980). What is suppressed during binocular rivalry? *Perception, 9,* 223–31.

Blake, R., Yu, K., Lohkey, M., & Norman, H. (1998). Binocular rivalry and visual motion. *Journal of Cognitive Neuroscience, 10,* 46–60.

Blakemore, C., & Campbell, F.W. (1969). On the existence of neurons in the human visual system selectively sensitive to the orientation and size of retinal images. *Journal of Physiology, 203,* 237–60.

Bonneh, Y.S., Cooperman, A., & Sagi, D. (2001). Motion-induced blindness in normal observers. *Nature, 411,* 798–801.

Breitmeyer, B.G. (1984). *Visual Masking: An Integrative Approach.* Oxford: New York.

Campbell, F.W., and Green, D.G. (1965). Optical and retinal factors affecting visual resolution. *Journal of Physiology, 181,* 576–93.

Chaudhuri, A. (1990). Modulation of the motion aftereffect by selective attention. *Nature, 344,* 60–2.

Changeuz, J.-P. (1985). *Neuronal Man.* New York: Pantheon Books.

Crick, F. (1994). *The Astonishing Hypothesis: the Scientific Search for the Soul.* New York: Scribner.

Crick, F., & Koch, C. (1995). Are we aware of neural activity in primary visual cortex? *Nature, 375,* 121–3.

Culham, J.C., Dukelow, S.P., Vilis, T., Hassard, F.A., Gati, J.S., Menon, R.S. *et al.* (1999). Recovery of fMRI activation in motion area MT following storage of the motion aftereffect. *Journal of Neurophysiology, 81,* 388–93.

Damasio, A. (1999). *The Feeling of What Happens: Body and Emotion in the Making of Consciousness.* New York: Harcourt Brace.

Dodd, J.V., Krug, K., Cumming, B.G., & Parker, A.J. (2001). Perceptually bistable three-dimensional figures evoke high choice probabilities in cortical area MT. *Journal of Neuroscience, 21,* 4809–21.

Edelman, G.M. (1992). *Bright Air, Brilliant Fire: on the Matter of the Mind.* New York: Basic Books.

Freeman, A., Nguyen, V.A., & Alais, D. (2005). The nature and depth of binocular rivalry suppression. In D. Alais, & R. Blake (ed.), *Binocular Rivalry and Perceptual Ambiguity.* Cambridge, MA: MIT Press.

Frisby, J.P. (1980). *Seeing: Illusion, Brain and Mind.* Oxford, UK: Oxford Press.

Gazzaniga, M. (1992). *Nature's Mind.* New York: Basic Books.

Gibson, J.J., & Radner, M. (1937). Adaptation, after-effect and contrast in the perception of tilted lines. *Journal of Experimental Psychology, 20,* 453–67.

Goodale, M.A., & Milner, A.D. (1992). Separate visual pathways for perception and action. *Trends in Neuroscience, 15*, 20–5.

Gur, M., & Snodderly, D.M. (1997). A dissociation between brain activity and perception: chromatically opponent cortical neurons signal chromatic flicker that is not perceived. *Vision Research, 37*, 377–82.

He, S., & MacLeod, D.I. (2001). Orientation-selective adaptation and tilt after-effect from invisible patterns. *Nature, 411*, 473–6.

He, S., Cavanagh, P., & Intriligator, J. (1997). Attentional resolution. *Trends in Cognitive Sciences, 1*, 115–21.

He, S., Cavanagh, P., & Intriligator, J. (1996). Attentional resolution and the locus of visual awareness. *Nature, 383*, 334–7.

He, S., Cohen, E.R., & Hu, X. (1998). Close correlation between activity in brain area MT/V5 and the perception of a visual motion aftereffect. *Current Biology, 8*, 1215–18.

He, S., & Cavanagh, P. (1996). *Orientation Selective Adaptation, but not Direction Selective Adaptation is Unaffected by Blocking Focused Attention.* Annual meetings of the Association for Research in Vision and Ophthalmology, Sarasota, FL.

He, S., Carlson, T., & Chen, X. (2005). Parallel pathways and temporal dynamics. In D. Alais, & R. Blake (ed.), *Binocular Rivalry and Perceptual Ambiguity*. Cambridge MA: MIT Press.

Huk, A.C., Ress, D., & Heeger, D.J. (2001). Neuronal basis of the motion aftereffect reconsidered. *Neuron, 32*, 161–72.

Humphrey, G.K., Goodale, M.A., Corbetta, M., & Aglioti, S. (1995). The McCollough effect reveals orientation discrimination in a case of cortical blindness. *Current Biology, 5*, 545–51.

Juan, C.H., Campana, G., & Walsh, V. (2004). Cortical interactions in vision and awareness: hierarchies in reverse. *Progress in Brain Research, 144*, 117–30.

Kawamoto, A.H., & Anderson, J.A. (1985). A neural network model of multistable perception. *Acta Psychologica, 59*, 35–65.

Kim, C.-Y., & Blake, R. (2004). Color promotes interocular grouping during binocular rivalry, *Journal of Vision, 4(8)*, 240a (abstract).

Kim, C-Y., Grossman, E., & Blake, R. (2002). Biologically relevant events are undetectable during suppression phases of binocular rivalry Program No. 161.12. *2002 Abstract Viewer/Itinerary Planner.* Washington, DC: Society for Neuroscience, (Online).

Kohler, I.W. (1940). *Dynamics in Psychology*. New York: Liveright.

Lamme, V.A., & Roelfsema, P.R. (2000). The distinct modes of vision offered by feedforward and recurrent processing. *Trends in Neuroscience, 23*, 571–9.

Lamme, V.A. (2001). Blindsight: the role of feedforward and feedback corticocortical connections. *Acta Psychologica, 107*, 209–28.

Lee, S.H., & Blake, R. (2002). V1 activity is reduced during binocular rivalry. *Journal of Vision, 2*, 618–26.

Lehky, S., & Blake, R. (1991). Organization of binocular pathways: Modeling and data related to rivalry. *Neural Computation, 3*, 44–53.

Lehmkuhle, S.W., & Fox, R. (1975). Effect of binocular rivalry suppression on the motion aftereffect. *Vision Research, 15*, 855–9.

Lennie, P. (1998). Single units and visual cortical organization. *Perception, 27*, 889–935.

Leopold, D.A., & Logothetis, N.K. (1996). Activity changes in early visual cortex reflect monkeys' percepts during binocular rivalry. *Nature, 379*, 549–53.

Leopold, D.A., & Logothetis, N.K. (1999). Multistable phenomena: Changing views in perception. *Trends in Cognitive Sciences, 3*, 254–64.

Leopold, D.A., Wilke, M., Maier, A., & Logothetis, N. (2002). Stable perception of visually ambiguous patterns. *Nature Neuroscience, 5*, 605–9.

Levi, D.M., Hariharan, S., & Klein, S.A. (2002a). Suppressive and facilitatory interactions in peripheral vision: peripheral crowding is neither size invariant nor simple contrast masking. *Journal of Vision, 2*, 167–77.

Levi, D.M., Klein, S.A., & Hariharan, S. (2002b). Suppressive and facilitatory spatial interactions in foveal vision: Foveal crowding is simple contrast masking. *Journal of Vision, 2*, 140–66.

Logothetis, N.K. (1998). Single units and conscious vision. *Philosophical Transactions of the Royal Society of London – Series B: Biological Sciences, 353*, 1801–18.

Logothetis, N. (2002). The neural basis of the blood-oxygen-level-dependent functional magnetic resonance imaging signal. *Philosophical Transactions of the Royal Society, London B, 357*, 1003–37.

Logothetis, N.K., & Schall, J.D. (1989). Neuronal correlates of subjective visual perception. *Science, 245*, 761–3.

Mack, A. (2003). Inattentional blindness: looking without seeing. *Current Directions in Psychological Science, 12*, 180–4.

Marcel, A. (1983). Conscious and unconscious perception: an approach to the relations between phenomenal experience and perceptual processes. *Cognitive Psychology, 15*, 238–300.

Mather, G. (1980). The movement aftereffect and a distribution-shift model of coding the direction of visual movement. *Perception, 9*, 379–92.

McCollough, C. (1965). Color adaptation of edge-detectors in the human visual system. *Science 149*, 1115–6.

Movshon, J.A., & Lennie, P. (1979). Pattern-selective adaptation in visual cortical neurones. *Nature, 278*, 850–2.

Mueller, T.J. (1990). A physiological model of binocular rivalry. *Visual Neuroscience, 4*, 63–73.

Murch, G.M. (1972). Binocular relationships in a size and color orientation specific aftereffect. *Journal of Experimental Psychology, 93*, 30–4.

Nawrot, M., & Blake, R. (1991). A neural network model of kinetic depth and stereopsis. *Visual Neuroscience, 6*, 219–27.

Nishida, S., Ashida, H., & Sato, T. (1997). Contrast dependence of two types of motion aftereffect. *Vision Research, 37*, 553–64.

Nguyen, V.A., Freeman, A.W., & Wenderoth, P. (2001). The depth and selectivity of suppression in binocular rivalry. *Perception & Psychophysics, 63*, 348–60.

O'Shea, R.P., & Crassini, B. (1981). Interocular transfer of the motion aftereffect is not reduced by binocular rivalry. *Vision Research, 21*, 801–4.

Orbach, J., Ehrlich, D., & Heath, H.A. (1963). Reversibility of the Necker cube: I. An examination of the concept of "satiation and orientation". *Perceptual and Motor Skills, 17*, 439–58.

Pascual-Leone, A., & Walsh, V. (2001). Fast backprojections from the motion to the primary visual area necessary for visual awareness. *Science, 292*, 510–2.

Pasley, B., Mayes, L.C., & Schultz, R. (2004). Subcortical discrimination of unperceived objects during binocular rivalry. *Neuron, 42*, 163–72.

Polonsky, A., Blake, R., Braun, J., & Heeger, D.J. (2000). Neuronal activity in human primary visual cortex correlates with perception during binocular rivalry. *Nature Neuroscience, 3*, 1153–9.

Rajimehr, R. (2004). Unconscious orientation processing. *Neuron, 41*, 663–73.

Rajimehr, R., Montaser-Kouhsari, L., & Afraz, S.R. (2003). Orientation-selective adaptation to crowded illusory lines. *Perception, 32*, 1199–210

Rajimehr, R., Vaziri-Pashkam, M., Afraz, S.R., & Esteky, H. (2004). Adaptation to apparent motion in crowding condition. *Vision Research, 44*, 925–31.

Ramachandran, V.S. (1991). Form, motion and binocular rivalry. *Science, 251*, 950–1.

Ramachandran, V.S., & Blakeslee, S. (1998). *Phantoms in the Brain.* New York: Morrow and Company.

Raymond, J.E., Shapiro, K.L., & Arnell, K.M. (1992). Temporary suppression of visual processing in an RSVP task: an attentional blink? *Journal of Experimental Psychology: Human Perception & Performance, 18*, 849–60.

Rees, G., Frith, C.D., & Lavie, N. (1997). Modulating irrelevant motion perception by varying attentional load in an unrelated task. *Science, 278*, 1616–19.

Ress, D., & Heeger, D.J. (2003). Neuronal correlates of perception in early visual cortex. *Nature Neuroscience, 6*, 414–20.

Ro, T., Breitmeyer, B., Burton, P., Singhal, N.S., & Lane, D. (2003). Feedback contributions to visual awareness in human occipital cortex. *Current Biology, 13*, 1038–41.

Robson, J.G. (1966). Spatial and temporal contrast-sensitivity functions of the visual system. *Journal of the Optical Society of America, 56*, 1141–2.

Rose, D., & Lowe, I. (1982). Dynamics of adaptation to contrast. *Perception, 11*, 505–28.

Sheinberg, D.L., & Logothetis, N.K. (1997). The role of temporal cortical areas in perceptual organization. *Proceedings of the National Academy of Sciences, U S A, 94*, 3408–13.

Sobel, K.N., Blake, R., & Raissian, T. (2004). Binocular rivalry suppression *does* impede buildup of the motion aftereffect. *Journal of Vision, 4(8)*, 243a (abstract).

Sperry, R.W. (1970). An objective approach to subjective experience: further explanation of a hypothesis. *Psychological Review, 77*, 585–90.

Tadin, D., Lappin, J.S., Gilroy, L.A., & Blake, R. (2003). Perceptual consquences of centre-surround antagonism in visual motion processing. *Nature, 424*, 313–15.

Toet, A., & Levi, D.M. (1992). The two-dimensional shape of spatial interaction zones in the parafovea. *Vision Research, 32*, 1349–57.

Tong, F., & Engel, S.A. (2001). Interocular rivalry revealed in the human cortical blind-spot representation. *Nature, 411*, 195–9.

Tong, F., Nakayama, K., Vaughan, J.T., & Kanwisher, N. (1998). Binocular rivalry and visual awareness in human extrastriate cortex. *Neuron, 21*, 753–9.

Tootell, R.B., Reppas, J.B., Dale, A.M., Look, R.B., Sereno, M.I., Malach, R. *et al.* (1995). Visual motion aftereffect in human cortical area MT revealed by functional magnetic resonance imaging. *Nature, 375*, 139–41.

Van der Zwan, R., Wenderoth, P., & Alais, D. (1993). Reduction of a pattern-induced motion aftereffect by binocular rivalry suggests the involvement of extrastriate mechanisms. *Visual Neuroscience, 10*, 703–9.

Van der Zwan, R., & Wenderoth, P. (1994). Psychophysical evidence for area V2 involvement in the reduction of subjective contour tilt aftereffects by binocular rivalry. *Visual Neuroscience, 11*, 823–30.

Wade, N.J., & Wenderoth, P. (1978). The influence of colour and contour rivalry on the magnitude of the tilt aftereffect. *Vision Research, 18,* 827–36.

Wiesenfelder, H., & Blake, R. (1990). The neural site of binocular rivalry relative to the analysis of motion in the human visual system. *Journal of Neuroscience, 10,* 3880–8.

Wiesenfelder, H., & Blake, R. (1992). Binocular rivalry suppression disrupts recovery from motion adaptation. *Visual Neuroscience, 9,* 143–8.

Williams, D.R. (1985). Aliasing in human foveal vision. *Vision Research, 25,* 195–205.

Wilson, H.R. (1999). *Spikes, Decisions and Actions.* Oxford: Oxford Press.

Wohlgemuth, A. (1911). On the after-effect of seen movement. *British Journal of Psychology. (Supplement), 1,* 1–117.

11

Attentional Modulation
of Motion Adaptation

DAVID ALAIS

11.1 Introduction

In varying degrees, it has long been suspected that attention can affect perform-ance on behavioural and psychophysical tasks. Traditionally, however, attention was thought to be a higher-level phenomenon, existing in the 'cognitive' rather than the low-level 'sensory' realm. One result that was seminal in changing this way of thinking was published by Chaudhuri (1991). His paper 'Modulation of the motion aftereffect by selective attention' showed that the duration of a motion aftereffect (MAE) was dramatically reduced if a subject's attention, rather than being focused on the adapting motion, was instead engaged in a demanding distractor task. The task he used was an alphanumeric discrimination task requiring observers to detect a particular digit in a rapid stream of letters and digits presented as a quasi-fixation point at the centre of a window containing a translating adaptation stimulus (Fig. 11.1). He reported a three-fold reduction in MAE duration in this condition, relative to a no-distractor condition. The significance of Chaudhuri's result was its suggestion that even the encoding of stimuli as simple as translational movement (often presumed to be a pre-attentive attribute) were not immune from attentional influence. A decade or so later, other psychophysical studies have appeared showing attentional modulation of various types of motion adaptation (Shulman 1993; Lankheet &

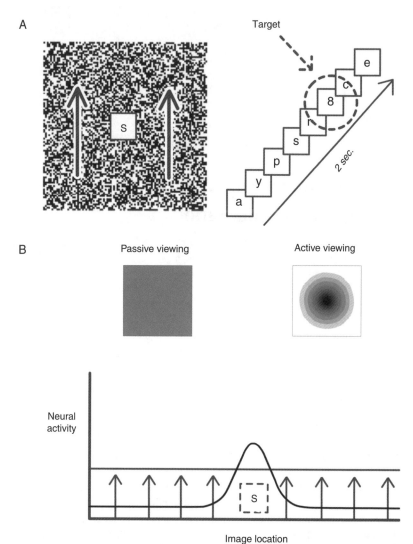

FIG. 11.1 An illustration of Chaudhuri's (1991) experiment. (A) Observers fixated the central square while the surrounding texture drifted at a speed of 5 deg/sec. After 60 seconds of motion adaptation, the pattern stopped and the subject was required to indicate the duration of the ensuing motion aftereffect (MAE) with a key-press the moment the MAE ceased. The MAE was measured under conditions of active and passive attention. In the active attention condition, the central square contained a single-character alphanumeric stream presented at 4 Hz. Subjects were instructed to focus on the stream of characters and to press a button each time a numeral was presented. In the passive attention condition, subjects were not required to do the character detection task and were instructed to treat the alphanumeric stream simply as a fixation point. Differences in MAEs were markedly different between the conditions, with durations in the active attention condition about three times shorter than those

in the passive condition. Apart from the attentional state of the observer, all aspects of the two conditions were identical. (B) One explanation of Chaudhuri's finding is in terms of a spotlight or zoom-lens of attention. With no directed focus of attention, the neural response to the adapting motion is approximately uniform across the spatial extent of the adapting stimulus. However, introducing the very demanding distractor task requires a tight focussing of attention around the character window, boosting neural activity for that region and attenuating the neural response to the surrounding motion. With the strength of the MAE being related to level of motion activation during adaptation, this necessarily produces a reduced aftereffect.

◄───

Verstraten 1995; Alais & Blake 1999), as well as modulation of adaptation to other basic visual attributes such as orientation (Spivey & Spirn 2000) and stereoscopic depth (Rose *et al.* 2003).

The implication of Chaudhuri's finding appeared to be that attention could influence neural activity at the lowest cortical level, that is, at the level of the primary visual cortex where direction-selective neurons respond to linear movement of the kind used by Chaudhuri (Hubel & Wiesel 1968). To fully understand these results, however, particularly their relevance to the likely level of attentional influence, we need to consider attentional processes and the origins of the motion aftereffect (MAE) in more detail. A decade or so after the appearance of Chaudhuri's paper, advances in neuroimaging and neurophysiology have seen our knowledge of the neural bases of attention and motion processing increase dramatically. This chapter will review these recent advances and discuss how they impact on psychophysical studies showing attentional modulation of motion adaptation.

11.2 Attention: Early or Late Selection?

Attention is generally defined as a process of selection in which cognitive resources are allocated to a certain spatial location or object. Historically, one of the major debates in attention has concerned whether selection occurs at an early or a late stage. Dichotomous views on this fundamental question emerged early in the attentional literature (Broadbent 1958; Deutsch & Deutsch 1963). The early-selection model holds that rudimentary visual processing occurs automatically or 'pre-attentively' but that attentional selection to an element of the pre-attentive map is needed to realize a complete percept of that element (Moray 1959; Treisman 1969; Neisser & Becklen 1975; Treisman & Gelade 1980; Broadbent 1982). On this view, unattended aspects of the pre-attentive map have an impoverished representation at the perceptual level. In contrast, the late-selection model (Moray 1959; Deutsch & Deutsch 1963) proposes a much greater role for pre-attentive processes which analyse the visual scene and identify objects almost completely prior to the stage of attentional selection. Attention then serves to select from an array of fully represented objects and percepts the one(s) most suited to the task or action to be executed (Treisman 1969; Neisser & Becklen 1975).

Chaudhuri's (1991) finding of attentional modulation of motion adaptation appeared to provide a challenge to the late-selection hypothesis by showing that processes which had been presumed to be low-level and pre-attentive (translational motion detection in cortical area V1) could be influenced by the attentional state of the observer. The implication that motion processing was less active when attention was directed to competing stimuli strongly suggested an early level of attentional selection. Of course, the strength of this conclusion depends on where in the visual processing hierarchy the MAE occurs. As the next section will show, our understanding of the MAE has moved on from adaptation of low-level detectors sensitive to movement as a feature or attribute to a view of motion processing as more distributed and involving a range of cortical areas.

11.3 The Locus of the MAE

The significance of Chaudhuri's finding for models of attentional processing depends upon where in the visual hierarchy the MAE arises. Early accounts suggested the MAE could occur early in visual cortex. Sutherland (1961) formulated an opponent-motion model of the MAE incorporating neural fatigue in which adaptation of one direction in a pair of opponent motion units led to a reduced response for that direction and therefore the relative dominance of the opponent direction. Soon after this model was proposed, Barlow and Hill (1963) observed the phenomenon of neural adaptation to motion in rabbit retinal ganglion cells. Later, findings by Hubel and Wiesel (1968) showed the existence of direction-selective cells in primate primary visual cortex and all the pieces appeared to fall in place for a complete account of the MAE at the lowest cortical level. Clearly, on this account, Chaudhuri's (1991) data would indicate attentional selection at an early level.

Consistent with early neurophysiological evidence of a low-level site for the MAE, behavioural findings from visual search experiments also implied a low-level site for motion. Several investigators measured reaction times for observers to detect moving targets presented in the presence of distractor elements. The results of these studies showed clearly that reaction times in such a context did not depend on the number of elements in the distractor set (Nakayama & Silverman 1986; Dick et al. 1987; McLeod et al. 1988; Horowitz & Treisman 1994). Reaction times that do not vary as a function of distractor set size are indicative of parallel processing. These findings therefore suggested that motion was a preattentive attribute, detected automatically without the need for a time-consuming serial search. Although parallel, preattentive processing need not necessarily point to a low-level site for motion, this conclusion was consistent with theories of motion processing in that most models have traditionally regarded motion as being pre-attentive. That is, these models are essentially based on a feed-forward assumption (Marr 1982) and do not directly include a role for attention (Adelson & Bergen 1985; van Santen & Sperling 1985; Wilson 1992).

In more recent years, however, our understanding of cortical motion processing has expanded dramatically. A large network of motion-sensitive areas lying beyond the primary visual cortex has been implicated in motion processing. This began with the discovery in the early 1970s in extrastriate cortex of the middle temporal (MT) area, also termed V5 (Zeki 1974). MT was shown to receive direct projections from area V1 and to be highly specialized for motion processing (Maunsell & Van Essen 1983; Albright 1984; Rodman & Albright 1987). One of the distinctive features of MT is that it has large receptive fields which pool input from many V1 cells. In this way, it is capable of taking an array of distinct local motion signals and integrating them to produce a response which reflects the net global motion (Newsome & Paré 1988; Britten & Newsome 1998). The high degree of motion specialization in area MT led to the proposal that MT was a distinct motion-processing module in the brain (Zeki 1993). It is now clear, however, that motion processing involves a network of areas much larger than just V1 and MT. For example, other cortical areas which receive projections from V1 and which respond to translational movement include areas V2, V3, and V3A. In addition, there are also several areas lying beyond MT which respond to movement, such as areas MST, FST, and VIP (Gegenfurtner et al. 1997; Singh et al. 2000; Vanduffel et al. 2001). In light of the distributed network of cortical areas involved in motion processing, it is difficult to maintain the idea that the MAE results exclusively from adaptation of direction-selective units in primary visual cortex. Instead, a distributed hierarchical model of the MAE is much more realistic (Nishida & Ashida 2000).

The arrival of functional neuroimaging techniques provided new insights into the cortices involved in motion processing and the motion aftereffect. A study by Tootell et al. (1995) involving prolonged adaptation to movement followed by a stationary test pattern found that MT activity was elevated during the stationary test phase and that the decay of this activity corresponded closely to that of the illusory movement perceived during the MAE. Other cortical areas responsive to movement either showed less activity elevations or none at all. The data appeared to point strongly to area MT as the site of the MAE. Another endorsement of MT as the site of the MAE came from Culham et al. (1999), who investigated the phenomenon of MAE storage. Storage occurs when, instead of a static test pattern, a period of darkness follows the cessation of motion adaptation. Remarkably, if this period is as long as, or even longer than, the normal duration of the MAE, presentation of the test pattern will still evoke a MAE whose duration is similar to that which would be elicited by a test pattern presented immediately after adaptation. Culham et al. examined MAE storage in an fMRI experiment. The elevated activity levels observed during motion adaptation dropped sharply during storage (to a level only slightly above a control sequence) but rose again steeply once the MAE test pattern was presented. Because the pattern of MT activity in Culham *et al.*'s study correlates closely with perception of the MAE and the related 'storage' phenomenon, it provides further support for MT being the likely site of the MAE.

Other authors have also argued for MT as the critical area corresponding to the perceived movement in the MAE (He *et al.* 1998). However, there are aspects of these papers that are difficult to reconcile with the fundamental effect of adaptation on neurons, which is to attenuate their responses. Indeed, in a recent single-unit paper specifically examining motion adaptation in MT cells (Kohn & Movshon 2003) it was established that MT cells in fact markedly decrease their firing rate following adaptation to motion. This creates a discrepancy: fMRI studies have reported elevations in MT activity during perception of the MAE while Kohn and Movshon's study shows attenuation of MT activity? An fMRI study of the MAE by Huk *et al.* (2001) proposes that attention might be the key to explaining why elevations of MT activity were reported in earlier fMRI studies of the MAE. They offer two possible reasons for this. First, they note that because the MAE is an illusory motion, it is likely to grab an observer's attention, and second, that observers were required to direct their attention to this motion in order to judge its presence (Hautzel *et al.* 2001) or cessation (Culham *et al.* 1999; Taylor *et al.* 2000). These factors are likely to have caused elevations in MT due to attention rather than to motion adaptation (evidence for attentional modulation of MT appears in the following two sections). Huk *et al.* attempted to quantify the extent to which MT elevation during the MAE could be attributed to attention, and drew the conclusion that activity elevations in previous reports can be solely attributed to attention. When appropriate attentional controls were introduced, they found significant direction-selective decreases in activity as a result of adaptation in MT, but also in several areas prior to MT (e.g. V1, V2, V3, V3a, and V4v). The findings of Huk *et al.*, then, do not support the claim that MT is the single critical area underlying the MAE. Instead, they point to a distributed process, beginning as early as primary visual cortex and involving numerous areas beyond this level.

11.4 Neuroimaging Evidence for Distributed Processes in Motion and Attention

A considerable body of neuroimaging evidence now exists concerning the cortical areas involved in both attention and motion processing. Concerning attention, the evidence points clearly to its being a distributed process. Attentional effects can be observed as low as the primary visual cortex, and as high as frontal cortices. Early evidence for higher-level involvement came from clinical studies showing that damage to fronto-parietal areas produced attentional deficits such as neglect (Posner *et al.* 1984; Vallar & Perani 1986) and from single-unit neurophysiological studies demonstrating attentional modulation in frontal cortical areas (Wurtz & Mohler 1976). With the advent of neuroimaging techniques, attention-related activation in frontal and parietal areas was confirmed (Corbetta *et al.* 1993; Nobre *et al.* 1997) in a functional context.

There are also findings of attentional modulation in early cortical areas, including primary visual cortex. Examples can be found in single-unit neurophysiological studies (Motter 1993; Luck *et al.* 1997; Ito & Gilbert 1999) and, more recently, neuroimaging studies. In one fMRI study specifically concerning motion, subjects performed a motion discrimination task alternatively in one or other visual hemifield. As observers changed their focus of attention from one hemifield to the other, brain activity in the primary visual area of the contralateral hemisphere modulated correspondingly, increasing by about 25 per cent during attention phases compared to non-attention phases (Gandhi *et al.* 1999). Corroborating evidence for this result comes from other fMRI studies which have also shown attention-modulated activity in V1 during motion tasks (Watanabe *et al.* 1998; Somers *et al.* 1999; Huk & Heeger 2000; Seiffert *et al.* 2003). In none of these studies was attentional modulation of cortical activity unique to V1; in most cases attentional effects were also reported in V2, V3a, MT, and other areas.

Together, these findings highlight the extent to which attention is a distributed process. This in turn limits the extent to which Chaudhuri's original result can be interpreted in terms of attention acting at an early versus a late level. The reason is that demonstrable attentional modulations in early visual areas may in fact result from reentrant processing feeding back from higher areas (to be discussed further in Section 11.6). Nonetheless, it does appear that lower and higher cortical levels do differ in that high-level areas are involved at a more general level in the planning of behavioural responses and the guiding of action while lower areas are activated selectively for specific features or attributes relating to the task. However, even at this lower, attribute-specific level there is considerable distribution of processes, with motion-specific attentional effects consistently observed in at least areas V1, V2, V3a, and MT. Congruent with this, the most recent neuroimaging studies examining the MAE point to these same areas as underlying the MAE (Huk *et al.* 2001; Seiffert *et al.* 2003). Thus, even if it is not appropriate to analyse Chaudhuri's results exclusively in terms of early versus late selection, we can at least propose that the MAE and attentional modulations concerning motion tasks activate largely common (though distributed) cortical areas in relatively early, attribute-specific areas.

11.5 Kinds of Attentional Selection

The traditional and most intuitive way to view attentional selection has been in terms of spatial selection. Metaphors such as the 'spotlight' of attention (Eriksen & Eriksen 1974; Egeth & Yantis 1997) convey this meaning very clearly. Eriksen and Eriksen's original observation was that the difficulty of identifying a target letter in the presence of distractor letters was dependent on the distance of the distractors from the target, and it was this that prompted the spotlight metaphor. This notion has a good deal of psychophysical (Eriksen &

Eriksen 1974; Posner 1980) and neurophysiological support (Connor *et al.* 1997; Luck *et al.* 1997; Bisley & Goldberg 2003). However, spatial selection appears not to be the only way that attention can operate.

In many early experiments on spatial attention, selection of spatial locations was confounded with selection of features or objects within those spatial locations. In studies that have teased apart these possibilities, evidence has been found to support attentional selection being made on the basis of whole objects or of features/attributes of particular objects. One early psychophysical study to highlight the importance of features showed that observers could attend to a cluster of letters provided they all shared the same movement (Driver & Bayliss 1989). In another study using a pair of transparently superimposed motions, it was shown that observers could selectively attend to one of the motions even though both occupied the same spatial location (Alais & Blake 1999). Studies such as these highlight the process of feature-based selection and neurophysiological support for such a process has been found in early extrastriate cortex in primates (Treue & Martinez-Trujillo 1999; Saenz *et al.* 2002). Additional evidence comes from neuroimaging studies. The first clear demonstration was a PET study by Corbetta *et al.* (1990). They presented an array of elements that differed in shape, colour, or velocity and had subjects attend selectively to a particular feature. The result was that different patterns of cortical activity were observed for each selected attribute, including activity in areas specific for the representation of each attribute. Similar results have been observed in several fMRI studies (Beauchamp *et al.* 1997; O'Craven *et al.* 1997).

As well as selection operating on the basis of features, it appears it can also operate by selecting entire objects. In an fMRI study, O'Craven *et al.* (1999) transparently superimposed two visual objects, a face and a house. Each of these objects is independently represented in different cortical areas (houses in the parahippocampal place area, faces in the fusiform face area), and attention to one of the objects led to increased activity in the appropriate cortical area. If the face stimulus (for example) was made to oscillate slightly while the other was static, and subjects attended to the face, then increases in activity were seen both in the fusiform face area and in motion sensitive areas. However, the activity increase seen in motion sensitive areas was much weaker when movement was added to the unattended object. These results indicate object-based selection because both objects shared the same retinal location, yet the effect of adding motion to one of them was dependent on whether or not it was attended. These results also suggest that selecting an object entails selection of the features that comprise the object, in this example, the face and its movement.

11.6 Attentional Mechanisms and Motion Adaptation

It was noted above that attention is a distributed process, occurring at many cortical levels including higher-level areas subserving intention and action. Given the extensive cortical feedback projections from prefrontal and parietal cortex to the dorsal and ventral streams (Barbas 1988; Ungerleider *et al.* 1989; Van Essen *et al.* 1992), a feedback network that projects back as far as V1 (Felleman & Van Essen 1991; Mignard & Malpeli 1991), one proposal is that attention can be directed from these higher areas to lower areas underlying the specific spatial and featural representation required for a given task. In this way, early anatomical structures can be modulated by temporally late feedback, as suggested by studies of event-related potentials (Olson *et al.* 2001). Throughout the cortex, feedforward signals tend to flow from the lower area's layers II and III to the higher area's layer IV, while reentrant signals tend to leave the higher area's layer V and terminate in the lower area's layer I or VI. A notable aspect of this loop is that reentrant fibres terminate in the lower area in a wider distribution than the neurons of the original ascending source. This pattern has been shown to exist between MT and V1 (Shipp & Zeki 1989; Hupé *et al.* 1998) and between V1 and LGN (Sillito *et al.* 1994). The advantages of diffuse feedback are two-fold. First, because some of the reentrant fibres return to the original ascending site, it provides a conduit for amplifying (or inhibiting) directly the original cells, and second, it provides a means of influencing those cells neighbouring a given group of cells. For example, this influence could be inhibitory if there were distractors surrounding an attended target, serving to make a target more visible. In a similar way, figure-ground segregation has been proposed to make use of this feedback arrangement (Hupé *et al.* 1998).

Another potential use for diffuse back projections might be to permit the shrinkage of receptive fields around a selected stimulus. Moran and Desimone (1985) proposed this idea after they noted that the response of V4 and IT neurons driven by two stimuli (one preferred, the other non-preferred) depended upon which one was attended to. If a non-preferred stimulus was attended, the cell's response was poor even though it was also being presented with a preferred (albeit unattended) stimulus. One possible interpretation of these data is that attention causes receptive fields to shrink around the attended target, which in this case would leave the preferred stimulus lying outside the receptive field's reduced extent. Similar results were subsequently reported in V4 and V2 (Luck *et al.* 1997; Reynolds *et al.* 1999), as well as in MT and MST (Treue & Maunsell 1996). Results such as these recall the proposal that attention acts as a spotlight with a 'zoom lens', a variant of the spot light metaphor (Eriksen & St James 1986) implying that the region of attentional selection can be tightly focused or diffuse. One interpretation of Chaudhuri's finding would be that the alphanumeric distractor task was difficult enough that attention needed to be very tightly focused, to the extent that motion processing in the surrounding region was greatly compromised.

One of the simplest ways in which attention could facilitate visual processes is simply to enhance the signals related to a particular task. The idea that attention could function as a signal enhancement operation has a long history among cognitive psychologists (Prinzmetal *et al.* 1997). It is perhaps the most parsimonious and intuitively appealing explanation of a host of findings showing improved performance and accuracy and reduced reaction times when attention is expressly directed at a particular task. In recent years, a good deal of evidence has appeared which supports this view. For example, neuroimaging studies have shown that when one object or spatial location rather than a competing one is selected, a corresponding enhancement of the neural signal for the selected stimulus is observed (Corbetta *et al.* 1991; O'Craven *et al.* 1997; Buchel *et al.* 1998; Somers *et al.* 1999).

Several neurophysiological studies have examined signal enhancement at the single-unit level for motion stimuli (Treue & Maunsell 1996; Seidemann & Newsome 1999; Treue & Martinez-Trujillo 1999). Treue & Martinez-Trujillo presented two moving targets in receptive fields of MT and MST neurons and trained behaving monkeys to attend to one of them. One target always moved in the null direction (that is, in the direction opposite the cell's preference), while the other moved in one of 12 directions (from which directional tuning curves could be calculated) (Fig. 11.2(A)). Compared with the tuning curve for a neutral comparison condition, a tuning curve of decreased response amplitude was observed when attention was directed to the null direction. In contrast, response amplitude was boosted when the non-null directions were attended (Fig. 11.2(B)). Importantly, the stimuli in all conditions were identical, with only the attentional state of the monkey differing. When the tuning curves are compared, they are found to vary in amplitude with little or no variation in tuning bandwidth. Modulations of response amplitude by attentional state can be effectively modelled by a multiplicative factor which boosts or attenuates response as a function of the behavioural relevance of a stimulus. Similar findings have been reported for orientation tuning curves in area V4 (McAdams & Maunsell 1999).

An important aspect of Treue and Martinez-Trujillo's results is that the activity of MT units is greater when attention is directed to the preferred direction even when the attended stimulus is located far from the receptive field being recorded. Thus, attention-related enhancement of neural gain can operate across discrete spatial locations on the basis of feature identity (Saenz *et al.* 2002) rather than non-selectively boosting all neural responses within a spatially limited region of attention. It is notable that large multiplicative changes in firing rate are generally only observed when a selection is made between two competing stimuli (Treue & Maunsell 1996; Reynolds *et al.* 1999), consistent with the 'biased competition model' proposed by Desimone and Duncan (1995). Given this, it may be the case that attention-related gain changes of a multiplicative kind result from attentional processes acting on divisive inhibitory processes that several researchers have proposed to underlie competitive neural interactions (Carandini *et al.* 1997; Simoncelli & Heeger 1998).

In addition to a multiplicative model, attention could also exert an additive influence on neural response. This possibility is supported by neuroimaging studies which show elevations in baseline firing rates when no stimulus is present. For example, Ress *et al.* (2000) found that cueing subjects to expect a stimulus led to elevations in baseline response even in conditions where no stimulus was presented. The baseline elevation was observed in V1 and was limited to the

A   B

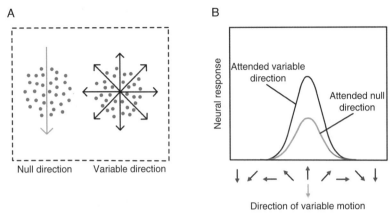

Null direction   Variable direction

Direction of variable motion

FIG. 11.2 Mechanisms of attention. Attention has been shown to boost the gain of neurons responsive to an attended feature. (A) The paradigm used by Treue and Martinez-Trujillo (1999) to demonstrate an atttentional boost of neural gain in single units in monkey MT/MST. Two stimuli are presented within a single receptive field (large dashed square): one moving in the anti-preferred (null) direction and another moving variously in one of 12 directions. The monkey maintains fixation on a point outside the receptive field and direction tuning curves are recorded under two conditions: once when the monkey attends to the anti-preferred direction, and again when it attends to the variable direction. (B) An illustration of typical tuning curves measured with this paradigm. The tuning curve shows a greater response when the variable stimulus is attended, showing that even the preferred direction needs to be attended in order to produce a maximal response from the cell. This effect can be modelled as a multiplicative gain change since the amplitude of the neuron's response increases but not its selectivity to the attended feature. In other words, the bandwidth of the tuning curve is approximately constant despite large changes in maximum response. A second possible mechanism of attentional modulation (not shown) is an additive process. This has been demonstrated in neuroimaging experiments where a cue indicating a stimulus soon to appear leads to increased levels of baseline activity prior to the appearance of the stimulus (Shulman et al. 1999; Ress et al. 2000).

attended spatial location, which argues against the response being a general increase in arousal in anticipation of the stimulus. These effects have also been observed for motion-sensitive areas in extrastriate cortex (MT/MST), where baseline increases are found when observers are presented with a non-motion cue which indicates the probable direction of a forthcoming motion stimulus (Shulman et al. 1999). Kastner et al. (1999) have also reported retinotopically localized boosts in baseline firing rate in V2 and V4 when subjects anticipated the presentation of a stimulus. These baseline shifts can be modelled as an additive factor, and thus both additive and multiplicative effects of attention can be observed.

Note that both effects could potentially coexist, as they are not mutually exclusive alternatives.

11.7 Attentional Modulation of Motion Adaptation: Psychophysics

Chaudhuri's (1991) paper sparked a lot of interest in the link between motion adaptation and attention. As already noted in the Introduction, one reason for this was that it suggested a much earlier role for attention in sensory processing than had been previously supposed. Another reason was that it contradicted an early monograph on the MAE. Wohlgemuth (1911) stated that the duration of MAEs were unaffected by concurrent distractor tasks during adaptation. Employing tasks such as mental arithmetic, Wohlgemuth reported that MAEs were 'as marked and long-lasting' (p. 83) with or without attentional distraction. Whatever the reason, Chaudhuri's study provoked a good deal of research from other investigators which will be reviewed in this section. These studies can be grouped into two categories based on their experimental designs. The first group of studies to be reviewed uses an 'opposed attribute' paradigm in which two equal and opposite stimulus attributes are presented, one of which is to be attentionally selected. The second group of studies to be discussed employs a 'distractor' paradigm, as used in Chaudhuri's (1991) original study, in which attention is drawn away from an adaptor stimulus by a demanding attentional task.

11.7.1 Motion Studies Using the 'Opposed Attributes' Paradigm

Among the first papers to appear following Chaudhuri's were two studies by Shulman (1991, 1993). The attentional task in these papers differed in an important way from Chaudhuri's. Rather than distract the observers' attention from a single translational adapting stimulus as Chaudhuri had done, Shulman presented two equal and opposite rotary motions and had observers attend to one of them. In the first study, two counter-rotating squares were presented, each centred on the same spatial location and counter-rotating in depth around a vertical axis (Fig. 11.3). After a period of adaptation to these stimuli, subjects viewed a square test stimulus whose direction of rotation was ambiguous. Normally, following adaptation to equal and opposite directions, the test stimulus would be bistable – equally likely to be perceived as rotating clockwise or anti-clockwise (Petersik et al. 1984). However, by having subjects attend to one of the squares during adaptation (their task was to detect perturbations in the square's form) it was shown that the direction of rotation during testing was reliably perceived to be opposite to the direction attended during adaptation. This study is also informative in terms of object-based attention in that attending to the rotating object to detect form perturbations also yielded an attentional effect on one of its other attributes, that of motion. Shulman's second study (1993) involved a very similar set of experiments except that rotation was in the picture plane rather than in depth. Again, an ambiguous test stimulus was reliably perceived to rotate in the direction opposite to that attended during adaptation.

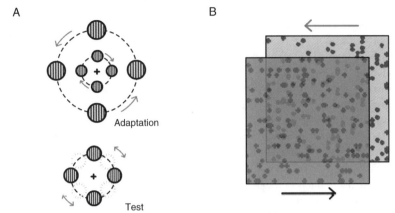

FIG. 11.3 Two examples of the 'opposed attributes' paradigm. (A) Adaptation and
test stimuli similar to those used by Shulman (1993). During adaptation, observers
were presented with sets of grating patches which rotated around the perimeter of a
virtual circle. One set of four equally-spaced grating patches rotated clockwise around
a large outer circle, while another set of four rotated anticlockwise around a small
inner circle. The grating patches were vertically oriented, with the attentional task
being, to detect occasional orientation shifts in one of the grating patches in either the
outer or inner set. Following adaptation, a test pattern of ambiguous rotation direction
was presented. It comprised four vertical grating patches spaced around a circle of
intermediate size whose location advanced by 45 deg each frame, thereby creating an
ambiguous direction of rotation. When the inner (clockwise) adapting patches were
attended, the test pattern tended to be perceived in anticlockwise rotation. Attending to
the outer (anticlockwise) patches tended to produce clockwise rotation in the test pattern.
(B) An illustration of the kind of stimuli used by Lankheet and Verstraten (1995).
Observers were presented with two transparent sheets of random dots moving in
opposite directions at the same speed. Adaptation to these stimuli will not normally
produce a motion aftereffect because equal and opposite adapting stimuli should produce
equal and opposite MAEs which would therefore cancel each other. However, by
attending to one of the motion components during adaptation, significant MAEs were
observed in the direction opposite the attended direction.

Lankheet and Verstraten (1995) explored attentional modulation of motion
adaptation in a similar paradigm. Instead of opposing two rotary motions, they
superimposed two translational motion signals that were equal and opposite in
magnitude. Normally, adaptation to equal and opposite linear motions would
null each other, producing no perceived aftereffect in a directionally ambiguous
test pattern. However, just as Shulman (1991, 1993) had found, attending to one
of the components during adaptation produced significant MAEs. To avoid the
asymptotic and criterion-related problems associated with measuring MAE
duration, they measured MAE strength by quantifying the amount of real motion
required to null the illusory motion of the aftereffect. One important aspect that

differentiates these papers from Chaudhuri's (1991) original observation is that they employ a feature-based attentional task, rather than a task designed to tightly constrict the focus of attention at the cost of the surrounding area. That is, both motion signals were spatially coextensive and the attentional selection was of a direction of motion within that region. Thus, these studies demonstrate selection of a particular feature from the visual field rather than a simple focusing of attention on a particular spatial region, which might potentially encompass a variety of features.

Another important aspect of the 'opposed motions' paradigm is that attentional selection, rather than the attenuation of motion adaptation implied by Chaudhuri's result, appears instead to strengthen the attended motion. This is presumably because that motion becomes enhanced in some way as a result of having been attentionally selected. A study by Alais and Blake (1999) explored this 'attentional boost' hypothesis further. Their study also utilized two superimposed linear motions but it varied the 'opposed motions' paradigm by pairing various motion directions and by combining a strong and a weak motion vector. Various directional separations were tested ranging from 0° to 360° in 45° intervals, and the weak motion vector consisted of 1-second periods of weakly coherent motion randomly inserted into a long period of purely random motion (Fig. 11.4). Attention was directed to the weak motion and the subjects' task was to detect the randomly inserted pulses of weak motion. The dependent measure was the direction of the MAE, the idea being to exploit the fact that MAE direction following bivectorial adaptation is uni-vectorial, in the direction opposite to the vector sum of the adapting directions. Alais and Blake's hypothesis was that if attention were to boost the responses of neurons representing the attended motion, as indicated by neurophysiological and neuroimaging studies (Gandhi et al. 1999; Treue & Martinez-Trujillo 1999; Saenz et al. 2002), then shifts in MAE direction should occur consistent with an increased weighting of the attended direction. The pattern of the results they obtained was consistent with this interpretation, supporting the gain hypothesis (Treue & Maunsell 1996; McAdams & Maunsell 1999) in which attention serves to boost the gain (without altering the bandwidth) of the neurons tuned to the attended feature.

One possible limitation of the experiments by Lankheet and Verstraten (1995) and Alais and Blake (1999) is that they are unable to determine whether the presumed boost of the attended component was accompanied by an attenuation of the unattended component due to the withdrawal of attention. In the Alais and Blake study, attenuation of the unattended component is less likely to have been a major factor because of the design of their stimulus. They used a strong motion component which was continuously present and a second weak motion component which was only intermittently present (several 1-second bursts inserted randomly over time). Since the directional component to be attended was only intermittently present, for most of the adaptation period the subject's attention by default fell upon the strong motion component (nominally, the 'unattended' component). Nevertheless, the issue of whether the attentional boost of the selected component is accompanied by an attenuation of the unattended component cannot be ruled out entirely from either study.

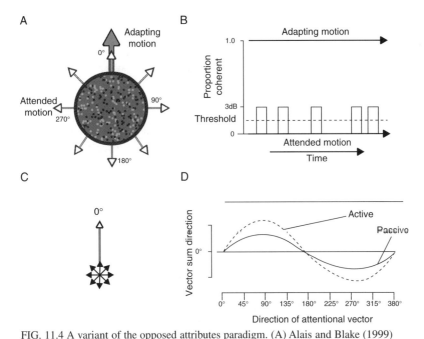

FIG. 11.4 A variant of the opposed attributes paradigm. (A) Alais and Blake (1999)
used stimuli similar to those shown here. Two sets of translating dots were
superimposed during a period of adaptation, one of which was to be attended. The
stimulus is similar to that of Lankheet and Verstraten (1995) but differs in important
ways: the two motions were not equal and opposite, and sometimes only one motion
was present. The motion to be attended was composed of light gray dots which on a
given trial drifted in one of eight directions with respect to the second motion component defined by the darker dots. (B) The strength of the 'attended' motion was weak
(just above detection threshold) whereas the strength of the other motion was maximal
(thus the 'adapting' motion). Importantly, the adapting motion was always present
while the attended motion was randomly presented for 1-second bursts. Between
bursts, the dots of the attended motion underwent incoherent motion so that no global
direction was present. Eight bursts of weak attended motion were inserted during the
32-second adaptation period and four during subsequent 16-sec periods of top-up
adaptation. The observer's task was to detect the weak motion inserts within the
1-second period of presentation. (C) The strong adapting motion and the eight directions of weak attended motion can be represented as vectors in a velocity space.
Pairing the adapting motion with any of the attended motions will produce a MAE
direction that is largely opposite the adapting motion, but with small directional deviations depending on the direction of the weaker attended motion paired with it. (D) The
directional deviations in the MAE will exhibit a sinusoidal pattern around the direction
opposite the adapting motion, with an amplitude determined by the relative strength of
the attended motion. If the attentional gain hypothesis is correct, the amplitude of this
sinusoidal deviation should be larger in the active attention condition relative to the
passive viewing condition. Alais and Blake's (1999) data confirmed this prediction.

An experiment by von Grünau *et al.* (1998) employed stimuli known as plaids to empirically separate the effects of attended and unattended components. Plaids are constructed by superimposing two gratings with different directions of motion, and they can be perceived either as a coherent pattern with a single direction or as two gratings sliding transparently over each other. When transparent, the gratings appear slightly segregated in depth and exhibit bistable behaviour over time, with one grating sometimes appearing to be the 'nearer' one and at other times the second grating appearing to be nearer. In their experiment, the plaid parameters were chosen so as to create a plaid that was almost exclusively transparent. Observers were asked to attend to one of the motion components, which had the effect of making it appear in a nearer plane than the other, and the observers' task was to keep it there throughout an adaptation period by strongly attending to it. To test the resulting MAE, a counterphase grating was used which could be oriented to match either the attended grating or the ignored grating. Relative to a no-attention baseline condition, the findings were that the MAE was stronger for the attended component and weaker for the unattended component. These results confirm that attending to one component when two are present not only entails a boost for the attended component (Lankheet & Verstraten 1995; Alais & Blake 1999), but also point to an attentional 'cost', the attenuation of the unattended component.

In a study using a simpler, single-component motion stimulus, Mukai and Watanabe (2001) found that simply attending to a single array of translating random dots was sufficient to boost the strength of its MAE, relative to a no-attention control condition. As in Lankheet and Verstraten's (1995) study, the MAE was measured using a motion nulling method in which coherent motion in the direction opposite the MAE is added to incoherent random dots to find the motion strength required to null the illusory movement of the MAE. Mukai and Watanabe attempted to go further and determine whether attention was a monocular or binocular process. Since monocular neurons are only found in primary visual cortex, this approach could possibly shed light on the cortical level at which attention exerts its influence. They did so by seeing whether attention acted on monocular or binocular components of the MAE. For this they compared conditions where MAEs were adapted and tested in the same eye with those adapted in one eye and tested in the other. The latter is an 'interocular transfer' condition designed to reveal the binocular component of the MAE, and, by subtraction from the monocular MAE, the magnitude of the purely monocular component is obtained. By measuring the effect of attention on monocular MAEs of various strengths, the authors claim that the binocular (top-down) influence of attention adds linearly with monocular (bottom-up) components of the MAE. In contrast, if linear translational motion is replaced by an expanding motion, then attention boosts MAEs equally irrespective of whether they are tested in the adapted or unadapted eye. This pattern of results for both types of MAE suggests that attention in this case is a fully binocular process.

11.7.2 Motion Studies Using the 'Distractor' Paradigm

In a series of papers, Georgiades and Harris (2000a,b; 2002a,b) returned to the original 'alphanumeric stream' distractor task employed by Chaudhuri to examine the spatial spread of attention. In their first paper (2000a), subjects adapted to a translating grating (12 deg wide and 9 deg high) while the size of the blank central window containing the alphanumeric stream varied across conditions from 0.5, 3.0, or 7.3 deg in diameter. The characters of the alphanumeric stream appeared with a fixed height and rate (0.2 deg; 1.2 Hz), and so the main factor of interest was the increasing distance between the central character stream and the inner edge of the adapting motion (Fig. 11.5(A)). In a standard non-attention condition (subjects fixated an unchanging 'zero', effectively a fixation point), there was a weak tendency for MAE duration to decrease as the size of the blank centre increased, likely due to the reduced area of adaptation. When subjects were actively engaged in the distractor task, MAE durations were

A

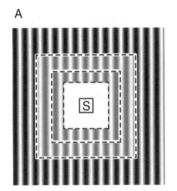

B

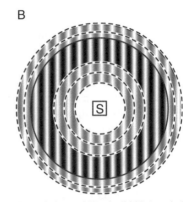

FIG. 11.5 Spatial spread of attentional focus. (A) Georgiades and Harris (2000a) varied the size of a blank window containing an alphanumeric stream centred within a larger drifting grating. Character size and task difficulty were constant. Strong decreases in MAE duration were measured in the active attention condition (relative to passive) regardless of the size of the central window, replicating Chaudhuri (1991). There was a slight tendency for this decrease to lessen as window size increased, suggesting that the attenuation of motion processing in the region surrounding the attentional focus is less pronounced as distance increases. The weakness of the trend might be due to the reducing area of adapting grating as the inner window increases. (B) In a second version of this experiment, Georgiades and Harris changed the adapting grating to an annular form so that increases in the size of the inner window could be offset by increasing the outer radius so as to maintain a constant area of adapting grating. This experiment confirmed, with a stronger trend, the finding that MAEs from areas more distant from the attentional focus are less attenuated by attentional focus on the distractor task. In sum, it appears that the reduction in motion processing in the region surrounding the distractor task (the 'cost' of attention) is localized to a certain extent and gradually recovers with increasing distance from the attentional focus.

lower overall (a main effect of attention, replicating Chaudhuri) but no interaction between MAE duration and window size was observed. In a second experiment, the form of the adapting grating was annular instead of square so that grating eccentricity could be varied (Fig. 11.5(B)). For fixed-area annuli with inner diameters of 1.2, 2.7, 3.8 deg, they found that MAE durations in the active attention condition increased slightly with increasing diameter of the annulus (2000a). While the effect is not strong, possibly a result of the small range of eccentricity they used, it does suggest that the region of attenuated processing surrounding the focal point of attention recovers slightly as distance from the attentional focal point increases. Similar results are obtained when MAE speed instead of MAE duration is used as the dependent measure (Georgiades & Harris 2000b).

Support for a shallow gradient of recovery from attenuation in the area surrounding a spatial focus of attention comes from another study to employ Chaudhuri's alphanumeric distractor task (Takeuchi & Kita 1994). These authors conducted a study very similar to Chaudhuri's original experiment with the difference that they compared motion adaptation stimuli of various sizes (5, 10, and 20° radius). They confirmed Chaudhuri's original finding of attenuated MAEs of translational motion during active attention, but only for radii of 5 or 10°. For the motion stimulus with a radius of 20°, no attenuation of MAE duration was observed during active attention to the alphanumeric distractor. Thus, the MAE attenuation reported originally by Chaudhuri does indeed appear to be limited in spatial extent. There is also some evidence to suggest that the influence that stationary surrounding patterns can exert on motion adaptation (Strelow & Day 1975) can also be modulated by attention (Georgiades & Harris 2002a). Together, these findings are broadly consistent with conclusions from other approaches to attention (such as visual search) that the 'spotlight' of attention, while spatially limited, is nonetheless quite broad and blurred (Egly & Homa 1984; LaBerge & Brown 1989). The term 'blur' in this case means that attentional effects are strongest at the centre of focus and dissipate with radial distance.

11.7.3 Non-motion Studies Using the 'Distractor' Paradigm

In addition to attentional modulation of motion adaptation, there are several reports of attention modulating other forms of adaptation. In a variant of his 1991 study described above, Shulman (1992) presented subjects with two superimposed Schroder staircases, one upright, the other inverted (Fig. 11.6(A)). The Schroder staircase is a simple, two-dimensional line drawing of stairs whose perspective is ambiguous so that the implied three-dimensionality of the staircase is perceptually bistable and therefore reverses over time. In Shulman's experiment, a small upright staircase was embedded in a larger inverted staircase. The staircases differed slightly in colour and subjects were instructed to direct their attention to one of the staircases during adaptation in order to detect small color changes. Following a period of adaptation to these stimuli,

A

B

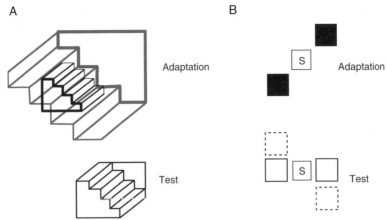

FIG. 11.6 Adaptation also influences figural aftereffects. (A) In the classical Schroder staircase figure (shown here as the test figure), a set of stairs is sketched in the form of a simple line drawing. In the absence of other pictorial cues, the only indication to the implied three-dimensionality of the stairs is perspective, and in this case it supports two possible viewpoints. For this reason, the figure is bistable and extended viewing of the test figure will produce intermittent alternations in perspective. Shulman (1992) superimposed two Schroder-like staircases (see adaptation figure), with each of them slightly altered to support a single (and opposing) viewpoint. This was achieved by removing the far surface from each perspective and by highlighting the near surface. Observers were instructed to attend to one of the staircases during adaptation in order to detect occasional changes in its colour (one staircase was red, the other green). This tended to make the attended perspective more dominant during adaptation, with the result that the normally ambiguous Schroder figure used for the test stimulus was seen predominantly in the perspective opposite the perspective of the attended staircase. (B) A version of the figural aftereffect used by Yeh *et al.* (1996). Adaptation to a pair of inducing elements aligned obliquely along a virtual line through the fixation point causes a test pattern composed of horizontally aligned elements to be perceived along the opposite oblique. When an alphanumeric stream task was located at the fixation point, the magnitude of the effect was reduced. However, in a divided attention task where observers directed their attention equally to each of the inducers, the effect is not reduced.

subjects were tested with a single staircase of ambiguous perspective and asked to indicate which perspective was perceived. When subjects directed their attention to one of the adapting staircases in order to detect colour changes, their test judgements of perspective were always opposite the perspective of the attended figure. Thus, the attentional condition produced results similar to those that would have been obtained had the adaptation been to a single, unambiguous staircase (which would have stabilized the ambiguity of a Schroder staircase in the perspective opposite that of the adapting staircase).

Another example of attentional modulation of non-motion adaptation comes from Yeh *et al.* (1996). Their study utilized the so-called figural aftereffect (Kohler & Wallach 1944). To produce the effect, subjects adapt to two small squares located on either side of fixation and aligned along a virtual oblique line (like a tilted horizon) (Fig. 11.6(B)). The aftereffect is seen in a test stimulus composed of two horizontally aligned squares, which appear displaced towards an alignment along the opposite oblique. As an attentional task, Yeh *et al.* used an alphanumeric distractor task similar to Chaudhuri's. The result they report is analogous to Chaudhuri's in that when the distractor task was located at fixation, the figural aftereffect was greatly reduced, as if a tight focus of attention excluded full processing of the inducing elements lying beyond fixation. This presumably reduced the salience of the inducers to the point where they were not sufficient to create an impression of a virtual oblique. However, when a dual task was used in which separate alphanumeric streams were located on each inducing element, requiring subjects to divide their attentional focus equally between the inducers, the figural aftereffect was not reduced. In this case, the inducing elements would not be attenuated because they would benefit from the allocation of attention, allowing adaptation to a salient virtual oblique to occur. Interestingly, there was no increase in effect size during divided attention, as might be predicted by the gain hypothesis. The probable reason for this is that the orientation of the virtual line is not altered by the salience of the inducers.

Another study to show attentional modulation of adaptation in a non-motion context was conducted by Rose *et al.* (2003). Their study employed the stereoscopic depth aftereffect (Blakemore & Julesz 1971) and an alphanumeric distractor task. The authors compared the magnitude of the stereoscopic depth aftereffect for attentional conditions of various levels of difficulty and reported a dependency on task difficulty, with demanding distractor tasks reducing the aftereffect more than easier tasks.

Attention has also been found to modulate the magnitude of the direct tilt aftereffect (Spivey & Spirn 2000), a result that links attentional modulation to V1 activity more directly than does modulation of the MAE. Spivey and Spirn presented two superimposed gratings, one tilted slightly leftward of vertical and the other slightly rightward, and asked observers to attend to one of them while keeping their gaze steady on a central fixation point. Normally, adaptation to gratings oriented with equal and opposite tilt around vertical would produce no orientation aftereffect in a vertical test grating. However, when subjects directed their attention to one of the gratings during adaptation their judgements of the test stimulus generally indicated a tilt away from the attended orientation, consistent with the gain hypothesis mentioned above in which the response to an attended feature is boosted by attentional selection. The authors, however, caution that the effect was usually weak and in some cases, absent. This may be due to the rather small orientational shifts the tilt aftereffect generally produces, but might also indicate that attentional gain in primary visual cortex, the presumed site of the tilt aftereffect, is less than typically observed in extrastriate areas (Treue & Maunsell 1996; McAdams & Maunsell 1999; Treue & Martinez-Trujillo 1999).

11.8 A Theoretical Framework for Attentional Modulation

In light of the many reports concerning attentional modulation of adaptation to motion and other stimuli that have appeared since Chaudhuri's (1991) original study, what sort of theoretical framework could account for these findings? One model that lends itself well to accounting for results from both paradigms is Lavie's (1995) attentional load theory. This theory proposes that the degree of processing of unattended stimuli depends on the amount of resources dedicated to the attentional task. It is a flexible theory, in that it could resemble the early-selection or the late-selection models. If a distractor task were made very demanding so as to necessitate a good deal of attentional resources, little residual capacity would be left to process other stimuli, as in an early-selection model. In contrast, if attentional demands were made low, leaving sufficient resources to process stimuli other than the attentionally selected one, then the model would resemble a late-selection model. In Chaudhuri's experiments, the presentation of the alphanumeric task at a rate of 4 Hz and a strict emphasis on not making more than 5 per cent errors was presumably demanding enough to substantially engage attentional resources, consequently leaving the processing of the surrounding motion stimulus severely impoverished. This is significant because, as has now become clear, without attention expressly directed at a stimulus, we can be virtually blind to it. Studies of inattention (Mack & Rock 1998) and change blindness (Rensink et al. 1997; Simons & Levin 1999) illustrate this point. In keeping with this, Chaudhuri reported very large attenuation effects when comparing the active and passive conditions: an average three-fold reduction in MAE duration.

The level of attentional demand then provides a framework for understanding the Chaudhuri result and the many other studies inspired by it. Indeed, Rees et al. (1997) tested this notion explicitly in a psychophysical paradigm very similar to Chaudhuri's original one which was conducted in conjunction with fMRI scanning. They measured the amount of activity generated in area MT by a motion stimulus while subjects were engaged on a distractor word-task of variable difficulty. The low-load condition required subjects to detect words presented in upper-case letters, while the more complex high-load condition required subjects to detect words that were bisyllabic. Their fMRI results showed that the amount of cortical activity generated by the motion stimulus, which was always irrelevant to the subject's task, depended on the difficulty of the distractor task. As predicted by their attentional load theory, an easy task was found to produce more MT activity than a difficult task. Their fMRI data were complemented by psychophysical measurements which demonstrated that the higher-load distractor did indeed result in reduced MAE durations relative to the low-load distractor. This result has been confirmed in a recent psychophysical investigation employing the same alphanumeric distractor task as Chaudhuri used (Rose et al. 2003). Task difficulty was varied by changing the presentation rate of the alphanumeric stream and their results showed that the higher rate of presentation attenuated aftereffect duration more than did the slower rate. Moreover, this model is not restricted to visual processing. Attentional demands from other sensory modalities could take up attentional resources and leave visual processing impoverished. Berman and Colby (2002) investigated visual motion adaptation and MAEs using fMRI. They compared attentional distractor tasks that were either visual or auditory and found that both were effective in reducing activation in the visual system's motion-specialized area, MT. This was observed during the motion adaptation phase, and in both cases this elicited reduced MAE durations. This points to a single attentional system with limited resources that is supramodal and from which both visual and auditory processing draw.

11.9 Evaluating Psychophysical Approaches to Attentional Modulation

There are several important points of difference between Chaudhuri's original 'distractor' paradigm and the 'opposed attributes' paradigm used in many of the studies that followed. In both kinds of experiment, two stimuli are typically present, however, in the 'distractor' paradigm, attention is allocated to one stimulus while the effect of attention is measured on the other (unattended) stimulus which surrounds it. The characteristic result is one of attenuation in which adaptation to the surrounding stimulus is weakened in the active 'distractor' condition compared to the passive condition. This is presumed to be indicative of a less vigorous sensory processing of the unattended surrounding stimulus when attentional resources are allocated to a competing task. It also indicates a spatial role for attention as the attenuation can be conceived of as a loss of cortical processing due to a tight focusing of the attentional spotlight on the demanding alphanumeric task. It is noteworthy, too, that the distractor task in this type of experiment is of a completely different kind to the stimulus whose adaptation is being measured. For example, in Chaudhuri's study, alphanumeric detection is fundamentally different to detection of translational motion and involves different cognitive and cortical processes. The fMRI data of Rees *et al.* (1997), in a modification of Chaudhuri's paradigm, indicate this very clearly.

The 'opposed attributes' paradigm differs significantly from the 'distractor' paradigm in that two stimuli of the same kind are presented in spatial superposition. Generally, the stimuli are opposed in some way, for example in motion (Lankheet & Verstraten 1995) or orientation (Spivey & Spirn 2000). In this type of experiment, one of the two stimuli is selected attentively, although the other will continue to activate the same portion of the retina. Consequently, this paradigm emphasizes feature-based rather than spatially-based selection. The attentional effect in this case is twofold. First, the selected stimulus contributes more strongly to the resulting measure of adaptation, implying a more vigorous response to the attended stimulus during adaptation, and second, there is an attenuation of the non-selected stimulus. Because the stimuli are opposed within a feature dimension and are nominally equal in strength, their adaptations would be expected to null each other. This is indeed what happens in a passive viewing condition. However, when one is attentionally selected, a non-null aftereffect obtains whose sign is consistent with a boost in the cortical response to the attentionally selected stimulus and/or an attenuated response to the unattended stimulus.

Overall, a general definition of the role of attention would be that it serves to improve performance or sensitivity on a given task. This is most clearly seen in the 'opposed attributes' paradigm, where a non-null result is indicative of an attentional boost in the strength of one of the competing attributes (and/or an attenuated response to the unattended stimulus). By contrast, if this is not evident in the 'distractor' paradigm, the reason is simply that it is not performance on the attended stimulus that is being measured. However, if the number of errors (for example, false alarms or misses) in the passive viewing condition were to be measured and compared with that obtained in the condition where subjects actively attended the alphanumeric stream, clear differences would be expected to result. Indeed, without paying particular attention to the rapid alphanumeric stream, it is difficult to see how anything other than a high error rate could possibly result. In Chaudhuri's experiment, the criterion for the inclusion of subjects' data was set rather high (at least 95 per cent correct), which the subjects were able to meet only if they paid close attention to the task.

11.10 Summary

Our knowledge of attentional modulation of basic perceptual processes such as motion processing was spawned by a seminal paper by Chaudhuri (1991). His finding that MAE durations were dramatically reduced if an observer's attention during adaptation was engaged on a demanding second task pointed to strong modulatory effects of attention at the earliest stages of cortical processing. Numerous psychophysical studies subsequently appeared supporting this observation and extending it to other basic visual attributes, and neurophysiological and neuroimaging studies provided confirmation that attention indeed exerted modulatory effects at early stages of visual cortex. Two basic psychophysical approaches emerged for studying attention: the 'distractor' paradigm, which Chaudhuri had developed, and the 'opposed attributes' paradigm, in which one member of an opposed pair of stimuli is attentionally selected. The 'opposed attributes' paradigm involves adaptation to two overlapping stimuli with equal and opposite attributes, such as opposed motions or tilts. Normally, this would produce no net aftereffect, however, if one of the stimuli is attended during adaptation, significant aftereffects are elicited. This illustrates the important points that attention can select a single object or attribute among several sharing the same spatial location, and that once selected, the cortical response to that object is boosted while that of the non-selected stimulus is attenuated. Chaudhuri's distractor paradigm illustrates other important points. His finding was that exposure to a translating motion stimulus elicits a weaker MAE when the subject is engaged in a demanding second task during adaptation. The weaker MAE presumably results from a reduced neural response to the stimulus during the adaptation phase. This implication, rather surprisingly at the time, suggested that the encoding of basic attributes such as motion was neither prior to the realm of attention nor entirely automatic. In other words, even a salient motion stimulus requires some amount of directed attention if it is to optimally activate motion detectors.

References

Adelson, E.H., & Bergen, J.R. (1985). Spatiotemporal energy models for the perception of motion. *Journal of the Optical Society of America Series A, 2*, 284–99.

Alais, D., & Blake, R. (1999). Neural strength of visual attention gauged by motion adaptation. *Nature Neuroscience, 2*, 1015–8.

Albright, T.D. (1984). Direction and orientation selectivity of neurons in visual area MT of the macaque. *Journal of Neurophysiology, 52*, 1106–30.

Barbas, H. (1988). Anatomic organization of basoventral and mediodorsal visual recipient prefrontal regions in the rhesus monkey. *Journal of Comparative Neurology, 276*, 313–42.

Barlow, H.B., & Hill, R.M. (1963). Evidence for a physiological explanation of the waterfall phenomenon and figural after-effects. *Nature, 200*, 1345–7.

Beauchamp, M.S., Cox, R.W., & DeYoe, E.A. (1997). Graded effects of spatial and featural attention on human area MT and associated motion processing areas. *Journal of Neurophysiology, 78*, 516–20.

Berman, R.A., & Colby, C.L. (2002). Auditory and visual attention modulate motion processing in area MT+. *Brain Research: Cognitive Brain Research, 14*, 64–74.

Bisley, J.W., & Goldberg, M.E. (2003). Neuronal activity in the lateral intraparietal area and spatial attention. *Science, 299*, 81–6.

Blakemore, C., & Julesz, B. (1971). Stereoscopic depth aftereffect produced without monocular cues. *Science, 171*, 286–88.

Britten, K.H., & Newsome, W.T. (1998). Tuning bandwidths for near-threshold stimuli in area MT. *Journal of Neurophysiology, 80*, 762–70.

Broadbent, D.E. (1958). *Perception and Communication.* London UK: Pergamon.

Broadbent, D.E. (1982). Task combination and the selective intake of information. *Acta Psychologica, 50*, 253–90.

Buchel, C., Josephs, O., Rees, G., Turner, R., Frith, C.D., & Friston, K.J. (1998). The functional anatomy of attention to visual motion. A functional MRI study. *Brain, 121*, 1281–94.

Carandini, M., Heeger, D.J., & Movshon, J.A. (1997). Linearity and normalization in simple cells of the macaque primary visual cortex. *Journal of Neuroscience, 17*, 8621–44.

Chaudhuri, A. (1991). Modulation of the motion after-effect by selective attention. *Nature, 344*, 60–2.

Connor, C.E., Preddie, D.C., Gallant, J.L., & Van Essen, D.C. (1997). Spatial attention effects in macaque area V4. *Journal of Neuroscience, 17*, 3201–14.

Corbetta, M., Miezin, F.M., Dobmeyer, S., Shulman, G.L., & Petersen, S.E. (1990). Attentional modulation of neural processing of shape, color, and velocity in humans. *Science, 248*, 1556–9.

Corbetta, M., Miezin, F.M., Dobmeyer, S., Shulman, G.L., & Petersen, S.E. (1991). Selective and divided attention during visual discriminations of shape, color, and speed: functional anatomy by positron emission tomography. *Journal of Neuroscience, 11*, 2383–402.

Corbetta, M., Miezin, F., Shulman, G., & Petersen, S. (1993). A PET study of visualspatial attention. *Journal of Neuroscience, 13*, 1202–26.

Culham, J.C., Dukelow, S.P., Vilis, T., Hassard, F.A., Gati, J.S., Menon, R.S., & Goodale, M.A. (1999). Recovery of fMRI activation in motion area MT following storage of the motion aftereffect. *Journal of Neurophysiology, 81*, 388–93.

Desimone, R., & Duncan, J. (1995). Neural mechanisms of selective visual attention. *Annual Review of Neuroscience, 18*, 193–222.

Deutsch, J.A., & Deutsch, D. (1963). Attention: some theoretical considerations. *Psychological Review, 70*, 80–90.

Dick, M., Ullman, S., & Sagi, D. (1987). Parallel and serial processes in motion detection. *Science, 237*, 400–02.

Driver, J., & Baylis, G.C. (1989). Movement and visual attention: the spotlight metaphor breaks down. *Journal of Experimental Psychology: Human Perception and Performance, 15*, 448–56.

Egeth, H., & Yantis, S. (1997). Visual attention: control, representation, and time course. *Annual Review of Psychology, 48*, 269–97.

Egly, R., & Homa, D. (1984). Sensitization of the visual field. *Journal of Experimental Psychology: Human Perception and Performance, 10*, 778–93.

Eriksen, B.A., & Eriksen, C.W. (1974). Effect of noise letters upon the identification of a target letter in a non-search task. *Perception and Psychophysics, 16*, 43–9.

Eriksen, C.W., & St James, J.D. (1986). Visual attention within and around the field of focal attention: a zoom lens model. *Perception and Psychophysics, 40*, 225–40.

Felleman, D.J., & Van Essen, D.C. (1991). Distributed hierarchical processing in the primate cerebral cortex. *Cerebral Cortex, 1*, 1–47

Gandhi, S.P., Heeger, D.J., & Boynton, G.M. (1999). Spatial attention affects brain activity in human primary visual cortex. *Proceedings of the Academy of Sciences USA, 96*, 3314–9.

Gegenfurtner, K.R., Kiper, D.C., & Levitt, J.B. (1997). Functional properties of neurons in macaque area V3. *Journal of Neurophysiology, 77*, 1906–23.

Georgiades, M., & Harris, J. (2000a). The spatial spread of attentional modulation of the motion aftereffect. *Perception, 29*, 1185–201.

Georgiades, M., & Harris, J. (2000b). Attentional diversion during adaptation affects the velocity as well as the duration of motion after-effects. *Proceedings of the Royal Society of London. Series B, 267*, 2559–65.

Georgiades, M., & Harris, J. (2002a). Effects of attentional modulation of a stationary surround in adaptation to motion. *Perception, 31*, 393–408.

Georgiades, M., & Harris, J. (2002b). Evidence for spatio-temporal selectivity in attentional modulation of the motion aftereffect. *Spatial Vision, 16*, 21–31.

von Grunau, M.W., Bertone, A., & Pakneshan, P. (1998). Attentional selection of motion states. *Spatial Vision, 11*, 329–47.

Hautzel, H., Taylor, J.G., Krause, B.J., Schmitz, N., Tellmann, L., Ziemons, K. *et al.* (2001). The motion aftereffect: more than area V5/MT?: evidence from 15O-butanol PET studies. *Brain Research, 892*, 281–92.

He, S., Cohen, E.R., & Hu, X. (1998). Close correlation between activity in brain area MT/V5 and the perception of a visual motion aftereffect. *Current Biology, 8*, 1215–18.

Horowitz, T., & Treisman, A. (1994). Attention and apparent motion. *Spatial Vision, 8,* 193–219.

Hubel, D., & Wiesel, T. (1968). Receptive fields and functional architecture of monkey striate cortex. *Journal of Physiology, 195,* 215–43.

Huk, A.C., & Heeger, D.J. (2000). Task-related modulation of visual cortex. *Journal of Neurophysiology, 83,* 3525–36.

Huk, A.C., Ress, D., & Heeger, D.J. (2001). Neuronal basis of the motion aftereffect reconsidered. *Neuron, 32,* 161–72.

Hupé, J.M., James, A.C., Payne, B.R., Lomber, S.G., Girard, P., & Bullier, J. (1998). Cortical feedback improves discrimination between figure and background by V1, V2 and V3 neurons. *Nature, 394,* 784–7.

Ito, M., & Gilbert, C. (1999). Attention modulates contextual influences in the primary visual cortex of alert monkeys. *Neuron, 22,* 593–604.

Kastner, S., Pinsk, M.A., De Weerd, P., Desimone, R., & Ungerleider, L.G. (1999). Increased activity in human visual cortex during directed attention in the absence of visual stimulation. *Neuron, 22,* 751–61.

Kohler, W., & Wallach, H. (1944). Figural aftereffects: An investigation of visual processes. *American Philosophical Society, 88,* 269–357.

Kohn, A., & Movshon, J.A. (2003). Neuronal adaptation to visual motion in area MT of the macaque. *Neuron, 39,* 681–91.

LaBerge, D., & Brown, V. (1989). Theory and measurement of attentional operations in shape identification. *Psychological Review, 96,* 101–24.

Lankheet, M.J., & Verstraten, F.A. (1995). Attentional modulation of adaptation to two-component transparent motion. *Vision Research, 35,* 1401–12.

Lavie, N. (1995). Perceptual load as a necessary condition for selective attention. *Journal of Experimental Psychology: Human Perception and Performance, 21,* 451–68.

Luck, S., Chelazzi, L., Hillyard, S., & Desimone, R. (1997). Neural mechanisms of spatial selective attention in areas V1, V2, and V4 of macaque visual cortex. *Journal of Neurophysiology, 77,* 24–42.

Mack, A., & Rock, I. (1998). *Inattentional Blindness.* Cambridge MA: MIT Press.

Marr D (1982). *Vision.* New York: W.H. Freeman and Co.

Maunsell, J.H., & Van Essen, D.C. (1983). Functional properties of neurons in middle temporal visual area of the macaque monkey. I. Selectivity for stimulus direction, speed, and orientation. *Journal of Neurophysiology, 49,* 1127–47.

McAdams, C.J., & Maunsell, J.H. (1999). Effects of attention on orientation-tuning functions of single neurons in macaque cortical area V4. *Journal of Neuroscience, 19,* 431–41.

McLeod, P., Driver, J., & Crisp, J. (1988). Visual search for a conjunction of movement and form is parallel. *Nature, 332,* 154–5.

Mignard, M., & Malpeli, J.G. (1991). Paths of information flow through visual cortex. *Science, 251,* 1249–51.

Moran, J., & Desimone, R. (1985). Selective attention gates visual processing in the extrastriate cortex. *Science, 229,* 782–4.

Moray, N. (1959). Attention in dichotic listening: affective cues and the influence of instructions. *Quarterly Journal of Experimental Psychology, 11,* 56–60.

Motter, B. (1993). Focal attention produces spatially selective processing in visual cortical areas V1, V2, and V4 in the presence of competing stimuli. *Journal of Neurophysiology, 70,* 909–19.

Mukai, I., & Watanabe, T. (2001). Differential effect of attention to translation and expansion on motion aftereffects (MAE). *Vision Research*, *41*, 1107–17.

Nakayama, K., & Silverman, G.H. (1986). Serial and parallel processing of visual feature conjunctions. *Nature*, *320*, 264–5.

Neisser, U., & Becklen, R. (1975). Selective looking: attending to visually specified events. *Cognitive Psychology*, *7*, 480–94.

Newsome, W.T., & Paré, E.B. (1988). A selective impairment of motion perception following lesions of the middle temporal visual area (MT). *Journal of Neuroscience*, *4*, 2201–11.

Nishida, S., & Ashida, H. (2000). A hierarchical structure of motion system revealed by interocular transfer of flicker motion aftereffects. *Vision Research*, *40*, 265–78.

Nobre, A., Sebestyen, B., Gitelmen, D., Mesulam, M., Frackowiak, R., & Frith, C. (1997). Functional localization of the system for visuospatial attention using positron emission tomography. *Brain*, *120*, 515–33.

O'Craven, K.M., Rosen, B.R., Kwong, K.K., Treisman, A., & Savoy, R.L. (1997). Voluntary attention modulates fMRI activity in human MT-MST. *Neuron*, *18*, 591–8.

O'Craven, K.M., Downing, P.E., & Kanwisher, N. (1999). fMRI evidence for objects as the units of attentional selection. *Nature*, *401*, 584–7.

Olson, I., Chun, M., & Allison, T. (2001). Contextual guidance of attention. Human intracranial event-related potential evidence for feedback modulation in anatomically early, temporally late stages of visual processing. *Brain*, *124*, 1417–25.

Petersik, A., Shepard, A., & Malsch, R. (1984). A three-dimensional motion aftereffect produced by prolonged adaptation to a rotation simulation. *Perception, 13*, 488–97.

Posner, M. (1980). Orienting of attention. *Quarterly Journal of Experimental Psychology*, *32*, 2–25.

Posner, M., Walker, J., Friedrich, F., & Rafal, R. (1984). Effects of parietal lobe injury on covert orienting of visual attention. *Journal of Neuroscience*, *4*, 1863–74.

Prinzmetal, W., Nwachuku, I., Bodanski, L., Blumenfeld, L., & Shimizu, N. (1997). The Phenomenology of Attention. *Conscious Cogn. 6*, 372–412.

Recanzone, G., Wurtz, R., & Schwarz, U. (1997). Responses of MT and MST neurons to one and two moving objects in the receptive field. *Journal of Neurophysiology*, *78*, 2904–15.

Rees, G., Frith, C., & Lavie, N. (1997). Modulating irrelevant motion perception by varying attentional load in an unrelated task. *Science*, *278*, 1616–19.

Rensink, R.A., O'Regan, J.K., & Clark, J. (1997). To see or not to see: the need for attention to perceive changes in scenes. *Psychological Science*, *8*, 368–73.

Ress, D., Backus, B.T., & Heeger, D.J. (2000). Activity in primary visual cortex predicts performance in a visual detection task. *Nature Neuroscience*, *3*, 940–5.

Reynolds, J.H., Chelazzi, L., & Desimone, R. (1999). Competitive mechanisms subserve attention in macaque areas V2 and V4. *Journal of Neuroscience*, *19*, 1736–53.

Rodman, H.R., & Albright, T.D. (1987). Coding of visual stimulus velocity in area MT of the macaque. *Vision Research*, *27*, 2035–48.

Rose, D., Bradshaw, M.F., & Hibbard, P.B. (2003). Attention affects the stereoscopic depth aftereffect. *Perception*, *32*, 635–40.

Saenz, M., Buracas, G.T., & Boynton, G.M. (2002). Global effects of feature-based attention in human visual cortex. *Nature Neuroscience*, *5*, 631–2.

Seidemann, E., & Newsome, W.T. (1999). Effect of spatial attention on the responses of area MT neurons. *Journal of Neurophysiology*, *81*, 1783–94.

Seiffert, A.E., Somers, D.C., Dale, A.M., & Tootell, R.B. (2003). Functional MRI studies of human visual motion perception: texture, luminance, attention and after-effects. *Cerebral Cortex, 13*, 340–9.

Shipp, S., & Zeki, S. (1989). The Organization of Connections between Areas V5 and V1 in Macaque Monkey Visual Cortex. *European Journal of Neuroscience, 1*, 309–32.

Shulman, G.L. (1991). Attentional modulation of mechanisms that analyze rotation in depth. *Journal of Experimental Psychology: Human Perception and Performance, 17*, 726–37.

Shulman, G.L. (1992). Attentional modulation of a figural aftereffect. *Perception, 21*, 7–19.

Shulman, G.L. (1993). Attentional effects of adaptation of rotary motion in the plane. *Perception, 22*, 947–61.

Shulman, G.L., Ollinger, J.M., Akbudak, E., Conturo, T.E., Snyder, A.Z., Petersen, S.E. *et al.* (1999). Areas involved in encoding and applying directional expectations to moving objects. *Journal of Neuroscience, 19*, 9480–96.

Sillito, A.M., Jones, H.E., Gerstein, G.L., & West, D.C. (1994). Feature-linked synchronization of thalamic relay cell firing induced by feedback from the visual cortex. *Nature, 369*, 479–82.

Simoncelli, E.P., & Heeger, D.J. (1998). A model of neuronal responses in visual area MT. *Vision Research, 38*, 743–61.

Simons, D.J., & Levin, D.T. (1997). Change Blindness. *Trends in Cognitive Sciences, 1*, 261–67.

Singh, K.D., Smith, A.T., & Greenlee, M.W. (2000). Spatiotemporal frequency and direction sensitivities of human visual areas measured using fMRI. *Neuroimage, 12*, 550–64.

Somers, D.C., Dale, A.M., Seiffert, A.E., & Tootell, R.B. (1999). Functional MRI reveals spatially specific attentional modulation in human primary visual cortex. *Proceedings of the Academy of Sciences USA, 96*, 1663–8.

Spivey, M.J., & Spirn, M.J. (2000). Selective visual attention modulates the direct tilt aftereffect. *Perception and Psychophysics, 62*, 1525–33.

Strelow, E.R., & Day, R.H. (1975). Visual movement aftereffect: evidence for independent adaptation to moving target and stationary surround. *Vision Research, 15*, 117–21.

Sutherland, N. (1961). Figural after-effects and apparent size. *Quarterly Journal of Experimental Psychology, 13*, 222–28.

Takeuchi, T., & Kita, S. (1994). Attentional modulation in motion aftereffect. *Japanese Psychological Research, 36*, 94–107.

Taylor, J.G., Schmitz, N., Ziemons, K., Grosse-Ruyken, M.L., Gruber, O., Mueller-Gaertner, H.W. *et al.* (2000). The network of brain areas involved in the motion aftereffect. *Neuroimage, 11*, 257–70.

Tootell, R.B.H., Reppas, J.B., Dale, A.M., Look, R.B., Sereno, M.I., Malach, R. *et al.* (1995). Visual motion aftereffect in human cortical area MT revealed by functional magnetic resonance imaging. *Nature, 375*, 139–41.

Treisman, A. (1969). Strategies and models of visual attention. *Psychological Review, 76*, 282–99.

Treisman, A., & Gelade, G. (1980). A feature integration theory of attention. *Cognitive Psychology, 12*, 97–136.

Treue, S., & Martinez-Trujillo, J.C. (1999). Feature-based attention influences motion processing gain in macaque visual cortex. *Nature, 399*, 575–9.

Treue, S., & Maunsell, J.H. (1996). Attentional modulation of visual motion processing in cortical areas MT and MST. *Nature, 382*, 539–41.

Ungerleider, L.G., Gaffan, D., & Pelak, V.S. (1989). Projections from inferior temporal cortex to prefrontal cortex via the uncinate fascicle in rhesus monkeys. *Experimental Brain Research, 76*, 473–84.

Vallar, G., & Perani, D. (1986). The anatomy of unilateral neglect after right-hemisphere stroke lesions: A clinical/CT-scan correlation study in man. *Neuropsychologia, 24*, 609–22.

Vanduffel, W., Fize, D., Mandeville, J.B., Nelissen, K., Van Hecke, P., Rosen, B.R. *et al.* (2001). Visual motion processing investigated using contrast agent-enhanced fMRI in awake behaving monkeys. *Neuron, 20*, 565–77.

Van Essen, D.C., Anderson, C.H., & Felleman, D.J. (1992). Information processing in the primate visual system: an integrated systems perspective. *Science, 255*, 419–23.

van Santen, J.P., & Sperling, G. (1985). Elaborated Reichardt detectors. *Journal of the Optical Society of America, Series A, 2*, 300–21.

Watanabe, T., Harner, A.M., Miyauchi, S., Sasaki, Y., Nielsen, M., Palomo, D. *et al.* (1998). Task-dependent influences of attention on the activation of human primary visual cortex. *Proceedings of the Academy of Sciences USA, 95*, 11489–92.

Watson, J.D.G., Myers, R., Frackowiak, R.S.J., Hajnal, J.V., Woods, R.P., Mazziota, J.C., *et al.* (1993). Area V5 of the human brain: evidence from a combined study using positron emission tomography and magnetic resonance imaging. *Cerebral Cortex, 3*, 79–94.

Wilson, H.R., Ferrera, V.P., & Yo, C. (1992). A psychophysically motivated model for two-dimensional motion perception. *Visual Neuroscience, 9*, 79–97.

Wohlgemuth, A. (1911). On the after-effect of seen movement. *British Journal of Psychology: Monograph Supplement, 1*, 1–117.

Wurtz, R., & Mohler, C. (1976). Enhancement of visual responses in monkey striate cortex and frontal eye fields. *Journal of Neurophysiology, 39*, 766–72.

Yeh, S.-L., Chen, I.-P., De Valois, K., & De Valois, R. (1996). Figural aftereffects and spatial attention. *Journal of Experimental Psychology: Human Perception and Performance, 22*, 446–60.

Zeki, S.M. (1974). Functional organization of a visual area in the posterior bank of the superior temporal sulcus of the rhesus monkey. *Journal of Physiology, 236*, 549–73.

Zeki, S.M. (1993). *A Vision of the Brain*, Oxford UK: Blackwell Scientific.

Zeki, S., Watson, J.D.G., & Frackowiak, R.S.J. (1993). Going beyond the information given: The relation of illusory visual motion to brain activity. *Proceedings of the Royal Society of London. Series B, 252*, 215–22.

12

Adaptation and Perceptual Binding in Sight and Sound

DEREK H. ARNOLD AND DAVID WHITNEY

12.1 Introduction

Our brains have no direct access to information concerning the external environment. For instance, information concerning sight and sound is carried by propagations of physical energy carried by waves of differing length. To see and hear we have to convert these physical signals into neural events and determine correspondences between the consequent neural activity and the properties of our environment. We have a good understanding as to how we convert physical signals into simple neural events but very little understanding concerning the inferential processes that are set in train by this transduction. In fact, the little knowledge that we do possess often seems to pose more questions than answers.

Our abilities to see and hear are mediated by sensory systems that are, at least initially, independent. Despite this initial physical and functional segregation, our brains seem to effortlessly integrate information encoded by the different sensory modalities. The need to integrate information provided by independent analyses is most evident when we consider different sensory modalities, like vision and audition. However, the brain may also need to integrate different types of information from within a single sensory modality. Vision, for instance, appears to be marked by considerable functional segregation. The analysis of different stimulus attributes, like colour and motion, are independent (Zeki 1978;

339

Livingstone & Hubel 1988). If this characterization is accurate, a central difficulty that needs to be resolved by the brain is how to bind information provided
by initially independent systems. In vision, this dilemma has been referred to
as the perceptual binding problem.

Studies using adaptation have provided some profound insights into the
process of perceptual binding. Sensory adaptation can be induced by prolonged
exposure to a particular environmental property. For instance, the classical motion
aftereffect is induced by prolonged exposure to movement in a given direction. As
a consequence of the motion adaptation, subsequently viewed stationary stimuli
can appear to move in the opposite direction (Mather *et al.* 1998). Adaptation
can also be induced by exposure to combinations of properties initially encoded
by functionally independent processing systems, like vision and audition. After
this type of adaptation, the perceptual relationship between the different attributes can be systematically altered. Later in the chapter, we will discuss several
specific situations where this occurs. As the perceptual consequences of such
adaptation are persistent, they demonstrate that the different sources of information are not simply contributing, on-line, to a further independent analysis.
Instead, the information must become integrated, or bound, within a persistent perceptual code that is shaped by both, initially segregated, sources of information.

Studies using sensory adaptation have provided clear evidence that some kinds
of initially segregated information, like visual and auditory signals, can become
integrated. However, this does not mean that all sensory input must initially be
processed in isolation, or that all information that is processed independently is
necessarily integrated with other sources of information. These considerations
have prompted the proposal that perceptual binding within a single modality,
vision, might not be necessary (Lennie 1998). In this regard, adaptation studies
have also proven useful, demonstrating that perceptual binding within a single
sensory modality is both necessary and is qualitatively similar to the process of
perceptual binding between different modalities.

In this chapter we will first review some studies that have used adaptation as
a tool to examine how information from different sensory modalities, vision
and audition, becomes perceptually bound. We will then describe some studies
that have used adaptation to show that there is another form of the perceptual
binding problem that occurs within a single sensory modality – vision. Together,
the two forms of perceptual binding suggest that the brain uses a dynamic strategy
that weights the available cues according to their relative reliability when integrating information from multiple sources. This strategy provides a means of
adaptively binding information from within and across sensory modalities that,
in turn, allows us to effortlessly perceive possibly disparate information in spite
of vast changes in our environment.

12.2 Binding Different Sensory Modalities

While there has been considerable debate concerning the degree and form of functional segregation within the visual system, it is indisputable that the analysis of

vision and audition is, at least initially, mediated by independent sensory systems. Yet there are many examples of robust interaction between the two. For instance, we all experience a cross-modal interaction whenever we sit down in front of the television or at the cinema. While we watch, it does not seem as if the sources of sight and sound are spatially displaced, as they actually tend to be. Of course the same type of interaction has been evident for many centuries in puppet shows, an effect known as ventriloquism (Thomas 1941; Recanzone 1998).

Psychophysical studies of the ventriloquism effect have shown that the phenomenon tends to be marked by an illusory shift of the perceived position of the sound source toward that of the visual stimulus. This, it is argued, is to be expected as the visual modality is marked by greater spatial acuity (Welch & Warren 1980). Therefore, the ventriloquism effect could be thought of as an instance of a 'visual capture' of a different sensory modality (Hay et al. 1965).

If the ventriloquism effect were dependent upon the temporal coincidence of a visual and auditory stimulus, perhaps the effect could be attributed to some form of cognitive bias. Observers might be influenced by the more accurate visual spatial cue, regardless of whether or not they were instructed to attend to it (Bermant & Welch 1976). However, psychophysical studies using adaptation have shown that the sources of sight and sound do not always have to be concurrent for the effect to be observed. After prolonged exposure to a consistent auditory-visual spatial offset, the perceived position of the auditory stimulus can be shifted towards that of the visual stimulus, even when the visual stimulus is not present: a ventriloquism aftereffect (Canon 1970; Radeau & Bertelson 1977; Recanzone 1998; Lewald 2002).

The perceptual mediation of the ventriloquism-aftereffect, as opposed to the introduction of some form of cognitive bias (Canon 1970; Radeau & Bertelson, 1977; Lewald 2002) is further suggested by the fact that the phenomenon can be highly selective. If the adaptation and test tones are of the same frequency, a robust illusory spatial offset of a test tone can be observed. However, if the adaptation and test tones differ in frequency, no aftereffect is observed (Lewald 2002).

The fact that spatial judgements concerning audition are systematically shaped by our recent visual experiences (Canon 1970; Radeau & Bertelson 1977; Recanzone 1998; Lewald 2002) has some profound philosophical implications. It is conceivable that spatial judgements concerning vision and audition could be mediated by entirely independent mechanisms. The ventriloquism aftereffect demonstrates that this is not the case. Alternatively, it is conceivable that spatial judgements concerning vision and audition are mediated by a common mechanism that extracts information from earlier modality-specific analyses. Another alternative is that spatial judgements concerning vision and audition are mediated by relatively independent mechanisms that nevertheless influence one another. We cannot discriminate between the latter two possibilities on the basis of the ventriloquism aftereffect. However, the phenomenon places an important constraint upon them. In either case, the process whereby information from audition and vision interacts can cause persistent changes in a spatial code that can have perceptual consequences for some period of time thereafter.

The traditional ventriloquism effect demonstrates that the presence of a visual stimulus can cause human observers to make systematic errors of sound localization (Canon 1970; Radeau & Bertelson 1977; Lewald 2002). While proximity in ventriloquism tasks has typically been defined in spatial terms, it has recently been shown that the interaction is shaped by both spatial and temporal proximity. For instance, observers are less accurate when discriminating the temporal order of sight and sound sources when the sources are spatially proximate, as opposed to when they are separated (Bertelson & Aschersleben 2003). This finding is consistent with the premise that spatially proximate sources of sight and sound also tend to be perceived as being temporally proximate. However, unlike the spatial ventriloquism effect, it is unclear if the sound source is attracted by the visual, the visual by the sound, or if the attraction is mutual.

The ventriloquism effect and aftereffect demonstrate that vision can influence audition. The reverse influence is demonstrated by other phenomena. For instance, Fig. 12.1 depicts a schematic plot of two dots moving towards one another, becoming superimposed, and then continuing along their trajectories. Or does it depict two dots moving towards one another, becoming superimposed, and then bouncing away from one another? The plot itself is ambiguous and it depicts a perceptually ambiguous visual phenomenon, the stream/bounce illusion (Bertenthal *et al.* 1993).

In the stream/bounce illusion, two dots can be seen to either pass through, or to bounce off, one another (Bertenthal *et al.* 1993). If an auditory stimulus is presented at the point in time when the two dots 'contact' one another,

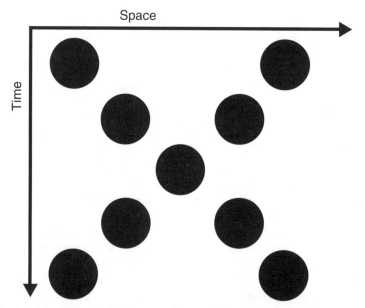

FIG. 12.1 Schematic depicting the stream/bounce illusion. Two dots move towards one another, become superimposed, and then move away from one another. The display is ambiguous and can be seen as two dots passing through or bouncing off one another.

observers are biased to see the two dots as 'bouncing' (Sekuler *et al.* 1997)[1]. It has been argued that this bias arises because the timing of the sound is ecologically consistent with a collision between the two dots (Sekuler *et al.* 1997).

A recent study has shown that the temporal tuning of this auditory–visual interaction is not fixed. In this study, observers were exposed to repeated presentations wherein the timing of a tone could precede, be simultaneous with, or lag the point at which the two dots became superimposed. Following repeated exposure to temporally offset tones, slightly offset tones became more effective at inducing a 'bouncing' percept. The direction of the effect was consistent with a shift in the point of subjective simultaneity, between sight and sound, toward that of the adapted offset (Fujisaki *et al.* 2004).

This demonstration is important for two reasons. First, it is a vivid demonstration of a situation wherein audition can influence vision. Second, it demonstrates that the interaction between the two modalities is not fixed, but can be changed by prolonged exposure to an altered environment. Similar conclusions have been reached by other recent studies that have explored interactions between audition and vision in relation to temporal rate perception. In one, it has been demonstrated that the presence of multiple auditory events can increase the perceived number of visual events (Shams *et al.* 2002). Another has demonstrated that audition can *drive* vision when it comes to rate perception (Recanzone 2003). There is a bias to perceive the rate of visual flicker as being similar to the rate of a concurrent auditory stimulus. Following prolonged exposure, or adaptation, to conflicting temporal rates of visual and auditory fluctuations, the altered perceptual rate of the visual stimulus will persist (for a period of time) even in the absence of the conflicting auditory information (Recanzone 2003).

Vision can influence (Canon 1970; Radeau & Bertelson 1977; Bertenthal *et al.* 1993; Lewald 2002), and be influenced by (Sekuler *et al.* 1997; Shams *et al.* 2002; Nishida *et al.* 2003; Recanzone 2003), audition across time and space. Furthermore, the interactions between vision and audition are dynamic. Through adaptation, the perceptual points of temporal (Nishida *et al.* 2003; Recanzone 2003) and spatial (Lewald 2002) correspondence between sight and sound can be shifted (also, see Bertelson *et al.* 2003 and Kitagawa & Ichihara 2002).

Why can adaptation systematically alter the correspondences that the brain determines between different sensory modalities? Why can adaptation influence cross-modal sensory binding? Elsewhere in this book, it has been argued that the effects of adaptation might be functional. For instance, prolonged exposure to an oriented grating may facilitate the subsequent detection of changes in spatial structure (Clifford, this volume). Cross-modal aftereffects might be indicative of similar functional processes. They raise the possibility that information processed in one modality might help to encode information more efficiently in a *different* modality – a potentially adaptive process. For instance, duplicate or overlapping information, like the visual images and sounds of a person speaking, could be

---

[1] See http://electra.psychol.ucl.ac.uk/derek/SB.htm for demonstrations.

encoded in such a manner that a degraded signal in one modality could be compensated by the duplicate information in the other[2]. This would not simply be an example of cross-talk between sensory modalities, but a consequence of an adaptive, multi-dimensional, analysis.

The sensory systems that mediate our senses of sight and sound are also marked by some substantial differences. For instance, auditory processing tends to be more sensitive to timing than visual (Welch & Warren 1980; Recanzone 2003). If observers are required to detect the longer of the two events, they are far more accurate if the two events are auditory as opposed to visual (Rousseau *et al*. 1983; Grondin *et al*. 1998). It would make sense therefore, when the brain has both visual and auditory cues concerning timing, to weigh the more accurate auditory cues more heavily than the less precise visual information (Welch & Warren 1980; Recanzone 2003). In contrast, the spatial precision of audition is relatively poor in comparison to vision. Consequently, if the brain has both visual and auditory information concerning spatial location it would make sense to weigh the visual information more heavily (Welch & Warren 1980; Recanzone 2003).

The patterns of interaction between sight and sound tend to be consistent with the premise that the brain weighs the most accurate information more heavily when determining a correspondence between – or binding-independent sources of information (Recanzone 2003; Welch & Warren 1980). As a consequence, when making judgements concerning timing, audition will tend to influence visual processing (Sekuler *et al*. 1997; Shams *et al*. 2002; Nishida *et al*. 2003; Recanzone 2003). When making judgements concerning location, vision will tend to influence audition (Canon 1970; Radeau & Bertelson 1977; Bertenthal *et al*. 1993; Lewald 2002).

Studies using adaptation have also shown that it is not even necessary for the two sources of information to be contemporaneous to observe the consequences of these interactions. Following prolonged exposure to conflicting visual and auditory cues, the less precise sensory modality will (for a time) continue to be influenced in the absence of any conflicting information from the other, more precise, sensory modality (Lewald 2002; Nishida *et al*. 2003; Recanzone 2003). This implies that our spatial and temporal judgements involve multidimensional analyses that maximize accuracy by weighting information according to the statistical precision of the input (Welch & Warren 1980; Recanzone 2003).

12.3 Correspondence between Visual Attributes: Is there a Visual Binding Problem?

Visual and auditory processing is mediated, at least initially, by independent sensory systems. The extent and form of functional segregation within the visual

---

[2] See Alais & Burr (2004) for a similar proposal and further evidence.

system, however, has been the focus of intense debate. A classical perspective suggests that the functional architecture of vision is marked by substantial functional segregation, with independent visual pathways analysing different visual properties (Livingstone & Hubel 1984, 1988; Casagrande 1994; Zeki 1993). The visual pathways have variously been divided into the 'magno' and 'parvo' (Livingstone & Hubel 1984, 1988; DeYoe & Van Essen 1988), the 'what' and 'where' (Mishkin & Ungerleider 1982), or the 'dorsal' and 'ventral' streams (Goodale & Milner 1992). Common to all of these characterizations is that one pathway (M/Where/Dorsal) is highly specialized for the analysis of motion whereas the other (P/What/Ventral) is heavily involved with the analysis of colour.

If this strict modular characterization of the visual system were correct, the functional architecture of the visual system would pose an additional problem of correspondence. How would we determine the correspondence between visual attributes processed within independent systems? While the modular view is supported by physiological and clinical evidence (Zihl *et al.* 1983; Newsome & Paré 1988; Zeki 1990; Cowey & Heywood 1997), an alternate perspective suggests that our perceptual experiences of colour and motion are actually mediated by a common visual pathway (Lennie 1998).

12.3.1 Psychophysical Evidence for a Modular Analysis

It has been proposed that, if visual analysis is modular and distributed over *space* within the brain, different visual analyses might also be distributed over *time* within the brain (Bartels & Zeki 1998). For instance, the analysis of different attributes (like colour and motion) may take different periods of time. If there is a relationship between the time required to analyse an attribute and the time course of perceptual experience, we might also expect awareness of physically coincident events to arise at different points in time (Bartels & Zeki 1998).

A recent series of psychophysical experiments purportedly demonstrated an asynchrony of visual consciousness (Moutoussis & Zeki 1997a,b). Observers were exposed to stimuli that oscillated in combinations of two attributes, such as colour (red/green) and direction of motion (up/down). The relative phase of the oscillations within the different attributes was manipulated and, as depicted in Fig. 12.2, observers were required to indicate the perceptual pairing that was predominant at each phasic relationship. Analogous experiments were also performed using stimuli oscillating in colour and orientation and in orientation and direction of motion.

The authors wanted to determine when different stimulus attributes (like colour and motion) are perceptually synchronous. Surprisingly, the pattern of results suggested that physically simultaneous features are not necessarily perceptually synchronous. The data suggested that colours and orientations were perceptually synchronous when the changes in colour lagged changes in orientation by 63 ms. Orientations and directions were perceptually synchronous when the changes in orientation lagged changes in direction by 52 ms and colours and directions of motion were perceptually synchronous when changes in colour lagged direction by 118 ms (Moutoussis & Zeki 1997b).

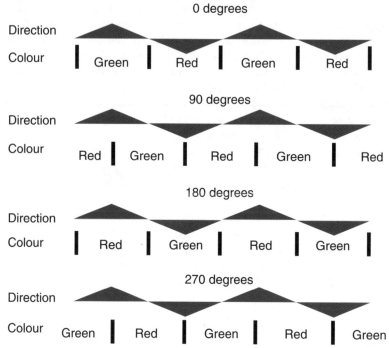

FIG. 12.2 Depiction of four phasic relationships between colour and motion.
At a phasic relationship of 0°, the colour green is always paired with upward motion
and red with downward. At a phasic relationship of 180°, this situation is reversed.
At phasic relationships of 90° and 270°, both upward and downward motions are
paired equally with red and green, such that no physical correlation exists between
the two stimulus attributes.

These data were originally interpreted as being indicative of a temporal hierarchy of functionally independent processing systems, with changes in colour
being processed faster (~63 ms) than changes in orientation that, in turn, are
processed faster (~52 ms) than changes in the direction of motion (Moutoussis
& Zeki 1997b).

The theoretical perspective of Moutoussis & Zeki (1997a,b) presumes a direct
correspondence between the time courses of neural activity and perceptual experience. This assumption has been the focus of intense debate for some time
(Dennett & Kinsbourne 1992; Whitney & Murkami 1998; Eagleman &
Sejnowski 2000; Johnston & Nishida 2001)[3]. Given that stimulus attributes

---

[3] For a detailed discussion of this issue, see also the entire June 2002 issue of the journal
Consciousness & Cognition.

such as contrast, salience, and luminance (Bolz *et al.* 1982; Gawne *et al.* 1996; Carandini *et al.* 1997; Maunsell *et al.* 1999) can impact upon the time course of neural activity, it has been suggested that it may be necessary to impose a process of temporal analysis by which any temporal ambiguities might be resolved (Eagleman & Sejnowski 2000; Rao *et al.* 2001). As a consequence, it is unclear if discrepancies between the physical and perceptual time courses of events arise because of asynchronous neural activity, or because of some form of interpretive process that is involved in the analysis of timing (Dennett & Kinsbourne 1992; Johnston & Nishida 2001; Nishida & Johnston 2002).

12.3.2 Using Contingent Adaptation to Explore the (A)synchrony of Vision

If you look at a coherently moving stimulus for a prolonged period of time and then look at a similar but stationary stimulus, the stationary stimulus typically appears to be drifting slowly in the opposite direction to the original stimulus. This phenomenon is known as the motion aftereffect. The direction of motion experienced during a motion aftereffect can become contingent upon the colour of the test stimulus (Favreau *et al.* 1972). For instance, if you view a circular stimulus wherein clockwise rotation is paired with the colour green and anticlockwise rotation with the colour red, a subsequently viewed stationary green stimulus can appear to rotate slowly in an anticlockwise direction while a stationary red stimulus may appear to rotate clockwise (Favreau *et al.* 1972). This situation is depicted in Fig. 12.3.

Some characteristics of the colour-contingent motion aftereffect suggested that, as a tool, it was uniquely suited to the analysis of the temporal properties of visual processing. One of the most distinguishing features of activity within extrastriate areas is that the activity can be elicited by appropriate stimulation of either eye. In contrast, colour contingent aftereffects are essentially monocular (McCollough 1964; Mayhew & Anstis 1972; Murch 1976; Potts & Harris 1979; Humphrey & Goodale 1998). This suggests that colour-contingent aftereffects are mediated at a relatively early point within the visual hierarchy.

The early mediation of colour-contingency is further suggested by the fact that the perceived hue of orientation-contingent coloured aftereffects is dependent upon the physical wavelength and not the perceived colour of the adapting stimulus (Thompson & Latchford 1986). This demonstrates that coloured aftereffects must be mediated at a point that precedes the neural site where colour constancy is achieved. In fact, a recent review of the empirical evidence regarding colour-contingency has identified V1 as the most probable neural correlate (Humphrey & Goodale 1998).

Perhaps the most desirable aspect of the colour-contingent motion aftereffect in the present context is that it is a measure of visual processing. The consequences of exposure to combinations of colour and motion become evident after a period of passive observation. Therefore, any interpretation of the effect is not complicated by philosophical considerations concerning the relationship between the

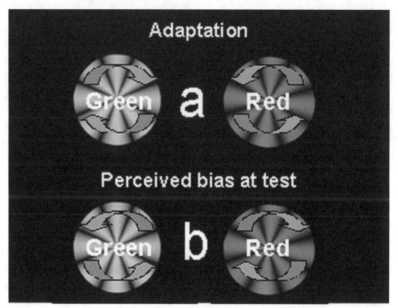

FIG. 12.3 Colour-contingent motion aftereffect: The perceptual consequences (b) of prolonged exposure to a stimulus that oscillates in both colour and direction of motion (a).

time courses of sensory processing and subjective perceptual experience (Dennett & Kinsbourne 1992; Eagleman & Sejnowski 2000; Johnston & Nishida 2001; Rao *et al*. 2001).

Like Moutoussis & Zeki (1997*a,b*), Arnold *et al*. (2001) exposed observers to a stimulus oscillating in both colour and direction, at a range of different phasic relationships. However, the observers were not required to make any perceptual decisions concerning the concurrent oscillations. Instead, for five minutes, observers first passively viewed a stimulus that oscillated between different directions of motion and between different colours. The perceptual consequences of this exposure were then explored. Observers were exposed to very slowly moving patterns, of different colour, and were required to determine the direction of rotation. These judgements were interspersed with additional five-second passages of additional passive adaptation. The results of the study demonstrated systematic differences between the perceptual biases caused by contingent adaptation and the physical correlations between the two stimulus attributes during passive adaptation. For instance, in some circumstances a robust perceptual contingency could be induced between a colour and direction of motion when the two attributes were actually negatively correlated during the period of adaptation (see Fig. 12.4).

To date, only two explanations have been proposed in relation to the temporal differences between colour and motion processing demonstrated within the context of contingent adaptation (Arnold *et al*. 2001). The phenomenon could be a consequence of a latency difference between the neural analyses of colour and

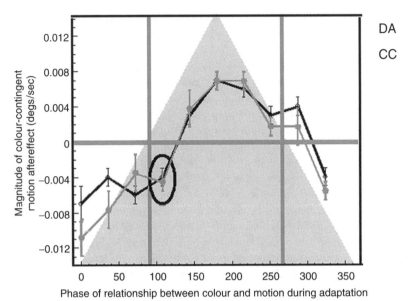

FIG. 12.4 Average colour-contingent motion aftereffects for two observers as a function of the phasic relationship between colour and motion during contingent adaptation. The bold horizontal line depicts points where no contingent aftereffects are evident. The bold vertical lines indicate points where no physical correlation exists between colour and motion. Data points lying above the horizontal line indicate phasic relationships where clockwise rotation becomes contingent upon the colour red. We have used the background shading within the frame to help depict the physical correlations between colour and motion during adaptation. At 0 and 360° along the horizontal axis, the background is entirely white, signifying that at these relationships clockwise rotation was always paired with the colour green. At 180° along the horizontal axis the background is entirely grey, signifying that at this relationship clockwise rotation was always paired with the colour red. If changes in colour and direction were processed in synchrony all data points lying between the two vertical lines should be of the same sign and lie above the horizontal line. This is not the case. For instance, at a phasic relationship of 108° (which is circled), clockwise rotation was physically paired with red for 300 ms and then with green for just 200 ms. Yet the contingent aftereffects observed were consistent with clockwise rotation becoming perceptually contingent with the colour green.

motion (Arnold *et al.* 2001). Alternatively, the effect might arise because of a difference between how the neural activities elicited by different attributes are distributed over time (Johnston & Nishida 2001; Nishida & Johnston 2002). Both proposals necessitate a high degree of, at least initial, independence between colour and motion processing. As there are systematic differences between the physical correlations between colours and motions and the perceptual contingencies that arise following passive exposure, systematic processing differences must exist between the visual system's treatments of the different attributes prior to or at the point within the visual hierarchy where perceptual contingency arises (Favreau *et al*. 1972).

The distributions depicted in Fig. 12.4 can be analysed to estimate the extent of the temporal offset between colour and motion processing (Arnold *et al*. 2001). In Fig. 12.5, the two distributions depicted in Fig. 12.4 have been fitted to polar plots and a centroid has been calculated to provide an estimate of the maximal processing correlation between colour and motion. These estimates suggest that the maximal processing correlation between colours and motions arises when changes in colour physically lag changes in direction. The temporal advantage for colour processing suggested by these analyses (58 ms for C.C. and 91 ms for D.A.) are smaller than but in the same direction as the asynchronies evident from perceptual pairing tasks using the same stimuli (135 ms for C.C. and 105 ms for D.A.) and the advantage of ~118 ms suggested by Moutoussis & Zeki (1997*a*,*b*). These data suggest that the perceptual asynchrony between colour and motion is at least in part accounted for by a difference in the temporal properties of processing at the level(s) at which the contingent aftereffect is mediated.

The suggestion that the visual brain is not marked by a high degree of functional specialization is seductive (Lennie 1998). It would resolve the inherent difficulty dictated by computational division: the need to integrate independent neural activity. However, the demonstration of temporal differences between the perceptual analyses of colour and motion (Arnold *et al*. 2001) suggests that, although a combinational code of colour and motion is formed, the analyses of colour and motion are also marked by a high degree of computational division.

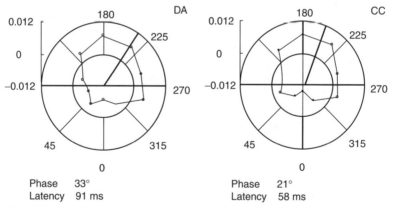

FIG. 12.5 Polar plots depicting the average colour-contingent motion aftereffects for observers C.C. & D.A. as a function of the phasic relationship between colour and motion during contingent adaptation, replotted from Fig. 12.4. Fitted centroids, a measure a central tendency, are indicated by bold black lines and are rotated clockwise by 21° for observer C.C. and by 33° for observer D.A. This is indicative of processing advantages for colour of ~58 ms and ~91 ms respectively.

Of course, this finding does not bring us any closer to understanding how the brain may determine correspondences between colour and motion. However, it does demonstrate that this correspondence can actually encapsulate characteristic differences between the two attributes that could only arise as a consequence of some degree of initial independence.

12.4 Correspondence between Cortical Activity and Perceived Position

Given that visual processing is marked by initial functional segregation and a subsequent re-integration (or binding) of visual information, how does the visual system determine the state of an attribute that can be signalled by multiple cues? The position of an object, for instance, could be signalled by variations in motion, luminance, colour, or by texture (Regan 2000). Does the visual system need to combine these cues? If so, how is this achieved? What can studies of adaptation tell us about these questions? To some degree, these questions may not have attracted the attention that they deserve because there seems to be an obvious cue, retinotopy, that the visual system can use to determine position.

12.4.1 Retinotopy

Our perception of a stable world suggests that there are mechanisms in the visual cortex that provide a systematic code for the relative positioning of objects. What sorts of information contribute to this coding and allow us to perceive the positions of objects in a consistent and accurate manner? Many visual areas of the brain are marked by retinotopic organization, such that each neuron responds to activation within a specific region of the retina and adjacent neurons are activated by the stimulation of adjacent regions (Daniel & Whitteridge 1961; Tootell *et al.* 1982; Sereno *et al.* 1995). The retinotopic organization of visual areas could provide a neural basis for the visual system's ability to consistently encode the positions of objects (Morgan 2003). However, adaptation to a luminance or texture pattern can cause illusory shifts in the positions of subsequently viewed stimuli (Whitaker *et al.* 1997; McGraw *et al.* 1999). Clearly, retinotopy is not sufficient to explain how we perceive the positions of objects.

Although retinotopy is insufficient to explain our perception of object position, perhaps it could help to explain why we perceive object positions as being relatively stable. That is, retinotopy might provide a means of stabilizing our perception of position, allowing us to perceive stationary images despite frequent movements of the eye and head. However, the classical motion aftereffect demonstrates that this idea is also flawed. Following prolonged exposure to a stimulus moving in a given direction, a subsequently viewed stationary stimulus can appear to contain *movement* in the opposite direction. However, while *movement* is perceived, the stimulus itself does not appear to shift in position in a manner that is consistent with the perceived *movement*, an apparently contradictory percept

(Mather *et al.* 1998). Thus, retinotopy is neither sufficient to explain our perception of position, nor our perception of stability or stationarity.

How then do we perceive the positions of objects? Clearly, retinotopic coding alone does not determine perceived position. Why is this?

12.4.2 The Problem of Perceiving Position

Perhaps one of the reasons that retinotopy alone does not determine perceived position is because of the nature of the problem facing the visual system. Given that the analysis of different visual attributes, like colour and motion, can be relatively independent, the visual system may have to first segregate and then recombine information at a later point of analysis. This functional segregation and subsequent reintegration of visual information seems to pose a dilemma when determining perceived position. Even if different attributes were initially analysed within independent retinotopically organized mechanisms, the very independence of the analyses (that may take differing periods of time to complete) would suggest that it is improbable that the different retinotopies would necessarily concur when recombined. Perhaps, then, apparent distortions of perceived position are indicative that the brain recombines sources of information that have provided slightly conflicting or incomplete positional cues? What can studies of adaptation tell us about these possibilities?

12.4.3 Is There a Correspondence Problem Between Motion and Position?

The classical motion aftereffect was originally taken as evidence that motion and position are processed by independent mechanisms (Wohlgemuth 1911; Gregory 1966; Nakayama 1985), since illusory motion could be perceived without a concurrent shift in the apparent location of the object. More recent evidence has qualified this dissociation, showing that the motion aftereffect can be accompanied by a shift in the apparent position of the test stimulus (Snowden 1998; Nishida & Johnston 1999; Whitaker *et al.* 1999; McGraw *et al.* 2002).

As the motion aftereffect is accompanied by a shift in apparent position, the possibility must be revived that the perceived motion and position of an object are coded by a single mechanism (e.g. Fu *et al.* 2002, 2004). However, Nishida & Johnston (1999) also showed that, although the apparent position of an object can be shifted when there is a motion aftereffect, there are important differences between the motion aftereffect and the illusory positional spatial shift that can accompany it. For instance, the rate of illusory positional change was more gradual than the speed of the illusory movement (Nishida & Johnston 1999). Further, the illusory position shift was visible immediately when the stimulus was presented, indicating that the perceived position of the pattern was not determined by the presence, or a build-up, of illusory motion. This suggests that perceived motion and spatial position are processed by relatively independent mechanisms.

The relationship between the neural codes for motion and position has been further clarified by another recent adaptation study (Whitney & Cavanagh 2003). If a static object is flashed at some distance away from a contemporary moving stimulus, it can appear to be shifted in the same direction as the physical movement (Whitney & Cavanagh 2000; Watanabe *et al.* 2002, 2003; Whitney 2002; Durant & Johnston 2004). This illusory shift is similar to the illusory spatial shift of an object that contains motion (Ramachandran & Anstis 1990; De Valois & De Valois 1991) in that it is an illusory positional shift in the direction of a contemporary movement. However, as depicted in Fig. 12.6, if the static object is flashed at some point in time following adaptation to movement, the direction of the illusory spatial shift is reversed (Whitney & Cavanagh 2003).

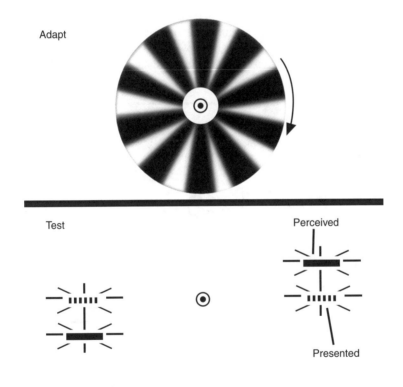

FIG. 12.6 Position shifts of stationary objects following adaptation to motion. After adaptation to a rotating radial grating (top), two stationary flashed lines that are physically aligned appear misaligned in a direction opposite that of the previously visible motion; i.e. in a direction consistent with that of the motion aftereffect (bottom). Note that the test flashes were separated from the motion of the grating by several degrees, and nothing else was visible on the screen during the test period. Therefore, there was no perceived or physical motion in the adapted region during the test period.

The illusory shift of a static flashed object following motion adaptation is similar to the illusory spatial shift that can accompany the motion aftereffect (Whitaker *et al.* 1997; Snowden 1998; Nishida & Johnston 1999): they are both illusory spatial shifts in a direction opposite that of a previous physical movement. However, the shift of a static flashed object (Whitney & Cavanagh 2003) differs from the illusory spatial shifts that can accompany the motion aftereffect (Whitaker *et al.* 1997; Snowden 1998; Nishida & Johnston 1999). First, as shown in Fig. 12.7, the object that appears shifted in position can be separated by some distance from the region of the visual field that was adapted to motion. Moreover, the shift is not necessarily accompanied by a contemporary perception of movement, illusory, or otherwise (Whitney & Cavanagh 2003). These factors make it difficult to argue that the mechanism that determines perceived position is the same mechanism that determines the perceived motion of a stimulus.

The observation that an illusory motion-induced spatial shift can occur in the absence of perceived motion (McGraw *et al.* 2002; Whitney & Cavanagh 2003) would be uninteresting if, given sufficient time, movement of the static flashed objects were experienced. However, as shown in Fig. 12.8, even when the static *flashed* objects were shown for ~300 ms, they still appeared to be stationary and

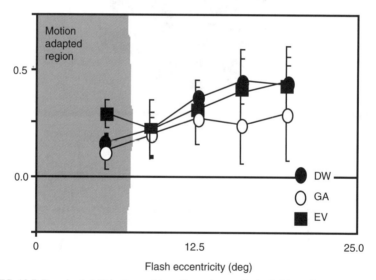

FIG. 12.7 Perceived shift in the position of a stationary flashed object after adaptation to motion. The perceived misalignment between the flashes (from Fig. 12.6) is plotted as a function of the eccentricity of each flash. The shaded area shows the location of motion adaptation (where the rotating grating was presented). Note that a misalignment was perceived between flashes whether they were presented inside or outside the motion-adapted (shaded) region, showing that the influence of motion on perceived position is not retinally specific. The perceived misalignment between the flashes increased slightly with eccentricity. The error bars show 95% confidence intervals.

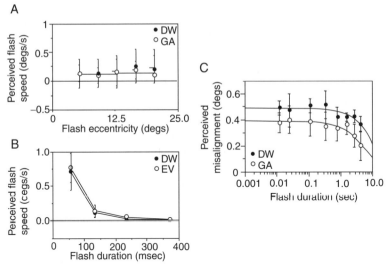

FIG. 12.8 Perceived speed of stationary flashed objects (from Fig. 6) after adaptation to motion. (A) The perceived speed of the (physically stationary) flashes is plotted as a function of their eccentricity. Flashes presented for 200 msec did not appear to move significantly. The error bars show 95% confidence intervals. The lines through the data show best linear fits [f(x) = 0.001*x + 0.11], for GA, and [f(x) = 0.007*x + 0.07], for DW. (B) The perceived flash speed is plotted as a function of the flash duration. The longer the flash was presented, the slower it appeared to move. Note that although flashes presented for longer than 300 ms appeared stationary when they were physically stationary, they still appear shifted in position. (C) Perceived misalignment as a function of flash duration. Error bars show 95% confidence intervals.

yet appeared to be shifted in position (Whitney & Cavanagh 2003). This demonstrates that, not only are the analyses of position and movement separable (Nishida & Johnston 1999), it is not actually necessary to experience the primary consequence of motion-processing (movement) at the point in time at which its influence upon a relatively independent visual attribute (perceived spatial position) is experienced.

12.5 Conclusions and Directions for Future Research

Information originating from different sensory modalities, like vision and audition, is first analysed within independent processing systems. However, studies of perceptual adaptation have demonstrated that the two sources of information can become integrated to determine a common perceptual consequence (Canon 1970; Radeau & Bertelson 1977; Recanzone 1998; Lewald 2002; Nishida *et al.* 2003). Relatively independent analyses also occur within the visual modality.

This might not pose a computational dilemma if the sources of information were never integrated (Lennie 1998). However, studies of adaptation have also demonstrated that initially independent sources of visual information become integrated to determine a common perceptual consequence (Whitaker *et al.* 1997; Snowden 1998; Nishida & Johnston 1999; Arnold *et al.* 2001; McGraw *et al.* 2002; Whitney & Cavanagh 2003).

Studies of visual adaptation have shown that although the analyses of motion and spatial position are relatively independent, the consequences of their interaction can continue to be evident for some period of time, even in the absence of one of the two attributes (McGraw *et al.* 2002; Whitney & Cavanagh 2003). This observation is consistent with what perceptual adaptation has revealed concerning one of the cross-modal phenomena that we described earlier, the ventriloquism aftereffect (Canon 1970; Radeau & Bertelson 1977; Recanzone 1998; Lewald 2002). In both instances, a perceptual bias in perceived position can persist in the physical and perceptual absence of the stimulus attribute that induced the shift.

Studies of adaptation suggest that the brain tends to weight the most accurate cue more heavily when determining correspondences between – or binding – independent sources of information originating from different sensory modalities (Welch & Warren 1980; Recanzone 2003). In vision, separable sources of information can also contribute to a common perceptual experience. Here too, it would make sense if the brain were to weight sources of information (Whitaker *et al.* 2004; McGraw *et al.* 2004). Further studies using adaptation may clarify how different sources of information contribute to common perceptual experiences and to identify the circumstances wherein different sources of information become integrated – or perceptually bound.

As different sources of information can be processed independently before they become integrated, there is a possibility that the initially independent analyses might require different periods of time to complete. It is also possible that any specific analysis might not always require the same amount of time to complete. These observations may help to explain why the point of subjective simultaneity between sight and sound can be shifted following adaptation to a temporal offset between repetitive sights and sounds (Nishida *et al.* 2003). If the brain needs to determine temporal correspondences between independent sources of information, it may be necessary to adopt a dynamic strategy. If this is true of cross-modal perceptual integration, it might also be true of intra-modal integration. For example, a shift in perceived simultaneity might arise following contingent adaptation to temporally offset colours and motions. If so, in which direction would the shift be?

The perceptual consequences of adaptation have provided a great deal of information about how the brain integrates independent sources of information. The effects of adaptation are conceptually important as they demonstrate that different sources of information are not simply contributing, on-line, to a further independent analysis. Instead, the information is integrated or bound in a manner that gives appropriate and persistent weighting to different sources of information.

Adaptation provides a means to isolate these different or even contradictory sources of information – to break the binding process – thereby providing deeper insight into which cues are, and are not, independently analysed. Furthermore, the visual illusions or perceptual mis-bindings that perceptual adaptation can produce provide a tantalizing insight into the manner in which the brain integrates different sources of information. Ultimately, it is this integration of independently processed sensory input that allows us to perceive the dynamic world as coherent rather than a scrambled cacophony of sight and sound.

References

Alais, D., & Burr D. (2004). The ventriloquist effect results from near-optimal bimodal integration. *Current Biology*, *14*, 257–62.

Arnold, D.H., Clifford, C.W.G., & Wenderoth, P. (2001). Asynchronous processing in vision: color leads motion. *Current Biology*, *11*, 596–600.

Bartels, A., & Zeki, S. (1998). The asynchrony of consciousness. *Proceedings of the Royal Society of London B*, *265*, 1583–5.

Bermant, R.I., & Welch, R.B. (1976). Effect of degree of separation of visual-auditory stimulus and eye position upon spatial interaction of vision and audition. *Perceptual Motor Skills*, *42*, 487–93.

Bertelson, P., & Aschersleben, G. (2003). Temporal ventriliquism: crossmodal interaction on the time dimension 1. Evidence from auditory-visual temporal order judgment. *International Journal of Psychophysiology*, *50*, 147–55.

Bertelson, P., Vroomen, J., & De Gelder (2003). Visual recalibration of auditory speech identification: a McGurk aftereffect. *Psychological Science*, *14*, 592–7.

Bertenthal, B.I., Banton, T., & Bradbury, A. (1993). Directional bias in the perception of translating patterns. *Perception*, *22*, 193–207.

Bolz, J., Rosner, G., & Wassel, H. (1982). Response latency of brisk-sustained (x) and brisk transient (y) cells in the cat retina. *Journal of Physiology*, *328*, 171–90.

Canon, L.K. (1970). Intermodality inconsistency of input and directed attention as determinants of the nature of adaptation. *Journal of Experimental Psychology*, *88*, 403–8.

Carandini, M., Heeger, D.J., & Movshon, J.A. (1997). Linearity and normalization in simple cells of the macaque primary visual cortex. *Journal of Neuroscience*, *17*, 8621–44.

Casagrande, V.A. (1994). A third parallel visual pathway to primate area V1. *Trends in Neuroscience*, *17*, 305–10.

Cowey, A., & Heywood, C.A. (1997). Cerebral achromatopsia: colour blindness despite wavelength processing. *Trends in Cognitive Neuroscience*, *1*, 133–9.

Daniel, P.M., & Whitteridge, D. (1961). The representation of the visual field on the cerebral cortex in monkeys. *Journal of Physiology*, *159*, 203.

Dennett, D.C., & Kinsbourne, M. (1992). Time and the observer: the where and when of consciousness in the brain. *Behavioural & Brain Sciences*, *15*, 183–247.

De Valois, R.L., & De Valois, K.K. (1991). Vernier acuity with stationary moving gabors. *Vision Research*, *31*, 1619–26.

DeYoe E.A., & Van Essen D.C. (1988). Concurrent processing in monkey visual cortex. *Trends in Neuroscience*, *11*, 219–26.

Durant, S., & Johnston, A. (2004). Temporal dependence of local motion induced shifts in perceived position. *Vision Research, 44*, 357–66.

Eagleman, D., & Sejnowski, T.J. (2000). Motion integration and postdiction in visual awareness. *Science, 287*, 2036–8.

Favreau, O.E., Emerson, V.F., & Corballis, M.C. (1972). Motion perception: a colour-contingent aftereffect. *Science, 176*, 78–9.

Fujisaki, W., Shimojo, S., Kashino, M., & Nishida, S. (2004). Recalibration of audio-visual simultaneity. *Nature Neuroscience, 7*, 773–8.

Gawne, T.J., Kjaer, T.W., & Richmond, B.J. (1996). Latency: another potential code for feature binding in striate cortex. *Journal of Neurophysiology, 76*, 1356–60.

Goodale, M.A., & Milner, A.D. (1992). Separate visual pathways for perception and action. *Trends in Neuroscience, 15*, 20–5.

Gregory, R.L. (1966). *Eye and Brain.* New York: McGraw-Hill.

Grondin, S., Meilleur-Wells, G., Ouellette, C., & Macar, F. (1998). Sensory effects on judgments of short-time intervals. *Psychological Research, 61*, 261–8.

Hay, J.C., Pick, H.L., & Ikeda, K. (1965). Visual capture produced by prism spectacles. *Psychological Science, 2*, 215–6.

Humphrey, G.H., & Goodale, M.A. (1998). Probing unconscious visual processing with the McCollough effect. *Consciousness & Cognition, 7*, 494–519.

Johnston, A., & Nishida, S. (2001). Time perception: Brain time or event time? *Current Biology, 11*, R427–R430.

Kitagawa, N., & Ichihara, S. (2002). Hearing visual motion in depth. *Nature, 416*, 172–4.

Lennie, P. (1998). Single units and visual cortical organization. *Perception, 27*, 1–47.

Lewald, J. (2002). Rapid adaptation to auditory-visual spatial disparity. *Learning & Memory, 9*, 268–78.

Livingstone, M.S., & Hubel, D.H. (1984). Specificity of intrinsic connections in primate primary visual cortex. *Journal of Neuroscience, 4*, 2830–5.

Livingstone, M.S., & Hubel, D.H. (1988). Segregation of form, color, movement, and depth: anatomy, physiology, and perception. *Science, 240*, 740–9.

Mather, G., Verstraten, F.A.J., & Anstis, S. (1998). *The Motion Aftereffect. A Modern Perspective.* Cambridge, MA: MIT Press.

Maunsell, J.H.R., Ghose, G.M., Assad, J.A., McAdams, C.J., Boudreau, C.E., & Noerager, B.D. (1999). Visual response latencies of magnocellular and parvocellular LGN neurons in macaque monkey. *Visual Neuroscience, 16*, 1–14.

Mayhew, J.E.W., & Anstis, S.M. (1972). Movement aftereffects contingent on colour, intensity and pattern. *Perception & Psychophysics, 12*, 77–85.

McCollough, C. (1964). Colour adaptation of edge-detectors in the human visual system. *Science, 149*, 1115–6

McGraw, P.V., Whitaker, D., Skillen, J., & Chung, S.T. (2002). Motion adaptation distorts perceived visual position. *Current Biology, 12*, 2042–7.

McGraw, P.V., Whitaker, D., Badcock, D.R., & Skillen, J. (2003). Neither here nor there: localizing conflicting visual attributes. *Journal of Vision, 3*, 265–73.

Mishkin M., & Ungerleider L.G. (1982). Contribution of striate inputs to the visuospatial functions of parieto-preoccipital cortex in monkeys. *Behavioural Brain Research, 6*, 57–77.

Morgan, M. (2003). *The Space Between our Ears.* London: Weidenfeld & Nicolson.

Moutoussis, K., & Zeki, S. (1997a). A direct demonstration of perceptual asynchrony in vision. *Proceedings of the Royal Society of London, B, 264*, 393–9.

Moutoussis, K., & Zeki, S. (1997b). Functional segregation and temporal hierarchy of the visual perceptive systems. *Proceedings of the Royal Society of London, B, 264,* 1407–14.

Murch, G.M. (1976). Classical conditioning of the McCollough effect: temporal parameters. *Vision Research, 16,* 615–9.

Nakayama, K. (1985). Biological image motion processing: a review. *Vision Research, 25,* 625–60.

Newsome, W.T., & Paré, E.B. (1988). A selective impairment of motion perception following lesions of the middle temporal visual area (MT). *Journal of Neuroscience, 8,* 2201–11.

Nishida, S., & Johnston, A. (2002). Marker location not processing latency determines temporal binding of visual attributes. *Current Biology, 12,* 359–68.

Potts, M.J., & Harris, J.P. (1979). Dichoptic induction of movement aftereffects contingent on colour and on orientation. *Perception & Psychophysics, 26,* 25–31.

Radeau, M., & Bertelson, P. (1977). Adaptation to auditory-visual discordance and ventriloquism in semirealistic situations. *Perception & Psychophysics, 22,* 137–46.

Rao, R.P., Eagleman, D.M., & Sejnowski, T.J. (2001). Optimal smoothing in motion perception. *Neural Computing, 13,* 1243–53.

Recanzone, G.H. (1998). Rapidly induced auditory plasticity: The ventriloquism aftereffect. *Proceedings of the National Academy of Sciences, 95,* 869–75.

Recanzone, G.H. (2003). Auditory influences on visual temporal rate perception. *Journal of Neurophysiology, 89,* 1078–93.

Regan, D. (2000). *Human Perception of Objects.* Sunderland, Massachusetts: Sinauer Associates.

Rousseau, R., Poirier, J., & Lemyre, L. (1983). Duration discrimination of empty time intervals marked by intermodal pulses. *Perception and Psychophysics, 34,* 541–8.

Sekuler, R., Sekuler, A.B., & Lau, R. (1997). Sound alters visual motion perception. *Nature, 385,* 308.

Sereno, M.I., Dale, A.M., Reppas, J.B., Kwong, K.K., Belliveau, J.W., Brady, T.J. *et al.* (1995). Borders of multiple visual areas in humans revealed by functional magnetic resonance imaging. *Science, 268,* 889–93.

Shams, L., Kamitani, Y., & Shimojo, S. (2002). What you see is what you hear. *Nature, 408,* 788.

Snowden, R.J. (1998). Shifts in perceived position following adaptation to visual motion. *Current Biology, 8,* 1343–5.

Thomas, G.J. (1941). Experimental study of the influence of vision on sound localisation. *Journal of Experimental Psychology, 28,* 167–77.

Thompson, P., & Latchford, G. (1986). Colour-contingent after-effects are really wavelength-contingent. *Nature, 320,* 525–6.

Watanabe, K., Nijhawan, R., & Shimojo, S. (2002). Shifts in perceived position of flashed stimuli by illusory object motion. *Vision Research, 42,* 2645–50.

Watanabe, K., Sato, T.R., & Shimojo, S. (2003). Perceived shifts of flashed stimuli by visual and invisible object motion. *Perception, 32,* 545–59.

Welch, R.B., & Warren, D.H. (1980). Immediate perceptual response to intersensory discrepancy. *Psychological Bulletin, 88,* 638–67.

Whitaker, D., McGraw, P.V., & Levi, D.M. (1997). The influence of adaptation on perceived visual location. *Vision Research, 37,* 2207–16.

Whitaker, D., McGraw, P.V., Keeble, D.R., & Skillen, J. (2004). Pulling the other one: 1st and 2nd-order visual information interact to determine perceived location. *Vision Research, 44,* 279–86.

Whitaker, D., McGraw, P.V., & Pearson, S. (1999). Non-veridical size perception of expanding and contracting objects. *Vision Research, 18,* 2999–3009.

Whitney, D. (2002). The influence of visual motion on spatial position. *Trends in Cognitive Sciences, 6,* 211–6.

Whitney, D., & Cavanagh, P. (2000a). Motion distorts visual space: shifting the perceived position of remote stationary objects. *Nature Neuroscience, 3,* 954–9.

Whitney, D., & Cavanagh, P. (2003). Motion adaptation shifts apparent position without the motion aftereffect. *Perception and Psychophysics, 65,* 1011–18.

Whitney, D., & Murakami, I. (1998). Latency difference, not spatial extrapolation. *Nature Neuroscience, 1,* 656–7.

Wohlgemuth, A. (1911). On the after-effect of seen movement. *British Journal of Psychology, (Supp.), 1,* 1–117.

Zeki, S. (1978). Functional specialization in the visual cortex of the monkey. *Nature, 274,* 423–8.

Zeki, S. (1990). A century of cerebral achromatopsia. *Brain, 113,* 1721–77.

Zeki S. (1993). *A Vision of the Brain.* Oxford: Blackwell.

Zhou, Y-X., & Baker, C.L. (1993). A processing stream in mammalian visual cortex neurons for non-Fourier responses. *Science, 261,* 98–101.

Zihl, J., Von Cameron, D., Mai, N., & Schmid, C.H. (1983). Selective disturbance of movement vision after bilateral brain damage. *Brain, 106,* 313–4

Index

RETURN TO: **FONG OPTOMETRY LIBRARY**

490 Minor Hall · 642-1020

LOAN PERIOD **1 MONTH**	1	2	3
	4	5	6

All books may be recalled after 7 days.
Renewals may be requested by phone or, using GLADIS,
type **inv** followed by your patron ID number.

DUE AS STAMPED BELOW.

This book will be hold
in OPTOMETRY LIBRARY
until _____ NOV 0 3 2005 _____
